# Medicine, Risk, Discourse and Power

This book critically explores from a comparative international perspective the role medicine plays in constructing and managing natural and social risks, including those belonging to modern medical technology and expertise. Drawing together chapters written by professional practitioners and social scientists from the UK, South America, Australia and Europe, the book offers readers an insightful and thought-provoking analysis of how modern medicine has transformed our understanding of both ourselves and the world around us; but in so doing, it has arguably failed to fully recognize and account for its unintended and negative effects. This is an essential read for social scientists, practitioners and policy makers who want to better understand how they can develop new ways of thinking about how modern medicine can promote social goods and enhance public health.

**John Martyn Chamberlain** is Associate Professor in Medical Criminology at the University of Southampton.

## Routledge Advances in Sociology

*For a full list of titles in this series, please visit www.routledge.com*

**136 Advances in Biographical Methods**
Creative Applications
*Edited by Maggie O'Neill, Brian Roberts and Andrew Sparkes*

**137 Social Cohesion and Immigration in Europe and North America**
Mechanisms, Conditions and Causality
*Edited by Ruud Koopmans, Bram Lancee and Merlin Schaeffer*

**138 Digital Publics**
Cultural Political Economy, Financialization and Creative Organizational Politics
*John Michael Roberts*

**139 Ideology and the Fight Against Human Trafficking**
*Reyhan Atasü-Topcuoğlu*

**140 Rethinking Serial Murder, Spree Killing, and Atrocities**
Beyond the Usual Distinctions
*Robert Shanafelt and Nathan W. Pino*

**141 The Re-Use of Urban Ruins**
Atmospheric Inquiries of the City
*Hanna Katharina Göbel*

**142 Reproductive Tourism in the United States**
Creating Family in the Mother Country
*Lauren Jade Martin*

**143 The Bohemian Ethos**
Questioning Work and Making a Scene on the Lower East Side
*Judith R. Halasz*

**144 Critical Theory and Social Media**
Between Emancipation and Commodification
*Thomas Allmer*

**145 Socio-Cultural Mobility and Mega-Events**
Ethics and Aesthetics in Brazil's 2014 World Cup
*Rodanthi Tzanelli*

**146 Seeing Religion**
Toward a Visual Sociology of Religion
*Edited by Roman Williams*

147 **European Citizenship and Social Integration in the EU**
*Jürgen Gerhards and Holger Lengfeld*

148 **International Migration and Ethnic Relations**
Critical Perspectives
*Edited by Magnus Dahlstedt and Anders Neergaard*

149 **Stigma and the Shaping of the Pornography Industry**
*Georgina Voss*

150 **Religious Identity and Social Change**
Explaining Christian conversion in a Muslim world
*David Radford*

151 **God, Politics, Economy**
Social Theory and the Paradoxes of Religion
*Bülent Diken*

152 **Lifestyles and Subcultures**
History and a New Perspective
*Luigi Berzano and Carlo Genova*

153 **Comedy and Social Science**
Towards a Methodology of Funny
*Cate Watson*

154 **Sociology of Economic Innovation**
*Francesco Ramella*

155 **Mobility, Modernity and the Slum**
The Real and Virtual Journeys of 'Slumdog Millionaire'
*Rodanthi Tzanelli*

156 **The Geography of Nostalgia**
Global and Local Perspectives on Modernity and Loss
*Alastair Bonnett*

157 **Transnational Students and Mobility**
Lived Experiences of Migration
*Hannah Soong*

158 **Aging in Contexts of Migration**
*Edited by Ute Karl and Sandra Torres*

159 **Twentieth Century Population Thinking**
A Critical Reader of Primary Sources
*Edited by Population Knowledge Network*

160 **The Synchronization of National Policies**
Ethnography of the Global Tribe of Moderns
*Pertti Alasuutari*

161 **Retail and the Artifice of Social Change**
*Steven Miles*

162 **Theorizing Social Memories**
Concepts and Contexts
*Edited by Gerd Sebald and Jatin Wagle*

163 **Addiction, Modernity, and the City**
A Users' Guide to Urban Space
*Christopher B.R. Smith*

164 **Medicine, Risk, Discourse and Power**
*Edited by John Martyn Chamberlain*

# Medicine, Risk, Discourse and Power

Edited by John Martyn Chamberlain

Routledge
Taylor & Francis Group
NEW YORK AND LONDON

First published 2016
by Routledge
711 Third Avenue, New York, NY 10017

and by Routledge
2 Park Square, Milton Park, Abingdon, Oxon OX14 4RN

*Routledge is an imprint of the Taylor & Francis Group, an informa business*



*Library of Congress Cataloging-in-Publication Data*
Medicine, risk, discourse and power / edited by John Martyn Chamberlain.
p. ; cm. — (Routledge advances in sociology ; 164)
Includes bibliographical references and index.
I. Chamberlain, John Martyn, 1972– , editor. II. Series: Routledge advances in sociology ; 164.
[DNLM: 1. Medicine. 2. Risk. 3. Sociological Factors. WB 100]
R729.8
610—dc23 2015025795

ISBN: 978-0-415-50269-6 (hbk)
ISBN: 978-1-315-65874-2 (ebk)

Typeset in Sabon
by Apex CoVantage, LLC



MIX
Paper from responsible sources
FSC www.fsc.org FSC® C013056

Printed and bound in Great Britain by
TJ International Ltd, Padstow, Cornwall

# Contents

# 1 An Introduction to Medicine, Risk, Discourse and Power

*John Martyn Chamberlain*

## INTRODUCTION

The study of modern medicine and the high levels of public trust and social status afforded to it, along with the economic and cultural rewards associated with this state of affairs, has long preoccupied social scientists. Over the last hundred years or so, sociologists have considered the causes and consequences of medical power within society, and more lately, they have considered its decline or, at the very least, just what new form it is transforming into. One particularly important element of this corpus of study has been the consideration of the rhetorical role played by medical knowledge and technology, alongside the diverse forms of clinical expertise which emerge as a result of its application in the health-care diagnosis and treatment context, in promoting risk identification and appraisal discourses that can serve to either promote or inhibit patient control over the medical encounter. Another body of literature linked to this considers the role played by medical discourse and power in enabling and legitimizing the greater surveillance and disciplinary control of populations, be they law abiding and healthy or otherwise. As this chapter will reinforce, both these viewpoints, along with the recognition of the practical value of medical knowledge and expertise for promoting public health and social welfare and community cohesion, are necessary for a fully developed understanding to emerge of the important social role medicine plays in enhancing our lives, both individually and collectively.

Although as we shall see, this has not always been the case; few sociologists today would consider medicine's role in transforming how we can live a healthy life to be beyond critique. It is the purpose of this book to contribute to the academic study of medicine through exploring the application of medical discourse and power through the lens of risk in various national contexts; including, Europe, the US and South America. In doing so, the authors collectively hope to elucidate the similarities and subtle differences which exist internationally in order to advance our understanding of the complex social role played by medicine internationally. In this chapter, I seek to set the scene for this by providing the reader with an introduction to the sociological study of medicine as a *profession* before moving on to situate the contents of each subsequent chapter against this background. To this end, the chapter first will outline the historical development of different sociological frameworks for studying medicine.

## THE SOCIOLOGY OF THE PROFESSIONS

> Our professional institutions are . . . an important stabilizing factor in our whole society
>
> Lynn (1963: 653)

Early sociological analysis of the professions was primarily concerned with the fact that certain occupational groups in society claimed to possess high ethical standards and indeed sought to place their clients' welfare and interests before their own. This explicit moral code governs the behavior of occupational members toward each other and society as a whole, as the Hippocratic Oath does in the case of medicine. This 'collectivity orientation' was seen by sociologists at the end of the nineteenth century to act as a stabilizing force to the excesses of the growing enterprise culture of capitalist-industrial society, whose primary concern was taken to be with profit (Turner 1995). Whether or not this viewpoint regarding capitalist society was correct, early sociologies focus on the altruistic connotations associated with the concept of professionalism reflected the concern of functionalist sociology with how social consensus and social order are maintained.

### Durkheim, Professionalism and Laissez-Faire Capitalism

Indeed, a founding father of functionalist sociology, Emile Durkheim (1957), viewed professional groups as important preconditions to the generation of social stability and consensus in society. Durkheim's concern with the professions as a stabilizing force to the excessive individualism of laissez-faire capitalism stems from his view of society as an organism constantly striving for equilibrium. He argued that individuals within preindustrial societies possessed shared values and beliefs that generated a social consensus called 'mechanical solidarity'. However, he argued that traditional forms of moral authority, which generated collective norms and values, were being undermined by a growing specialization within the division of labor. This was due to the increasingly complex nature of industrial society as the eighteenth and nineteenth centuries progressed. This produced a state of affairs which was causing alienation and anomie (i.e. antisocial individualism) amongst the general populace.

This worried Durkheim. He believed that when collective norms and values declined, social restraints similarly decayed. This could lead to a situation where: "nothing remains but individual appetites, and since they are by nature boundless and insatiable, if there is nothing to control them, they will not be able to control themselves" (Durkheim 1957: 11). All was not lost. Durkheim argued that a new form of 'organic solidarity' was emerging. This was based upon the recognition of the need for cooperation between individuals due to their growing functional interdependence within the social sphere as society became more complex. He held that the professions formed moral communities, which promoted values such as selflessness that engendered social consensus and 'organic solidarity'.

This viewpoint informed much of the subsequent sociological analysis of the professions until the 1960s. For instance, Tawney (1921) held that the economic individualism of capitalism was inherently destructive to the community interest and that the morality of professionalism could be used to counter its excesses. He stated that:

> The difference between industry as it exists today, and profession is, then, simple and unmistakable. The essence of the former is that its only criterion is the financial return, which it offers its shareholders. The essence of the later is that though men enter it for the sake of livelihood the measure of their success is the service which they perform, not the gains which they amass.
>
> (Tawney 1921: 94–95)

Similarly, Parsons (1949) emphasized the social altruism of professional groups by arguing they possessed a 'collectivity-orientation'. While Carr-Saunders and Wilson (1933: 497) held that the professions:

> inherent, preserve and pass on a tradition . . . they engender modes of life, habits of thought and standards of judgment which render them centers of resistance to crude forces which threaten steady and peaceful evolution . . . The family, the church and the universities, certain associations of intellectuals, and above all the great professions, stand like rocks against which the waves raised by these forces beat in vain.

This early functionalist hegemony regarding the sociological study of the professions also revealed itself in the work of authors who were concerned with identifying characteristics which taken together denote that an occupation is a profession. For example, Etzioni (1969) classified occupations into 'professions' and 'semi-professions' based upon characteristics such as length of training. Barber (1963: 671) held that professions possessed four essential attributes—a high degree of generalized and systematic knowledge, an orientation toward the interest of the community instead of individual self-interest, a high degree of self-control exercised by practitioners over behavior through the possession of a code of ethics internalized during a prolonged period of education and training, and, finally, a reward system of monetary and status rewards that are symbolic of work achievement not self-interested gain.

To this day, occupations such as medicine protest that they possess a 'service ideal' when they seek to justify collective privileges. Such as the principle of self-regulation and the individual social and economic rewards which come with the possession of professional status. Yet the core problem with the early functionalist approach to the sociological analysis of the concept of professionalism is that it takes uncritically the altruistic claims of occupations calling themselves professions at face value, while it also views the task of sociology as being to quantify and measure the concept, 'professionalism'. Furthermore, the functionalist approach to the analysis of professionalism was criticized for being largely ahistorical. It lacked consideration of the process by which occupations utilized their cognitive and altruistic resources to exercise power in order to initially gain and subsequently maintain the social and economic rewards associated with the possession of professional status (Johnson 1972). Sociologists were coming to realize that they were starting their analysis of the professions with the wrong question. As Hughes (1963: 656) wrote:

> in my studies I passed from the false question 'Is this occupation a profession?' to the more fundamental one 'What are the circumstances in which people in an occupation attempt to turn it into a profession and themselves into professional people?

Hughes was highlighting that classifying an occupation as a profession was what society did and it was not the task of sociology to do it in more scientific terms. Rather, its focus should be on investigating the socioeconomic and political circumstances out of which the concept of professionalism arose. This signaled the beginning of a more critical turn in the sociological study of the professions. In contrast to the functionalist viewpoint, this focused upon the material and symbolic benefits gained from the possession of an occupational monopoly over license to practice (McDonald 1995). According to this more critical viewpoint, professionalism is not a set of traits which jobs have in common, nor a distinct ethic, but a mode of occupational control (Moran and Wood 1993).

## Critiquing the Altruistic Foundations of Medical Privilege

> The professional rhetoric relating to community service and altruism may be in many cases a significant factor in molding the practices of individual professionals, but it also clearly functions as a legitimation of professional privilege.
>
> (Johnson 1972: 25)

As the quote illustrates, by the start of the 1970s, sociologists were turning away from the viewpoint that the professions transcended the unbridled self-interest they held to be symptomatic of modern society (McDonald 1995). Functionalist sociologists mostly accepted the altruistic claims to public service espoused by professions such as medicine. Indeed, they often endorsed the fact that this separated them from other occupational groups. However, the 1970s saw social scientists question increasingly the legitimacy of the self-espoused altruistic tendencies and 'value-neutral' knowledge claims of occupational groups which possessed professional status. In the context of the medical profession, they began to focus upon how medical professionalism has operated ideologically as an exclusive form of occupational control. This was seen to operate both at the microlevel of everyday interaction through the concept of clinical freedom at the bedside and the macro-institutional level through the principle of state-licensed self-regulation. They highlighted how poorly performing doctors, and in some cases even criminals, were being shielded from public accountability by the 'club rule' of mutual protectionism inherent within medicine's self-regulatory system.

A focus upon professional self-interest as opposed to professional altruism lay at the heart of the growing symbolic interactionist critique of the early functionalist view of the professions in American sociology. The interactionist viewpoint assumes reality is socially constructed in and through everyday social interaction. Consequently, it viewed professionalism as "an ascribed symbolic, socially negotiated status based on day-to-day interaction" (Allsop and Saks 2002: 5). Studies of the medical profession inspired by this viewpoint highlighted that professional principles of altruism, service and high ethical standards were less than perfect human social constructs rather than abstract standards which characterized a formal collectivity (McDonald 1995). Yet instead of focusing on the micro-individual level of the individual professional interacting within his or her work sphere, the growing critique of the professions primarily focused on the macro-organizational and societal level. This was largely informed by neo-Weberian sociology, as the next section of the chapter will demonstrate.

## The Neo-Weberian Perspective

The 1970s saw the growth of the neo-Weberian critique of the professions in general and medical dominance and power in particular. Weber focused upon trying to understand emerging new social patterns in the nineteenth century caused by the rise of industrial technology, the growth of scientific knowledge and the greater potential than ever before for participation by the general populace within the political sphere. Weber was a polymath interested in law, economics, politics, science, religion as well as sociology. A key unifying theme in his writing is the idea that the progressive rationalization of life was the main directional trend in Western civilization. By rationalization, Weber meant a process by which explicit, abstract, calculable rules and procedures (what he called 'formal rationality') increasingly replaced more traditional and personal social values and ways of life (what he called 'substantive rationality') at the organizational and institutional levels which govern social life (Gerth and Wright Mills 1946).

Though Weber did not specifically address the issue of the growth of the professions, his concept of rationalization is clearly tied to the development of modern scientific forms of expertise, and sociologists with a historical bent, such as Parry and Parry (1976), Berlant (1975) and Larkin (1983), primarily drew upon Weber's economic theory of monopolization when analyzing the initial growth and subsequent development of professions such as medicine (Weber 1978). In doing so, they highlighted collective preoccupations with pecuniary interests, securing economic and technical domains, as well as consolidating positions of high social status and power within the sociopolitical arena.

This was to be expected, as Weber views professionals as a privileged commercial class, alongside bankers and merchants. He holds that they seek to exclude competitors and reap economic and social rewards through pursuing strategies that enable them to monopolize the marketplace for their services by controlling market entry and supply. By engaging in collective social mobility (i.e. the formation of group organizations and political pressure groups), occupational groups such as medicine seek to obtain privileges from the political community to become what Weber (1978) called a legally privileged group and ensure the closure of social and economic opportunities to outsiders.

## FREIDSON AND MEDICAL POWER

A key early proponent of the neo-Weberian 'social closure' model was Freidson (1970). In 1970, Freidson published his landmark study of the American medical profession, *Profession of Medicine*. In line with Weber's 'social closure' perspective, Freidson held that medicine was a particularly powerful example of how professionalism operated ideologically as a form of occupational control to ensure control of the market for services. Freidson (1970) highlighted that the professions possessed three powerful interlocking arguments on which they justified their privileged status. First, the claim is that there is such an unusual degree of skill and knowledge involved in professional work that nonprofessionals are not equipped to evaluate or regulate it. Second, it is claimed that professionals are responsible—that they may be trusted to work conscientiously without supervision. Third, the claim is that the profession itself may be trusted to undertake the proper regulatory action on those rare occasions when an individual does not perform his work competently or ethically.

Freidson recognized that medical autonomy must be viewed as having limits as the state was involved in the organization and delivery of health care. Occupations must submit to its 'protective custody' to reap the social and economic rewards associated with being a profession. Nevertheless, the state largely left doctors alone to control the technical aspects of their work. This made it for him such a good example of what a profession is. He argued that:

> so long as a profession is free of the technical evaluation and control of other occupations in the division of labor, its lack of ultimate freedom from the state, and even the lack of control over the socio-economic terms of work, do not significantly change its essential character as profession.
>
> (Freidson 1970: 20)

Freidson discussed how medical professionalism operated ideologically as a form of occupational control at the microlevel of everyday interaction through the concept of clinical freedom at the bedside, as well as at the macro-institutional level through the principle of state-licensed self-regulation. The common link between the micro and macro aspects of medical autonomy for Freidson was the need for a doctor to exercise personal judgment and discretion in her work due to its inherently specialist nature (Freidson 1970, 1994, 2001). This state of affairs was legitimized by the scientific basis of modern medical expertise and public acceptance of medicine's altruistic claim that it put patient need first. Furthermore, Freidson argued that medicine's freedom to control the technical evaluation of its own work had led to it possessing a high level of dominance and control not only over patients but also over the work of other health-care occupations, such as nursing for example. Freidson (1970: 137) stated that medicine

> has the authority to direct and evaluate the work of others without in turn being subject for formal direction and evaluation by them. Paradoxically its autonomy is sustained by the dominance of its expertise in the division of labor.

Freidson concluded that the dominance of medicine in the health-care arena had a negative effect on the quality of health-care patients received. For Freidson, medicine was failing to self-manage satisfactorily its affairs and ensure that adequate quality control mechanisms to govern doctors' day-to-day activities were in place. Freidson (1970: 370) believed that the development of unaccountable, self-governing institutions surrounding medical training and work had led to the profession of medicine to possess:

> a self-deceiving vision of the objectivity and reliability of its knowledge and the virtues of its members. . . . [Medicine's] very autonomy had led to insularity and a mistaken arrogance about its mission in the world.

## The Dominance of the 'Social Closure' Model

Given the previous discussion, it is not surprising to learn then that the neo-Weberian viewpoint has dominated the sociological study of medicine since the 1970s. It encapsulates many of the socio-legal and political realities of the regulatory context with regards to the professions in general and medicine in particular, particularly in Western nation-states where occupational associations and peer-led colleges, such as the Royal College of Medicine in the United Kingdom, exercise considerable influence in regards to ensuring members adhere to professional practice standards. However, the neo-Weberian perspective is not beyond criticism. It can be accused of being as one sided as early functionalist accounts when they uncritically accepted the altruistic claims made by occupational groups such as medicine. For the neo-Weberian viewpoint does highlight how professions sought to obtain, protect and promote their self-interest over the interest of their clients. Nevertheless, it can be argued that it does so by neglecting that the day-to-day activities of a large number of health-care practitioners demonstrate that they possess a strong personal commitment to their work. Indeed, they often place their personal needs second to their professional commitments in order to ensure that patients receive the best quality of care possible. It could equally be argued, however, that the value of the neo-Weberian analysis lies in the fact that it reinforces the need for the general public and state to recognize that doctors need to be able to exercise discretion in their work and, indeed, can by and large be trusted to place their clients' interests before their own.

## Medicine and the State: The Invasion of Capital Into the House of Medicine

Despite its dominance in the sociological study of professional regulation, the neo-Weberian perspective was criticized by authors operating from a neo-Marxist viewpoint for failing to account for the entwined nature of the development of the modern state and professions such as medicine, as was touched upon earlier when discussing 'club governance' (Moran 1999, 2004). Indeed, although his *Profession of Medicine* was (and still is) regarded as a sociological classic, Freidson was criticized by neo-Marxist commentators for ignoring the political economy and under theorizing the relationship between medical and state power. Freidson's work does tend to assume that the professions are independent from or at least neutral vis-à-vis the class structure. In contrast, the neo-Marxist perspective of the professions argued that medical dominance in the health-care division of labor played a central role in the surveillance and reproduction of working-class labor on behalf of capital (Johnson 1977). As Johnson (1977: 106) notes:

> the professionalism of medicine—those institutions sustaining its autonomy—is directly related to its monopolization of 'official'

> definitions of illness and health. The doctor's certificate defines and legitimates the withdrawal of labor. Credentialism, involving monopolistic practices and occupational closure, fulfils ideological functions in relation to capital and reflects the extent to which medicine in its role of surveillance and the reproduction of labor power is able to draw upon powerful ideological symbols.

McKinley is typical of the neo-Marxist viewpoint when he states that "the House of Medicine under capitalism will never contribute to improvements in health unless such improvements facilitate an acceptable level of profit" (McKinley 1977: 462). According to neo-Marxists, there is no difference between the production of taken-for-granted capitalist commodities such as cars, fridges and clothes and the practice of the surgical techniques of modern medicine, such as open-heart surgery (Navarro, 1976). Both involve the search for profit. Large corporations involved in the production of medical supplies, particularly pharmaceutical therapies, profit from individual experiences of illness and disease (Navarro 1986).

Neo-Marxist commentators may agree with their neo-Weberian counterparts that medicine possessed substantial control over other health-care occupations and patients. Nevertheless, they also held that medical work was increasingly coming under direct bureaucratic-managerial surveillance and control operating on behalf of capital (McKinley 1977). The neo-Marxist sociologist Navarro (1976, 1986) argued that medical autonomy is tied to the needs of capital. He held that it only emerged because the increasingly scientific foundations to medical expertise were congruent with the interests and needs of nineteenth century industrialists, who were using the apparently neutral concept of science to justify the introduction of new factory-based, mass production methods. Navarro (1976) argued that there had been an invasion of the house of medicine by capital and consequently medical knowledge and technology could not be seen as separate from capitalism but rather were a part of it. Medical knowledge was not overlain onto capital ideology but rather modern medicine under capitalism is capitalist medicine (Navarro 1980). Navarro views medicine's essentially mechanistic view of the human body as being tied up with the capitalist mode of production. Neo-Marxists argue that medicine plays a key role in supporting the status quo in the capitalist system by reinforcing the idea that 'lifestyle choices' as well as 'natural processes' are responsible for personal and collective experiences of illness and disease. They hold that in adopting this approach, medicine camouflages alternative social and economic factors relating to worker exploitation under the capitalist system (McKinley 1977).

A key criticism of the neo-Marxist viewpoint is that, similar to functionalism, it seeks to explain medicine's position in society as stemming from the important social role it plays in maintaining the established social order. The main difference between the two perspectives is that neo-Marxists regarded this order as exploitative and ultimately offering no benefit to the individual worker. This is an overly simplistic viewpoint. In contrast, authors operating from the Foucauldian Governmentality perspective may, like their neo-Marxist counterparts, focus upon how health- and social-care professions such as medicine are deeply bound up with the process of governing populations. So much so that Governmentality authors such as Johnson (1995: 13) hold that, "the expert is not sheltered by the environing state, but shares in the autonomy of the state".

Yet the key difference between the respective neo-Marxist and Foucauldian perspectives is that while the neo-Marxist viewpoint sees this state of affairs as fundamentally repressive by arguing it sustains class-based inequalities, in contrast a Foucauldian viewpoint considers its productive affects. It does this by focusing upon the role professional expertise plays in promoting and sustaining an individual's capacity for engaging in self-surveillance and self-regulation (i.e. through acting on advice provided by his or her local general practitioner and other public health experts regarding appropriate dietary and exercise regimes) (Peterson and Bunton 1997). For the Governmentality perspective sees this as being part of the ability of expertise to render "the complexities of modern social and economic life knowable, practicable and amenable to governing" (Johnson 1995: 23). The chapter will now turn to discussing the Governmentality perspective and its contribution to the sociological study of the professions.

## Governmentality and the Revival of Liberalism

The 1970s and 1980s saw the renewal of liberalism as an economic and political ideology, with its emphasis on individualism, advocacy of 'rolling back the state' and belief in the ability of the discipline of the market to promote consumer choice, improve service quality and minimize risk. Classical liberalism emerged in the seventeenth and eighteenth centuries, through the works of a variety of writers, such as Thomas Hobbes, John Stuart Mills, Adam Smith, Thomas Locke, Jeremy Bentham and Herbert Spencer. It is possible to identify at the center of classical liberalism the underlying concept of possessive individualism (Macpherson 1962). Macpherson (1962) argues that for these thinkers, the individual and her capabilities prefigure the circumstance into which she is born. In short, her talents and who she is owes nothing to society, rather she owns herself, and she is morally and legally responsible for herself and herself alone. She is naturally self-reliant and free from dependence on others. She need only enter into relationships with others because they help her pursue her self-interests. According to this viewpoint, society is seen as a series of market-based relations made between self-interested subjects who are actively pursuing their own interests. Only by recognizing and supporting this position politically and economically will the greatest happiness for the greatest number be achieved. Classical liberalism is a critique of state reason, which seeks to set limits on state power.

It is against this background of the re-emergence of liberalism that sociologists concerned with the role and governance of expertise within society have recognized the importance of the work of Foucault and his concept of Governmentality in the analysis of the relationship between the professions and the state (Peterson and Bunton 1997). This highlights how individual subjectivities are neither fixed nor stable but rather are constituted in and through a spiral of power-knowledge discourses. These are generated by political objectives, institutional regimes and expert disciplines, whose primary aim is to produce governable individuals (Dean 1999).

At the end of the eighteenth century onward there was a steady growth in 'the dubious sciences', what Foucault calls the human sciences, particularly new scientific disciplines, such as psychiatry. Foucault holds that a key outcome of the rise of these new sciences was the more intensive use of 'dividing practices' to objectify an individual and his or her body via systems of notation, classification and standardization (Turner 1995). Foucault argues that through their examination and assessment techniques, experts produce normative classifications for subjective positions (normal, mad, sexually deviant, etc.), which increasingly became inscribed within the disciplinary regimes of society's organizational and institutional structures. There regimes spread throughout society as a whole as the dominance of the 'pastoral power' of Christianity started to decline and a more secular concern with 'the conduct of conduct', Governmentality, emerged from the sixteenth century onward (Foucault 1991).

Foucault first published his study of Governmentality in 1979 and further developed it as a concept within a series of lectures given at the College de France. Foucault discusses that from around the sixteenth century onward, an ever-growing number of treatises were published on the governance of the soul and the self, the family and the state. These were published against an increasingly complex background of technological development, rapid social change and political and intellectual upheaval. It should not be surprising to learn that events such as the Enlightenment, the Reformation, the rise of modern science and development of industrial capitalism collectively led to a growth in the writing of treatises which sought to answer fundamental problems of rule: "how strictly, by whom, to what end, by what methods etc" (Foucault 1991: 88). Foucault notes that these treatises focused more and more upon the idea that good governance entailed 'the right disposition of things' and had as its aim the common welfare and salvation of all. Governance came to involve securing the security, health, welfare and happiness of the population. The population comes to appear above all else as the ultimate end of government (Foucault 1991). Over time, governance would become increasingly tied into a liberalist conception of economics. Good government was economical, both fiscally and in its use of power.

Furthermore, the development of new forms of expertise, Foucault's dubious human sciences such as psychology, medicine and sociology, are tied up with this need to govern the population to ensure its betterment. This was because at an increasingly complex administrative and bureaucratic level, the population was seen as possessing its own regularities, its own rate of deaths and diseases, its cycles of scarcity and so on (Foucault 1991). Consequently, "novel forms of expertise in the fields of public health hygiene, mental health and mass surveillance emerged in concert with developing government policies and programmes . . . and were intimately involved in the construction of governable realms of social reality" (Johnson 1994: 142). The modern professions and their associated training and regulatory arrangements are emergent as an aspect of the formation of a liberal form of Governmentality that has as its target the population and its welfare, and which itself was emergent with the growth of capitalist-industrial economies across Europe during the nineteenth century.

Foucault notes that two other forms of power, sovereignty and discipline, are tied up with the development of the power of a population-focused form of governance, with its concern for 'the conduct of conduct', to enable the promotion of the security, health, wealth and happiness of individual subject-citizens. Sovereign 'command' power is exercised over subjects through the juridical and executive arms of government. Historically, sovereign power is related to monarchical rule, with its executive mechanisms of constitutions, laws and parliaments. Over time, these were made into more representative institutions through the development of democratic ideals, with allegiance to the monarch becoming transformed into allegiance to the rule of law (Foucault 1991). The power of discipline goes back to ancient religious, military and educational practices.

As Foucault noted in *Discipline and Punish* (1979), its expansion over the population during the seventeenth and eighteenth centuries is tied up with a growing administrative and institutional need to survey and make docile individual and collective bodies. Disciplined individuals have acquired habits of action and thought which enable them to act in appropriate and expected ways and to do so through the exercise of self-control (Foucault 1979). 'Good governance' is about how to best align the sovereign power of command and productive disciplinary power in order to achieve the primary object of securing the health, wealth and happiness of the population. This is why Foucault argues that the power of governance does not replace the power of discipline or sovereignty. Rather it recruits them. Indeed Foucault (1991: 102) argues that:

> we need to see things not in terms of the replacement of a society of sovereignty by a disciplinary society and the subsequent replacement of a disciplinary society by a society of government; in reality one has a triangle, sovereignty-discipline-government, which has as its primary target the population.

In short, the power of governance is where technologies of domination of individuals over one another have recourse to processes by which the individual acts upon himself and, conversely, where techniques of the self are integrated into structures of coercion (Foucault 1991). Governance retains and utilizes the techniques, rationalities and institutions characteristic of both sovereignty and discipline, but it also departs from them and seeks to reinscribe them. The object of sovereign power is the exercise of authority over the subjects of the state within a defined territory, e.g., the deductive practices of levying taxes, of meting out punishments. The objects of disciplinary power are the regulation and ordering of the numbers of people within that territory, e.g., in practices of schooling, military training or the organization of work. The new object of government, by contrast, regards these subjects and the forces and capacities of living individuals, as members of a population, as resources to be fostered, to be used and to be optimized (Dean 1999).

## The Contribution of the Governmentality Perspective

The Governmentality perspective makes a significant contribution to the sociological study of medicine. It highlights the key role professions, such as medicine, have played in the governance of the population. In doing so, it adopts a similar critical view of the emergence of professionalism as a form of regulatory control as the neo-Weberian perspective. It highlights how it is theoretically useful to collapse the 'commonsense' dichotomy of state-profession, which often exists in sociological accounts of the professions and the governance of expertise. For neoliberal 'mentalities of rule' are concerned with 'the conduct of conduct' as they seek to promote the autonomous self-actualized enterprising subject who, as an active citizen of a modern democracy, recognizes they are responsible for themselves. This means that modern government must seek to govern through the freedom and aspirations of their citizen-subjects so that they come to recognize and self-regulate their activities in such a way that they 'naturally' align with broader social, economic and political objectives. This requirement has led to a critical reconfiguration of the legitimate grounds on which 'good governance' can be practiced. With the 'field of medicine' becoming more than ever before simultaneously 'governed' and 'self-governing' as a consequence (Deleuze 1988). As illustrated by the reappropriation by medical elites of an emergent rationalistic-bureaucratic discourse of outcomes-based standard setting and performance appraisal in the face of its increasing use by 'outsiders', such as hospital management, to monitor the activities of doctors.

However, the Governmentality perspective suffers from the fact that, in a practical sense, professional groups and the state *are* different entities. And it is arguable that they should always be treated as such if sociological understanding is furthered regarding the role-institutionalized forms of expertise, such as medicine, play in the governance of the population. Certainly it is often necessary for practical reasons to demarcate professional expertise from the governing apparatus of the state. Particularly when analyzing empirically the effect of contemporary reforms on the principle of professional self-regulation in the eyes of professional practitioners themselves. It is the neo-Weberian 'social closure' perspective that is most useful here. For its account of the historical development of medicine's exclusive cognitive identity, which underpins its 'members only' stance concerning the issue of who should govern doctors, reflects the nature of the regulatory context and the form of the occupational culture of the medical profession, particularly in in the Anglo-American context.

## The Rise of the Risk Society

Finally, a key further development pertinent to the study of the medical profession is the emergence of risk as an organizing construct in the sociological study of medical discourse and power. For many social scientists, the re-emergence of liberalism from the 1980s coincided with a general social shift toward the conditions of late or high modernity. We certainly live in an increasingly interconnected, technologically advanced, globalized world where events and happenings occurring on the other side of the globe are immediately available for personal consumption (and arguably therefore immediately impact on the sociocultural and economic-political spheres). For social theorists such as Beck (1992) and Giddens (1990, 1991, 1999), a key defining feature of modern society—or late or high modernity as they call it—is that there has been:

> a social impetus towards individualization of unprecedented scale and dynamism . . . [which] . . . forces people—for the sake of their survival—to make themselves the center of their own life plans and conduct.
>
> (Beck and Beck-Gernsheim 2002: 31)

Both Beck and Giddens argue that as capitalist-industrial society gives way under the tripartite forces of technology, consumerism and globalization, there is a categorical shift in the nature of social structures, and, more importantly, the relationship between the individual and society. Here key sociological categories which have traditionally structured society increasingly lose their meaning. Hence social categories such as race, gender and class, for example, increasingly no longer serve to restrict people's social opportunities or define who they are as individuals to the extent they once did. Furthermore, as working conditions change, and the technology and communication revolutions continue at pace, more than ever before individuals are required to make life-changing decisions concerning education, work, self-identity and personal relationships in a world where traditional beliefs about social class, gender and the family are being overturned.

Now for many social theorists this state of affairs has led to a concern with dangerousness and risk entering center stage within society's institutional governing apparatus, alongside individual subject-citizen's personal decision-making process (Mythen 2004). One of the key risk theorists, Giddens (1990), talks about two forms of risk: external and manufactured risk. Put simply, external risks are those posed by the world around us and manufactured risks are created by human beings themselves. In essence, as Giddens explains, it is the difference between worrying about what nature can do with us—in the form of floods, famine and so on—and worrying about what we have done to the natural world via how we organize social life. But of course it is not that simple. Risk theorists argue that throughout human history, societies have always sought to risk-manage threats, hazards and dangers. But these management activities have by and large been concerned with natural external risks, such as infectious diseases and famine.

However, in today's technologically advanced society, individuals are seen to be both the producers and minimizers of manufactured risk (Giddens 1990). That is, within the conditions of high modernity, risks are seen to be solely the result of human activity (Mythen 2004). Hence manufactured risk takes over. Even events previously held to be natural disasters, such as floods and famine, are now held to be avoidable consequences of human activities that must be risk-managed (Lupton 2011). Hence society's governing institutions and expert bodies need to become ever more collectively self-aware of their role in the creation and management of risk (Beck and Beck-Gernsheim 2002). For individuals, meanwhile, uncertainties now litter their pathway through life to such an extent that it appears to be loaded with real and potential risks. So they must seek out and engage with a seemingly ever-growing number of information resources, provided by a myriad of sources, as they navigate through their world. In the risk society, we "find more and more guidebooks and practical manuals to do with health, diet, appearance, exercise, lovemaking and many other things" (Giddens 1991: 218).

Of course, this state of affairs all links in with the possessive liberalism view of individuals being responsible for themselves and, indeed, risk theorists such as Giddens and Beck talk about how we can see that since the 1960s and '70s there has been a growing cultural and political discourse of rights and responsibilities emerging which seeks to regulate the individual while also arguing for the need for greater personal freedom. This leads us into another key feature of high modernity, which is arguably central to the study of medicine. Namely, that within the risk society, a sense of growing (perhaps even mutual) distrust characterizes the relationship between the public and experts (Giddens 1999). At the same time, a pervasive and seemingly increasingly necessary reliance on an ever-growing number of experts appears to be a key feature of individuals' personal experiences of everyday life (Mythen 2004).

Interestingly, it was argued that this established the conditions for the public to challenge elitism and expert forms of knowledge. For under such changing social conditions, expert authority can no longer simply stand on the traditional basis of position and status. Not least of all because individuals' growing need to manage risk and problem solve their everyday lives, to make choices about who they are and what they should do means that personal access to the technical and expert knowledge of the elite becomes more urgent than ever before. The development of mass information sharing tools, such as the mobile phone, personal computer and the Internet, meant that knowledge and expertise were no longer the sole preserve of those elite few who had undergone specialist training. As Giddens (1991: 144–146) notes:

> technical knowledge is continually re-appropriated by lay agents . . . Modern life is a complex affair and there are many 'filter back' processes whereby technical knowledge, in one shape or another, is re-appropriated by lay persons and routinely applied in the course of their day-to-day activities . . . Processes of re-appropriation relate to all aspects of social life—for example, medical treatments, child rearing or sexual pleasure.

There is then a tension between experts and citizens, between those in power and those who are not, and this can perhaps most clearly be seen in relation to modern technological advancements, particularly in relation to the rise of surveillance technology. After all, surveillance is essential to the task of identifying and managing and controlling risk. Not least of all because under the neoliberal social conditions associated with high modernity, it is by their ability to successfully manage risk that state legitimizes its governing activities. Bound up with this, as we shall now turn to discuss, is the need for law-abiding citizens to allow the surveillance of their everyday lives to become a normalized feature of everyday existence

## EXPLORING MEDICINE AND RISK: A BRIEF OVERVIEW OF SUBSEQUENT CHAPTERS

I would argue that the preceding discussion reinforces that as both producer and user of the fruits of modern scientific research, medicine has played a key role in the dispersal of new forms of population discipline throughout modern society. Medicine has formed a key part of the development of the disciplinary apparatus of the modern state as it has increasingly sought to manage the risks associated with urban planning and environmental management, public health, social welfare and the problem of criminality. The profiling, care and treatment of a range of risk-laden, dangerous subpopulations, including the criminal, the mentally ill, as well as the serially violent and sexually abusive, are all subject in one way or another to modern advances in the technology of health-care delivery, medical diagnostic and surgical procedures and pharmacological regimes. All of which have been bequeathed to us by the success of modern biomedical science in conceptualizing, surveying, examining and treating the human body as it suffers from a range of illnesses and diseases on its sometimes all too short journey from the maternity ward to the mortuary table. And it is against this context that the following chapters explore different aspects of the application of medical knowledge and expertise.

In chapter two, "Sociology and Risk: A Link in Permanent (Re)Construction", Fiorella Mancini analyzes the genesis, distribution and management of social risk in complex societies against a concern with the individual life course. In doing so, the problem of risk imposes a new demand on the social sciences: with what analytical tools and methodologies can one read the social map of complex societies? Andy Alaszewski and Patrick Brown seek to answer this question in chapter three, "Time, Risk and Health", where they focus on *time* is a key element of social life. They begin by noting that time has been relatively neglected in social theory and in the study of health and risk. They show how interrogating understandings of time provides insights into how uncertainty and risk shape the ways in which organizations and individuals respond to illness. While individuals have their own personal 'my' time, if they want to engage with others, they need to recognize and align their personal time with others, and this alignment involves implicit agreements about and standardization of time between members of a community. The development of abstract times has implication for the ways in which individuals think about and organize their personal time and the ways in which time is used to organize activities in modern bureaucratic organizations. In this manner, the development of abstract time has created the possibility for individuals to view their own lives through the lens of risk.

Alaszewski and Brown note that in modern society, bureaucratic organizations play a key role in the creation and management of uncertainty; for example, hospitals claim to provide a safe environment which individuals can rely on during fateful moments when their very existence is under threat. Such organization use abstract time embedded in institutional routines to manage uncertainty. While such routines may appear to be rational and technically neutral, they do in practice contain irrational elements and are used as a form of social control. There is tension between the abstract time imposed by organizations and institutions and personal timings which form an important locus of power relations. Personal time is often colonized by those in more powerful positions and by organizations, while resistance to such colonization requires both determination and subterfuge.

Brown also further explores the need to develop new analytical approaches to examining medicine and risk in chapter four, which is entitled "Using Medicines in the Face of Uncertainty—Developing a Habermasian Understanding of Medicines Lifeworlds". This chapter introduces the concept of lifeworld as a useful basis for exploring how various social actors make sense of their health, illness and medicines (non-) use in light of background knowledge and assumptions. In this way, the lifeworld generates exciting analytical possibilities for interrogating how actors give meaning to medicines, how related risks and uncertainties come to be known or assumed away, and how such processes are structured amid broader social norms and taken-for-granted modes of acting in everyday life. One of the central purposes of the chapter is to extend this more Schutzian and culture-oriented approach toward a more Habermasian conceptualization. Habermas's lifeworld is three dimensional, encompassing cultural properties of common-lived experiences which lead medicine users (MUs) to assume truths, or question uncertainties, around medicines; MUs' particular membership and relative location within social groups and communities which shape the perceived legitimacy of using particular medicines or, in contrast, the legitimacy of particular risks attributed to medicines; and individual MUs' biographically acquired sense of self (identity), which becomes bound up with practices of medicines (non-) use in relation to experiences of authenticity. Applied to various case studies of medicines' use amid uncertainty, this more elaborate lifeworld conceptualization is then developed further in two key respects. First, in providing a 'thicker' grasp of socially embedded action around medicines and risks in that, far from a mere intellectual exercise of reflexivity toward knowledge and various truth-claims therein, this 'doing' is profoundly structured by actors' locations within particular social spaces and communities, not to mention their identities and biographies. So while individuals may challenge and rework mainstream perspectives of medicines and uncertainty in ways which resonate as authentic with their identities and biographies, the extent to which these views and actions are legitimated within social networks and communities are important to understanding the emancipation and/or vulnerability of such agency. Second, although analyzing medicines' use and risk practices in terms of actors' social locations within cultural communities recalls aspects of Mary Douglas's work, Habermasian approaches go much further by capturing the effects of an uncoupling of the political-economic from cultural processes within late modernity. By considering how the reproduction of lifeworlds—in terms of rationalizing cultural understandings, generating social cohesion and socializing individual identities—is impeded by system concerns of money and power, various important and insidious effects of power and institutionalized knowledge are rendered apparent

In chapter five, "Performing Risk and Power: Predictive Technologies in Personalized Medicine", Nadav Even Chorev similarly focuses on matters of power to explore how quantified predictions of risk and efficacy, produced and used by artifacts and humans in the field of personalized medicine, reflect the interests of powerful elites. To explore this topic, the chapter analyses a qualitative case-study analysis of the WINTHER (Worldwide Innovative Network THERapeutic) cancer clinical trial in which a personalized method to tailor treatment is applied. This trial does not test a new therapy but a personalized method by which to choose between various possible therapies. In order to achieve this goal, the trial makes use of computerized matches between the molecular characteristics of the participating patients and information on drugs. As part of the trial, an algorithm was developed to rank drugs according to their projected effectiveness for a specific patient based on analysis comparing the patient's gene expression in the tumor with that in the normal tissue. The investigators factor these results into their decision-making process on suitable treatment for the specific patient. This approach, it is argued, attests to a new development that has implications for the governmental understanding of risk as a form of power. Risk, according to this approach, is not only attached to the body by the external application of epidemiological assessments. Estimations of risk and uncertainty in this case are reached from within the individual body as well. This partly reverses the rationality of risk as conceptualized by governmental studies in which individual attributes disappear into large statistical distributions. By discussing a specific instance of clinical decision making, the chapter reveals how this partial reversal takes place in actuality. Information artifacts enact their performative capacity in the context of the trial while interacting with human actors and other discursive and nondiscursive elements. By producing predictive and probabilistic estimations of an uncertain future, they exert what is termed 'power to': the capacity to carry out actions. Yet when examined in the framework of the trial, this form of power gains a relational quality, usually ascribed to the domination of one actor over another or 'power over'.

Jeremy Dixon explores the complex relationships which exist between notions of 'power to' and 'power over' when he explores in chapter six two dominant themes within mental health care today—risk and recovery—in a piece entitled "Balancing Risk and Recovery in Mental Health: An Analysis of the Way in Which Policy Objectives Around Risk and Recovery Affect Professional Practice in England". Drawing on Governmentality theory, the chapter focuses on professional practice in England where there has been an increase in law and policy focused on risk management since the 1990s. It is argued that public concerns about the perceived risk that people with mental health problems are seen to pose to others has led to a range of 'safety-first' policies. These policies have promoted the use of standardized risk tools and coercive treatments in the community. However, a focus on risk only tells half the story, as the government has also introduced policy objectives promoting notions of recovery. Whilst the concept of recovery is contested, most definitions focus on the subjective experience of service users arguing that they should be able to define what recovery means to them. This poses an implicit challenge to mental health professionals seeking to frame and manage risk.

The chapter charts the tensions between these two sets of policy objectives. It is argued that service users are only enabled to define their own recovery in cases where professionals do not view their choices as 'risky'. The chapter concludes by examining the way in which mental health professionals currently assess and manage risk. It is argued that professionals have resisted the use of standardized risk tools. However, policy directives instructing professionals to minimize risk continue to frame professional practice. Consequently, professionals are only able to facilitate service users' recovery goals in limited circumstances.

In chapter seven, "Moving From Gut Feeling to Evidence: The Case of Social Work", Gemma Mitchell charts how the rise of evidence-based practice (EBP) in child and family social work has been underpinned by a techno-rational response to risk and uncertainty which persists despite a robust critique of EBP in both medicine and social work. This is the context in which social workers must make judgments and decisions about children and their families; a crucial part of which is sharing information with others. Although a vast amount of literature exists on the problems inherent in sharing knowledge between experts in other fields, there tends to be an assumption within this literature that those within the same field can share information in a fairly straightforward manner. The chapter challenges this assumption and explores how, when sharing risk knowledges, social workers use complex informal practices to respond to the disparity between the messy, uncertain reality of family life and what is deemed to be 'acceptable' evidence that can help promote change for children and their families. The findings are based on qualitative interviews with thirty-five qualified and unqualified social workers and document analysis of official rules and guidance.

Mitchell argues that 'deep expertise' is required in order to sharing risk knowledges within the same epistemic community. Deep expertise includes 1) acknowledging the importance of gut feeling to social work practice, which is a form of tacit knowledge; and 2) an ability to move from gut feeling to evidence which is accepted by the profession and also other groups, such as the police, health and education. She holds that social workers are able to facilitate this move by sharing their gut feeling with others using what she calls 'adequate explication'. Finally, she argues that a further sign of expertise in child and family social work is the ability to acknowledge the role of gut feeling within this epistemic community and reconcile this with the traditional EBP approach that underpins the official rules and guidance they must follow.

John Martyn Chamberlain explores the role of knowledge, power and professional jurisdictions in chapter eight, "Regulating for Safer Doctors in the Risk Society", which examines reforms in medical governance through the lens of Governmentality and risk society perspectives. In doing so, Chamberlain notes the central role played by science and medicine in the construction of regulatory order in the United Kingdom. This point is explored in a different context several thousand miles away by Renata Motta and Florencia Arancibia in chapter nine, "Health Experts Challenge the Safety of Pesticides in Argentina and Brazil". Motta and Arancibia assert that pesticides provide a good entry point to discuss the role of science and medicine in the construction of a regulatory order that legitimizes the dominant model of agrarian development in South America as well as in challenging it and constructing alternatives. The chapter addresses the problem of how the high and nonassessed negative health and environmental impacts of agrarian practices with intensive use of pesticides are ignored by science-based regulatory frameworks and constitutes issues of 'undone science'.

Through a comparative case study, Motta and Arancibia analyze the role of health professionals in challenging 'regulatory science' and producing knowledge that supports claims from local populations in their struggles against the unrestricted use of pesticides in Argentina and Brazil, two important global agrarian players. They argue that their analysis shows that even if producing 'undone science' is a critical first step in challenging the regulatory science's discourse that agrochemicals are safe, making these findings 'official' and changing current regulatory frameworks requires further struggle. Finally, in chapter ten, "Changing Discourses of Risk and Health-Risk—A Corpus Analysis of the Usage of the Term Risk in the *New York Times*", Jens O. Zinn and Daniel McDonald bring the collection of essays to a close by looking at the role of the media in reporting health risks. They argue that the development of social media, mobile devices and advancements in the digitization and storage of text, means 'big data' are offering new opportunities for social science research. They note that it is not only the production of new data in the present, but the digitization of old data such as (historical) newspaper archives which open unprecedented opportunities for sociologists to examine long-term social change. Against this background, they outline the findings of their research, which capitalizes on the increased availability of digitized newspaper archives in order to examine discursive changes in the meaning and use of risk in relation to the reporting of health issues, focusing on data from the *New York Times* (NYT) between the years 1987–2014. Zinn and McDonald note that there is a clear trend toward reporting the negative side of risk, a representation of risk as uncertain rather than controlled. They consider the consequences of this for the sociological analysis of health reporting and regulation. In doing so, they usefully end our exploration of medicine and risk by highlighting how this relationship is often mediated by other interest groups who may further misconstrue events. It is left to the reader to decide how best to respond to this state of affairs in their own professional practice.

## REFERENCES

Allsop, J. and Mulcahy, L. (1996) *Regulating Medical Work: Formal and Informal Controls* Milton Keynes: Open University Press.

Allsop, J. and Saks, M. (2002, editors) *Regulating the Health Professions* London: Sage Publications.

Barber, B. (1963) Some Problems in the Sociology of the Professions *Daedalas* 92: 669–689.

Beck, U. (1992) *Risk Society: Towards a New Modernity* London: Sage Publications.

Beck, U. and Beck-Gernsheim, E. (2002) *Individualization: Institutionalized Individualism and its Social and Political Consequences* London: Sage Publications.

Berlant, J.L. (1975) *Profession and Monopoly: A Study of Medicine in the United States and Great Britain* University of California Press.
Blake, C. (1990) *The Charge of the Parasols: Women's Entry to the Medical Profession* London: The Women's Press.
Carr-Saunders, A.M. and Wilson, P.A. (1933) *The Professions* The Clarendon Press.
Davies, C. (2004) Regulating the Health Care Workforce: Next Steps for Research *Journal of Health Services Research and Policy* 9 (1): 2–10.
Dean, M. (1999) *Governmentality: Power and Rule in Modern Society* London: Sage Publications.
Deleuze, G. (1988) *Foucault* Minneapolis, MN: University of Minnesota Press.
Dingwall, R. and Lewis, P. (1983, editors) *The Sociology of the Professions: Lawyers, Doctors and Others* London: McMillan.
Doyal, L. and Pennell I. (1979) *The Political Economy of Health* London: Pluto Press.
Drolet, M. (2004, editor) *The Postmodernism Reader* London: Routledge.
Durkheim, E. (1957) *Professional Ethics and Civic Morals* London: Routledge and Kegan Paul.
Elston, M.A. (1991) The Politics of Professional Power: Medicine in a Changing Medical Service, in Gabe, J., Calman, M, and Bury, M. (editors) *The Sociology of the Health Service* (pp 187–213) London: Routledge.
Elston, M.A. (2004) Medical Autonomy and Medical Dominance, in Gabe, J., Bury, M. and Elston, M.A. (editors) *Key Concepts in Medical Sociology* (pp 56–76). London: Sage Publications.
Engels, F. (1974) *The Condition of the Working Class in England* London: Progress Publishers.
Etzioni, A. (1969) *The Semi-Professions and Their Organization* New York: Free Press.
Freddi, G. and Bjorkman, J.W. (1989, editors) *Controlling Medical Professionals: The Comparative Politics of Health Governance* London: Sage Publications.
Freidson, E. (1970a) *The Profession of Medicine* New York: Dodds Mead.
Freidson, E. (1970b) *Professional Dominance: The Social Structure of Medical Care* New York: Atherton Press.
Freidson, E. (1985) The Reorganization of the Medical Profession *Medical Care Review* 42 (1): 1–20.
Freidson, E. (1994) *Professionalism Reborn: Theory, Prophecy and Policy* Cambridge: Polity Press.
Freidson, E. (2001) *Professionalism: The Third Logic* Cambridge: Polity Press.
Friedman, M. (1962) *Capitalism and Freedom* Chicago: University of Chicago Press.
Foucault. M. (1979) *Discipline and Punish: the Birth of the Prison* London: Allen Lane.
Foucault, M. (1991) Governmentality, in Burchell, G., Gordon, C., and Miller, P. (editors) *The Foucault Effect: Studies in Governmentality* (pp 11–27) London: Harvester Wheatsheaf.
Gabe, J., Bury, M. and Elston, M.A. (2004) *Key Concepts in Medical Sociology* London: Sage Publications.
Gerth, H.H. and Wright Mills, C. (1946) *Essays in Sociology* Oxford: Oxford University Press.
Giddens, A. (1990) *The Consequences of Modernity* Cambridge: Polity.
Giddens, A. (1991) *Modernity and Self-Identity: Self and Society in Late Modernity* Cambridge: Polity.
Giddens, A. (1999) Risk and Responsibility *Modern Law Review* 62 (1): 1–10.
Gladstone, D. (2000, editor) *Regulating Doctors* London: Institute for the Study of Civil Society.

Halliday, T. (1987) *Beyond Monopoly* Chicago: University of Chicago.
Hanlon, G. (1998) Professionalism as Enterprise *Sociology* 32 (1): 43–63.
Holmes, H. (1980) *Birth Control and Controlling Birth* Clifton, NJ: Humana Press.
Hughes, E. (1963) Professions *Daedalus* 92: 655–668.
Jamous, H. and Peliolle, B. (1970) Changes in the French University-Hospital System, in Jackson, J.A. (editor) *Professions and Professionalization* (pp 144–165) Cambridge: Cambridge University Press.
Johnson, T.J. (1972) *Professions and Power* London: Macmillan Press.
Johnson, T.J. (1977) Professions in the Class Structure, in Scase, R. (editor) *Class Cleavage and Control* (pp 156–177) London: Allen and Unwin.
Johnson, T.J. (1994) Expertise and the State, in Gane, M. and Johnson, T.J. (editors) *Foucault's New Domains* (pp 121–144) London: Routledge.
Johnson, T.J. (1995) Governmentality and the Institutionalization of Expertise, in Johnson, T., Larkin, G. and Saks, M. (editors) *Health Professions and the State in Europe* (pp 177–193) London: Routledge.
Johnson, T., Larkin, G. and Saks, M. (1995, editors) *Health Professions and the State in Europe* London: Routledge.
Jewson, N.D. (1974) Medical Knowledge and the Patronage System in Eighteenth Century England *Sociology* 8: 369–385.
Jewson, N.D. (1976) The Disappearance of the Sick-Man from the Medical Cosmology *Sociology* 10: 225–244.
Kuhlmann, E. (2006a) *Modernizing Health Care: Reinventing Professions, the State and the Public* Bristol: Policy Press.
Kuhlmann, E. (2006b) Traces of Doubt and Sources of Trust: Health Professions in an Uncertain Society Current *Sociology* 54: 607–619.
Kuhlmann, E. and Allsop, J. (2008) Professional self-regulation in a changing architecture of governance: Comparing health policy in the UK and German *Policy and Politics* 36 (2): 173–189.
Kullmann, E. and Saks, M. (2008) *Rethinking Professional Governance: International Directions in Healthcare* Bristol: Policy Press.
Larkin, G. (1983) *Occupational Monopoly and Modern Medicine* London: Tavistock.
Larkin, G. (1995) State Control and the Health Professions in the United Kingdom, in Johnson, T., Larkin, G. and Saks, M. (editors) *Health Professions and the State in Europe* (pp 87–103) London: Routledge.
Larson, M.S. (1977) *The Rise of Professionalism: A Sociological Analysis* Berkeley: University of California Press.
Light, D.W. (1998) Managed Care in a New Key: Britain's Strategies for the 1990s *International Journal of Health Sciences* 28 (3): 427–444.
Lloyd-Bostock, S. and Hutter, B. (2008) Reforming Regulation of the Medical Profession: The Risks of Risk Based Approaches *Health, Risk and Society* 10 (1): 69–83.
Lupton, D. (2011, third edition) *Medicine as Culture* London: Sage Publications.
Lynn, K. (1963) Introduction to the Professions *Daedalus* 92: 653–655.
Macpherson, C.B. (1962) *The Political Theory of Possessive Individualism* Oxford :Clarendon Press.
Marx, K. and Engels, F. (1958) *Selected Works Volume 1* London: Penguin.
McDonald, K.M. (1995) *The Sociology of the Professions* London: Sage Publications.
McKinlay, J.B. (1977) The Business of Good Doctoring or Doctoring as Good Business: Reflections on Freidson's views on the Medical Game *International Journal of Health Services* 7: 459–483.
McKinlay, J.B. and Arches, J. (1985) Towards the Proletarianization of Physicians *International Journal of Health Services* 15: 161–195.

McKinlay, J.B. and Stoeckle, J.D. (1988) Corporatization and the Social Transformation of Doctoring *Health Services* 18: 191–205.

Moran, M. (1999) *Governing the Health Care State; A Comparative Study of the United Kingdom, the United States and Germany* Manchester: Manchester University Press.

Moran, M. (2004) Governing Doctors in the British Regulatory State, in Gray, A. and Harrison, S. (editors) *Governing Medicine: Theory and Practice* (pp 133–155) Milton Keynes: Open University Press.

Moran, M. and Wood, B. (1993) *States, Regulation and the Medical Profession* Milton Keynes: Open University Press.

Murphy, R. (1988) *Social Closure* Oxford: Clarendon Press.

Mythen, G. (2004) *Ulrich Beck: A Critical Introduction to the Risk Society* London: Pluto.

Navarro, V. (1976) *Medicine under Capitalism* New York: Prodist.

Navarro, V. (1980) Work Ideology and Medicine *International Journal of Health Services* 10: 523–550.

Navarro, V. (1986) *Crisis, Medicine and Health: A Social Critique* New York: Tavistock.

Navarro, V. (1988) Professional Dominance or Proletarianization? Neither *Millbank Quarterly* 66 (2): 57–75.

Parry, N. and Parry, J. (1976) *The Rise of The Medical Profession: A Study of Collective Social Mobility* London: Croom Helm.

Parsons, T. (1949) *Essays in Sociological Theory* Glencoe Free Press.

Perkin, H. (1989) *The Rise of Professional Society: England Since 1980* London: Routledge.

Peterson, A. (1997) Risk, Governance and the New Public Health, in Peterson, A. and Bunton, R. (editors) *Foucault Health and Medicine* (pp 3–21) London: Routledge.

Peterson, A. and Bunton, R. (1997, editors) *Foucault Health and Medicine* London: Routledge.

Saks, M. (1995) *Professions and the Public Interest: Medical Power, Altruism and Alternative Medicine* London: Routledge.

Schubert, M.K. (1998) The Relationship Between Verbal Abuse of Medical Students and Their Confidence in Their Clinical Abilities *Academic Medicine* 73 (8): 907–909.

Tawney, R.H. (1921) *The Acquisitive Society* New York: Harcourt Brace.

Turner, B.S. (1995, second edition) *Medical Power and Social Knowledge* London: Sage Publications.

Vogel, D. (1986) *National Styles of Regulation: Environmental Policy in Great Britain and the United States* London: Cornell University Press.

Waring, J.J. (2005) Beyond Blame: Cultural Barriers to Medical Incident Reporting *Social Science and Medicine* 60: 1927–1935.

Weber, M. (1946, edited by Gerth, HH and Wright Mills, C) *Essays in Sociology* Oxford: Oxford University Press.

Weber, M. (1947) *The Theory of Social and Economic Organization* New York: Free Press.

Weber, M. (1978) *Economy and Society* London: The University of California Press.

# 2 Sociology and Risk

## A Link in Permanent (Re)Construction

*Fiorella Mancini*

### INTRODUCTION

One of the fundamental characteristics of contemporary societies—modern, liberal, capitalist, globalized—is the generalization and expansion of social risk, in which a variety of sociological analyses coincide as a by-product of economic and cultural transformations that have taken place in recent decades (Rosanvallon 1995, Douglas 1996, Lash 1997, Beck 1998a, Luhmann 1998, Alexander 2000, Leisering 2003, Castel 2004, Bauman 2009). The crisis of organized modernity (Wagner 1997) calls into question principal regulations that, through state, market and social organizations, had guaranteed access to minimal safety nets for the survival of a large portion of the population.

Against this background, this chapter examines three important approaches to social risk from current social theories with the aim of ordering a multifaceted and highly heterogeneous debate. Through the revision of the concept (and the dimensions) of risk, the reflexive, contractualist and life course approaches attempt to account for new contemporaneous complexities in the present stage of modernity whose transformations are in constant debate and reconstruction on both the theoretical and empirical level.

On the level of theoretical debate, concern has been expressed by questioning not only some of modernity's (and modernization's) meta-comprehensive premises but also the theoretical pillars of social development, the regulatory ability of industrial societies, class divisions and stratifications, processes of social rationalization and even the ideal of emancipation, which underlies political democracy, economic systems and science or knowledge.

On the empirical level, these socially comprehensive possibilities are challenged by endless economic, institutional and cultural changes. Hence current debates about social risks resolve this 'paradox of delusion' through a common denominator of social change: the transfiguration of modernity into a new (second, high, late, developed, multiple, incomplete, fluid, unfinished, etc.) stage in which a feeling of uncertainty predominates, emanates reflectively and, among other things, calls into question the map of structural social inequities. Processes related to the internationalization of local economies, the relative weakening of nation-states, globalization and trans-nationalization and the nature of social protections in general have given rise to the emergence of new patterns of collective (in)securities. Today the idea of an existence surrounded by a safety nucleus is questionable not only in social systems that are historically vulnerable but also in societies characterized by a reasonable management of social risks (Castel 2010).

This generalized reference suggests that modern systems are built on uncertainty insofar as they are societies unable to guarantee the protection of their individual members during the relatively prolonged periods of their lives. This extended observation notwithstanding, one also must acknowledge the differentiated ability of politics and institutional arrangements to generate alternative configurations and specific mechanisms for the administration, governance or management of risks. By extension, one also must recognize the diverse ways of experiencing, accepting and counteracting risks with socially and culturally discernable repercussions (Blossfeld 2003).

Nonetheless, the problem of risk is not exclusive to modern society: it doesn't emerge in the advent of modernity and isn't dealt with exclusively by sociology. Contingency management, for example, appears in Aristotle under the distinction essential/accidental, and, at least since the French Revolution, history has attempted to clarify that no other actor actually controls the course of events in its totality; rather, there are anonymous forces that define us beyond will and reason or with intention and consciousness. If the future were predetermined or independent of individual actions, the concept of risk clearly would have no meaning (Renn 1992, Zinn 2008b). The contingency that assumes a breach between reality and possibilities is what feeds the concept of risk its epistemological content.

Under these premises, the objective of this article is to analyze the problem of social risks in complex societies through three of contemporary sociology's complementary gazes that allow us to systemize some of the guiding principles of the discussion about mechanisms of construction and distribution, as well as the effects associated with risk. To this end, it is important to acknowledge that the primary attribute of the modern concept of risk is its eminently social, cultural and political character and that its sociological relevance lies in its capacity to set apart what is socially important. To function, societies permanently demand selection criteria. Currently, and in the face of the profound crisis of contemporary welfare systems, risk selections are essential for ordering, distinguishing and assuming what is most important for us to protect collectively versus what we can leave in the hands of fate and individual choice.

There are, however, three methodological limitations to this proposal. The reflexive, contractual and life course perspectives expounded on here are not unique or all-encompassing enough to specify the question of social contingency.[1] Their selection is based on the explanatory and heuristic usefulness in mounting a debate that is multidimensional, interdisciplinary and has an extensive theoretical trajectory from the perspective of conventional sociology. Second, the focus accommodated in this essay is eminently sociological and does not address the economic, historical, anthropological, psychological or ecological reproduction of social risks explored at length by each of these disciplines.[2] This suggests dividing the three perspectives from a common premise: social risks take place in a determined sociocultural, political and historical context, thus forming part of a concept more relative than universal (Zinn and Taylor Gooby 2006). Third, in the analysis proposed here, risks are embedded in social contexts where stratification is insufficient to account for the mechanisms of social reproduction of contemporary societies.

With these considerations in mind, the structure of the present text is as follows. In the first section, general contours are drawn for comprehending the concept of risk, which implies unraveling the operative rationality of risk and its teleological limitations. What characteristic does each school of thought acquire? What are its attributes? And, what type of action and subject does risk allow? These are some of the questions that will attempt to be answered here. The second section describes the notion of time specifically related to the concept of risk. Although the sociology of time has addressed in depth the particularities of social time, exegetic studies of the topic have ignored the temporal dimension of the problem. How time is to be understood in relation to the concept of risk is the question that guides this second segment. Section three distinguishes the types of risks recognized by each of the selected schools of thought. The questions addressed in this section are: risk of what and with respect to what? Ordering the sections in this way is useful insofar as it permits us to identify the differentiated nature and constitutive principles that generate and also question social risks and, by extension, demand different mechanisms of social transformation. Finally, section four identifies the socio-historical conditions of new social risks, including the causing factors observed by each perspective, because those are the mechanisms that allow us to locate the novelty of this social problem. What has changed in the social configuration of risks is the guiding question of this last section.

## RATIONALITY AND CONTINGENCY

Although there is relative consensus that risk is a social and historical construction (and therefore an indeterminate condition), in recent years a multiplicity of analyses in the social sciences has diversified the nature, heuristic reach, theoretical centrality and dimensions of this concept (Althaus 2005, Taylor-Gooby and Zinn 2006, Beriain 2008, Zinn 2008b, Lupton 2013). Since sociology deems risk one of the central characteristics of complex societies, there are at least three major theoretical approaches that currently attempt to specify its contents.[3]

The first, which I designate the reflexive approach, includes various authors (especially from the German and English schools) who position the problem of risk as the constitutive nucleus of their object of study, be it society, a system or the individual. This perspective reasons that risks are a generalized structural condition of contemporary societies and an internal characteristic of social systems (Bauman 1996, Giddens 1996, Lash 1997, Beck 1998a, Luhmann 1998). Socially constructed or mediated risk appears here as a condition that is no longer found exclusively in nature but also in human behaviors, conduct, freedom, relationships, organizations and in society itself (Ewald 1993, Lupton 2013).[4] The reflexive theory in particular recognizes that the concept of risk is ample, extending across all of society and directly related to processes of modernization; is a central and novel aspect of politically, socially and institutionally mediated subjectivity; can be managed through human intervention, reflection and social action; generates new and complex social conflicts; and, finally, is associated with notions of choice, responsibility and decision—thus a concept that resurfaces in direct relationship to processes of social individualization.

However, the second perspective, which I call the contractualist approach, is set forth primarily by the French school and emphasizes the normative, institutional and (to a degree) moral construction of risk. This second focus treats risks as the primary 'social question,' spatially and temporally limited to a specific state of national systems (Fitoussi and Rosanvallon 1997, Castel 2004). In this case, risk can only be defined collectively (Ewald 1993) and with explicit reference to the figure of the nation-state and the institutional systems by which it is comprised.

While there is no modernity without risks in the first school of thought, in the second there are no risks without the national historicity of all things social. Meanwhile, the third perspective is from the life course school and consists of authors from the North American and European schools, most notably from the University of Bremen. This approach holds that risk is not found in the structural condition of the modern individual (reflexive approach) or in the deliberate destructuralization of its ways of life (contractualist approach) but rather in the temporal intersection of institutional nonaffiliations and the subjectification of those new social ways (Mayer 2001, DiPetre 2002, Leisering 2003, Blossfeld 2003, Heinz 2003). The life course perspective has been well developed recently, not just in theoretical terms but also primarily through comparative empirical analysis. One of the relative advantages to this school's empirical research is precisely its focus on the life course, because with relative methodological ease, it allows for a temporal understanding of risk.

Establishing itself as a crucial lens through which to read contemporary modernity, the reflexive school converts risk into a structural criticism of itself (Millán 2009). For this focus, risk is 'the' condition of modern man (Beck 1998a), an inherent aspect of this phase of capitalism (Sennet 2000), an intrinsic component of modernity (Giddens 1996) and an attribute that is not necessarily desired but is tolerated and distributed as an existential condition (Cohen y Méndez 2000). Risk in this theory is explained as a quasi-anthropological category; it is an individual mechanism, although socially mediated. Hence for Beck (1998a), risk is like a quasi-subject produced by institutional contradictions that assume the function of delegitimizing modernity's traditional (obsolete) institutions.[5] In Giddens's case (1997), this individual condition is the result of the 'unanchoring' of social relations from their local and temporal context; it is the product of the detraditionalization process through which modern societies are passing. Risk arises when social relations must be restructured in intervals of indefinite time and space, or when they cease to be formed by traditional, socio-temporal values. As such, deinstitutionalization and detraditionalization are two fundamental changes found in the origin of expansion and generalization of new social risks.

In this perspective, reason that accompanies risk is more reflexive than instrumental insofar as it represents, among other things, an expansion and proliferation of options and decisions. In Beck, however, reason enables major possibilities for 'change,' because reflexivity is based on the critique of behavior toward social structure (with clear precedents in the Frankfurt school), while Giddens places more emphasis on the possibility of reproducing these structures and on the new regulation of the individual based on detraditionalization. This difference within the reflexive movement is rooted in Beck's notion that the individual reflects according to his/her distrust of previous social norms and structures, while Giddens's does so based on his/her own actions (Lash and Urry 1998). In other words, Beck's reflexivity is a type of compulsive and obligatory response in the face of new social risks; while in Giddens, it is the rise and transformation of reflexivity (via detraditionalization) that provokes a greater awareness of traditional risks. In the latter, reflectivity, like risk itself, is self-referential and a creator of narratives that are more biographical than social. Giddens's reflectivity regulates conduct; Beck's regulates new social forms. For Giddens, reflectivity functions as an adaptation strategy in the search for security, whether through resilience or even anticipation. In both authors, a reflexive individual is necessary to combat social risk; one who is capable of doubting his/her own existence (Giddens) or the institutional forms of his/her own creation (Beck).

For the reflexive approach, moreover, risk supposes a specific kind of social action as a preliminary measure, while accepting the human responsibility that this implies and that social action can produce unanticipated and undesirable results (Lupton 2013). Therefore, risk is a specific form of action, be it post-traditional (Giddens 1997) or instrumental/post-rational (Beck 1996), the latter of which only occurs once an action involving prior choice has been carried out. In this approach, new risks form part of the decisions that modern individuals make. In contrast to early modernity, contemporary society doesn't view risks simply as dangers, but rather as risks taken for the sake of personal choices or for the choices of others that tend to affect us or increase the amount of danger on our horizon (Millán y Mancini 2014).

This brand of critical realism from the reflexive perspective (Tulloch 2008, Lupton 2013), which finds that risks exist objectively but are mediated and politicized by social and cultural processes (and, by extension, differentiated by context), is shared by the symbolic cultural focus of Douglas (1996), for whom risk is a socially determined assortment of certain dangers. Only those dangers that are socially accepted and morally determined become problems of risk[6] as a consequence of an earlier choosing mechanism.[7] In other words, there is a possibility (more or less predictable) of future harm rooted in socially modified decisions made in the present. This is why, for this school of thought, risk could become a temporary form of reason that, unlike notions of uncertainty and contingency, leaves room for a possible solution.

Yet how does one explain the social dimension of this individual condition in reflexive theory? Once a mechanism of choice, here risk becomes an organizing principle of social organization (Giddens 1997, Lash 1997, Beck 1998), a measurement or a convention that makes it possible to socially determine fate (Kates and Kasperson 1983) and rationalize it. Risk is a social configuration that acquires individual experience in order to confront the uncertain,[8] temporarily distancing the experience of uncertain expectations (Beriain 1996, Luhmann 1998) and allowing—from the perspective of social acceptance and moral determination—collective constructs to be achieved (Douglas and Wildavsky 1982).

For the contractualist perspective, risk acquires a collective character. That is, more than an element of consciousness, risk is a historical configuration based on the connection to the kind of protection that societies normatively generate (Castel 2004). Risk, then, is a relative concept that necessarily makes use of a reference in order to define itself. An individual, a system or a collective can be at risk only with respect to a specific social, temporal and objective frame of reference. This is the basic premise of this theory, which can be summarized by Castel's (2004) well-known definition of social risks as those events that compromise an individual's capacity to secure his/her own social independence. In essence, risk is external and predictable, and its probabilities of occurrence can be estimated as well as the costs of its potential harms. If risk is an event external to the individual, it can be repaired, indemnified or compensated, because it can be mutualized and redistributed through familiar state, social or commercial technologies (Castel 2004).

Rosanvallon (1995) supports this notion that positions risk as a probabilistic dimension of the social by implicating collective mechanisms to assume it. Above all, risk is a 'social fact.' According to this perspective, the difference between risk and danger resides in the fact that social resources are only available for confronting the former of the two. Rosanvallon (1995) specifies that the concept of insurance, as passage toward modernity (Ewald

1999), is what permitted the historical shift from a subjective notion of behavior to the objective notion of risk and, on the social plane, left individuality behind on a secondary explanatory level.[9] The notion of risk facilitates a departure from the idea of individual culpability, because it allows for the collectivization and universalization of the consequences of behavior. So in this theory—and this is a fundamental difference with the reflexive school—only the collective is able to generate securities in the individual in complex and differentiated societies (Castel 2004). While, for the reflexive school, risk arises when identified as the contingent moment of choice, for the contractualist school, risk appears when the social action that precedes it falls outside of the control of the subject who endures it.[10]

In turn, the life course school identifies risk as a temporal and locatable point of intersection between alienation from institutions and the way in which individuals respond to these constraints. The theoretical nucleus of this perspective focuses on the consideration of risk as a problem of time (and of times) conditioned by institutional and cultural rules. Risk is treated here as a temporalized cultural representation of the destandardization of the social (Mayer 2001, DiPetre 2002, Blossfeld 2003).

In this case, more than an individual or social attribute, risk supposes a contingent personification of norms in order to determine the moment and sequence of transitions in biographical trajectories, which if recurring in an institutionalized manner (Heinz 2003) allow for the diffusion of a variety of temporalities in every individual. From this perspective, the multiplication of individual temporalities associated with risk is constructed institutionally and culturally, especially with regard to reference groups determined by gender, age or social sector. Risk, as temporal intersection between the institutional and the personified, evolves into a type of incentive system for the temporal orientation of individuals in their own biographies. Hence the importance this theory places on the knowledge of biographical experiences in the management of risks and the dynamic process of their perception throughout life (Taylor-Gooby and Zinn 2006).

For this perspective, there is a new social uncertainty in social groups that had been characterized historically as having a relatively stable and secure set of beliefs and expectations in terms of their biographical trajectories. The rationale of new risks is not what is of interest here, as it is for the reflexive school, but rather traditional risks that now compromise a new social sector. All of this happens for the first time in history in the most dynamic sectors of society, which, historically, have been the firm nucleus of the notion of security. From an epistemological point of view, a large portion of the life course theory rests on the phenomenological and hermeneutic studies of contemporary sociology, where what matters are the contextualized meanings of risk. Some of these authors (Furlong and Cartmel 1997, MacDonald and Marsh 2002, Mayock 2009, Pedrelli and Cebulla 2011, Shirani and Weller 2010, Mancini 2014) are less interested in the macro social aspects of the new conditions of modernity and more concerned with micro social experiences that are lived and interpreted within frameworks of common sense in any given context. A large part of this analytic perspective attempts to define how risk is constructed in moments of interaction between individuals, taking into account the social differentiation of risk, especially in terms of class, gender, nationality, age, etc. (Tulloch and Lupton 2003).

Although risk is a novel, constitutive element of complex societies in all three theories,[11] for the reflexive school it is a structural attribute of agency, as a result of reflexive rationale, that becomes a quotidian fact inseparable from societal functions; for the contractualist school, it is an event external to the individual, a product of the destabilization of the social; and from the life course perspective, it is an institutionally designed moment of inflection. In each case, these definitions would suggest that risk is a politically constructed reality that implies power to define it and symbolic production to reproduce, accept and tolerate it socially[12] (Mora Salas 2003a).

Unanswered questions remain in these three approaches, however. What possibilities does agency account for in response to these new social mechanisms? How do individuals resist in the face of risk? And, what options for responding are generated socially and individually for combating contemporary uncertainty (Lipper and Stenson 2010)? In addition to being an individual condition, normative construction or system of incentives, risk is also a sensation, a perception that can be revised and specified through temporal subjectification, as appropriation of the problem and its interpretation via symbolically and morally defined constructs. That which can occur (or not) in the future and be objectively defined (the risk of losing my job exists objectively outside my consciousness) is experienced, lived and perceived in the present according to particularities and subjective variations that, in turn, depend upon and fluctuate according to cultural, psychological, social, economic, gender, life course and other factors. The way each individual or social group appropriates future risk in the present depends on such constraints. Moreover, the perception of risk is conditioned by elements not necessarily associated with specific patterns of reason or reflexive behaviors. Cultural, symbolic, motivational, linguistic and even mythological modulations exist which impact the emergency (or nonemergency) of an individual consciousness of risk and its revision in light of experiences and perceptions of insecurity or uncertainty (Alexander 2000).

## RISK AND TIME

New social risks are constraining in the context of the temporal dimension of the social. If the notion of risk supposes a determined way of observing the future (Luhmann 1998), if it is the temporal dimension of the new capitalism (Sennet 2000) or a way of observing what is modern (Millán 2009), then it refers to a particularized way of dealing with time. This idea accommodates at least two observations: risk affects the chronological, organized perception of time and, in turn, is conditioned by the particularities that temporal reference acquires from any potential, dispositional or contingent problem.

For the reflexive perspective, risk fractures the continuity between past and future. In situations of risk, the individual and social past loses the ability to determine trajectories in the present—be it because of the weak ability of institutions to temporally integrate biographies or the process of detraditionalization—and the future becomes a projection of threats anchored in a temporal vacuum (Beck 1996, Giddens 1996). At the same time, if risk provokes a rupture between past and present, individual narratives become emotionally illegible (Sennet 2000) and socially indifferent. This fracture between experience and expectation impedes logical narration where one event leads to another and conditions it a previous moment. Narrative possibilities lack the temporal foundation necessary to construct biographical trajectories, and the concatenation of events becomes far more indefinite. In turn, this generates a state of disorder that increases uncertainty and entails a multitude of consequences, among which stands out what Castells (1995) refers to as lateral ambiguous movement or purely horizontal social displacement that, despite this, requires an indiscriminate use of time.

Due to the intervention of risk, social time loses its regulatory capacity to coherently guide biographical trajectories, which become diverse, plural (particularized), self-determining and more illegible per traditional institutional standards to the extent that the order as much as the achievement of events becomes more indeterminate. While the individual needs lasting narratives that will lend content to his/her character (Sennet 2000), his/her experience leads continuously to disjointed time.

At least initially, risk deters a routine construction of life, which is what gives time meaning. Hence social experience becomes temporally amorphous. On one hand, because situations of risk can easily disavow or inhibit a coherent organization of the present based on stable social models and, on the other hand, because they can interrupt the quotidian link between social and individual worlds (Wilson 1997, Cohen an Méndez 2000). To be unemployed, to go from one job to another, to have rotating work shifts, these are all events that contribute to chronological time's void of specific content, generating enormous possibilities for a type of social interaction that conceives time as meaningless. Therefore, for the authors of this school, everything that cannot be routinized generates anguish, fear or guilt as a by-product of the temporal alienation of individuals with traditional or classic social moorings.

Giddens, for example, opposes the concept of risk to that of ontological security, which implies a sense of continuity and order of events. This security is a necessary framework for organizing existence and clarifying the rules of abstract systems, whether on an unconscious level, a level of practical consciousness (like internalized social rules) or on the level of discursive consciousness (as clarification of the rules of abstract systems). In this context, risk management can be achieved only by applying these rules, whose function is to minimize uncertainty while generating order and routines (Giddens 1996). Without this protective mechanism, basic individual experience translates into anguish.[13] Routine as a temporary solution to problems of risk thereby acquires a cognitive reference (if every day I carry out the same activity, my self-awareness deepens) as well as emotional meaning (it reduces anxiety). Therefore, routine is a necessary reference for events and social roles. In modernity, the burden of managing these protective mechanisms falls primarily on the abstract system or discursive consciousness (in contrast to the past, when traditional systems were responsible). When these reductionist processes fail, when the temporal lines that define routine become socially imprecise—due to informational, technical, or decision-making problems—the result is an individual insecurity that becomes assimilated as practical consciousness for functioning. In other words, when traditional social institutions lose their regulatory capacity, as occurs in the current phase of modernity, the temporalization of risk becomes subjectivized or personalized (Lash 1997).

While for the reflexive perspective, risk fractures the continuity between past (as experience) and future (as expectation), in the contractualist and life course theories, risk can only exist in the link between past and present. According to the latter theories, risk in the context of virtual reality—it is not yet occurring and may not occur, yet has an effect on the present (Ewald 1999)—can only exist through filters constructed from previous experience (Franklin 1998). Risk as future is created based on past experience, which also allows for a certain degree of elasticity in the present, wherein insecurity settles in as part of daily life (Nolan 2005). In this case, Luhmann (1998), as well as Urry and Lash (1998), approximate this approach when they suggest that what produces anxiety is not a lack of trust in the future (as in Beck or Giddens), but rather *past experience*, which confuses expectations. Risk is a temporal observation of reality based on the past/future distinction as a horizon of possibilities (Luhmann 1998). Risk society is a temporal society that constructs its identity from continuous returns to the past. In the same vein, for Fitoussi and Rosanvallon (1997), the past is more important than the future in determining risk, because personal history is what crystalizes social differences and, by extension, what structurally conditions experiences of risk in the present, although, at the same, the future operates as the differentiation between those who believed they were equals.

From an institutional perspective, in these two theories, we participate in a change in risk on a temporal and spatial scale (Rosanvallon) in the sense that risk has lost its unifying character, meaning its capacity to socially regulate particular behaviors, be it through the internationalization of certain dangers (the notion of catastrophe) or the internalization and privatization of guilt and responsibility that resurface in an institutionalized manner. The erosion of social compromises that once unified risks spatially and temporally generates a change in orientation, which makes them more difficult to locate. This dislocation of risks presumably generates new mechanisms of temporal inequality that demand different moral devices or innovative normative frameworks capable of securing the right to a discontinuity of trajectories as an integral and nondisruptive part of the life course (Castel 2004). Social recognition of the discontinuous is a new institutional demand, because risk can imply being out of sync with the rhythms of society. Evidently, this produces a permanent problem participating in structured organizations (Presser 1998, Mills 2004), thus reducing the possibilities and opportunities for social interaction and leading to more unstructured social relations (Johnson 1997), which ultimately translates into greater problems of inclusion.

The problem of de-synchronization with the social world during experiences of risk undoubtedly leads to a problem of social inequality. In contrast to the reflexive school's generalization of risks argument, the life course perspective (Berger and Sopp 1993, Heinz and Marshall 2003) brings this to light through what it calls temporalized social inequality. Empirical research guided by this theory reveals how, within a set of discontinuous trajectories, there is—as a structural characteristic of determined social groups—a profound temporal inequality associated with the postponement of events for those who endure experiences with risk (Heinz 2003, Mills 2004).

Generally speaking, of the three perspectives, the one that has explored these temporal mutations the most is the life course perspective, which focuses on the historical changes that individual and social trajectories have suffered with respect to the management and administration of risks (Heinz and Marshall 2003, Mayer 2004a 2004b, Mills 2004). For this school, inserting the problem of risk into the observation of biographical trajectories assumes repairing the organization and narration of time throughout the life course. Risk modifies the distribution of time as much in trajectories directly affected (generally labor trajectories) as it does in other spheres of life (Mills 2004). In generalized and extended situations of risk, social time is redistributed, especially via abrupt fragmentations of trajectories. When disturbed by risk, social time loses its regulatory capacity to coherently guide biographical trajectories. Individuals that experience profound processes of uncertainty construct a disarticulate notion of time, which is likely to impede the possibility of lasting narratives that would give content, from the standpoint of subjectivity, to their own trajectory.

Finally, for the three perspectives, risk is affected by time to the extent that, from the moment that something did not occur temporally and may not occur, we act and make decisions in the present that can modify this contingency positively or negatively. This temporal influence on risk affects trajectories in material as well as subjective terms. To be able to uproot and cast oneself into the future, one must have a minimal degree of security at his/her disposal in the present (Castel 2004). What social consequences does this absence of expectations imply? When expectations are unstable over time, and the possibility of long-term calculations becomes difficult, what comes into play (what is 'at risk') is Castel's social independence, Beck's individual autonomy, Giddens's ontological security or the biographical illumination of Bertaux and Kohli (1984)—all of which are essential, constitutive elements of the social in this stage of modernity.

## TYPES OF RISK IN COMPLEX SOCIETIES

When the different theoretical perspectives mentioned here speak of risk, they do so in reference to different types. In each case, there is an attempt to classify differences based primarily on their nature and, therefore, on the social principles they interpellate. In the reflexive school in general, risks are distinguished according to the principle of basic security (Giddens 1996) or individual autonomy (Beck 1996). For the contractualists, the guiding principle for defining types of risk is solidarity (Rosanvallon 1995) or social security (Ewald 1999, Castel 2004). From the life course perspective, the central concept of distinction is the principle of social equality (Leisering 2003).

Within the reflexive perspective, Giddens's functional risk supposes constitutive principles associated with ontological security and tradition. For Beck, on the other hand, acting risk reverts back to the principles of modernity as a project of individual autonomy and the liberation of the subject from his/her social class. In this context, the process of reflexive individualization that accompanies the generalization and expansion of risks creates a type of historic opportunity to rescue these principles undermined by industrial society. Below the horizon of modernization-individualization-risk, the revision of biographical narratives permanently subjected to an individual and social scrutiny that imposes risk would lead to mechanisms for individual reaffirmation (*I am me*) and the social liberation of the individual. With important differences in nuance, the proponents of this theory agree that social rules resulting from normative or formal institutional criteria are increasingly less frequent, and individuals are instead the ones with the ability and obligation to set the (more or less new) rules of the game in their own lives (Giddens 1996, Beck 1998, Lash and Urry 1998, Luhmann 1998). This kind of institutionalized individualization[14] (Beck and Beck-Gernesheim 2002) indicates that people are increasingly called upon, in demand and made responsible as individuals in specific social and institutional contexts without being provided the necessary resources to respond appropriately to the complexity of risks as individual beings (Millán and Mancini 2014). The erosion of traditional sociocultural ways usually involves a loss of stability (Zinn 2008b) given that established values and consolidated standards no longer function as guidance for the individual, because every connection or position can be questioned as much in the affective sphere as in the labor or social sphere. In this context of broken connections, the individual is no longer integrated through more extensive and dense forms of sociability or by way of weighty institutions such as the state, but rather via institutions of average reach such as the welfare state or the market (Millán and Mancini 2014). Lacking the ties that once provided support, the individual is very dependent on those institutions, and this increases his/her risks, which are by-products of certain social policies, trends and/or patterns of consumption (Beck and Beck-Gernesheim 2002).

From this process of generalized individualization, the reflexive school identifies an enormous variety of social risks. Wilson (1997), for example, underscores the existence of extended risks on one hand and contained risks on the other. Extended risks are those observed in social environments that for various reasons reproduce some sort of culture of uncertainty and a high tolerance for risk. In contrast, contained or differential risks are those that are managed with a greater individual burden of guilt. The reflexive current also distinguishes between acceptable and unacceptable risks (Franklin 1998). The difference lies in the political character of the first group. The acceptable or normal risks are politically and culturally 'manufactured' (Beck 1998a), intercepted by modes of communication and, consequently, count on a degree of political legitimacy (Cohen and Méndez 2000) rooted in certain culturally and socially shared values. To quote Mary Douglas (1996), 'common values lead to common fears': individuals accept certain risks (and not others) on the basis of a determinate political adhesion to a particular way of being in society.

The contractualist or institutional school (Fitoussi and Rosanvallon 1997, Castel 2004) responds to the sociological provocation of the individualization of risks by reminding us that certainties are constructed socially or not at all: only via a high level of generalized reciprocity can social contingencies be compensated for. If the modern idea of 'the social' and 'the collective' loses its historical centrality, what remains is the complex problem of individually constructing securities and continuities in the diverse organizational forms of life. This approach clearly suggests that individualization is actually a politically deliberate and institutionalized process that has managed to personalize socio-historic categories—not by negating but rather by diversifying them—throughout the individual life course. The notion that risk is negotiated increasingly more often by family, social networks or 'the community' and less by formal institutions (Martinez Franzoni 2003) is also part of a set of institutional decisions and of an intense process of social intervention.

According to the contractualist and life course schools, there are controllable risks and uncontrollable risks (Castel 2004), depending on social options, choices, decisions and selections (Breen 1997). Uncontrollable risks are those that presume institutional reparations based on a certain level of generalized reciprocity that permits compensation or prevents contingencies. Risks can be shared socially through long-term pacts. The nature of these social agreements is more moral or political than economic, insofar as they are created based on principles of social citizenship and allow for the differentiation between internal and external risks (Castel 2004). Internal risks are directly related to social insecurity. They are the contingencies that can be controlled, because they are socialized and redistributed. External risks, on the other hand, are a type of insurmountable threat that falls outside of the reach of all social programs. This distinction allows, in normative and legal terms, for the possibility of a redistribution of social responsibility for the various types of contingencies. As such, internal risks are defined by principles of solidarity (Rosanvallon 1995), whose protection (be it through anticipation or compensation) becomes a right based on these social pacts. In contrast, existential risks, those external to the social system, involve greater individual responsibility and are directly associated with behavior.

From the life course perspective, Mills (2004) establishes empirically the existence of elective, voluntary risks, which assumes free and proactive agents, and forced risks. Based on a study of segmented labor markets, Ferrie (2001) also identifies the superposition of structural risks characteristic of the most socially marginalized sectors and new risks associated with the most dynamic sectors of the economy. Therefore, according to this theory, there would be risk associated with the equality of opportunities (structural or class risks) and risks that generate insecurity throughout life with no guarantee of equal opportunities (Leisering 2003). In this second category of risk, the frame of reference is not social equality that permits structural risks to be absorbed by social institutions, but security, whose assurance is mainly ascribed to the market. This distinction is attractive insofar as security related risks destandardize the life course—new risks—while those associated with equality deinstitutionalize the life course inasmuch as they are traditional risks that have been commercialized or individualized and impact new social groups.

A third difference for this theory originates amid structural risks lacking institutional and cultural mediation and variable risks that are filtered by institutional agreements on the national level (Blossfeld and Hofmeister 2005). Hence the comparative analysis of social risks plays an important role in this approach. One important thesis that breaks away from this school is that, with greater regulation of the life course by public institutions, there would be a greater continuity and standardization of trajectories, although this would occur in detriment to the process of individualization governed by higher standards of individual autonomy. Leisering (2003), for example, points out that, in societies with weak risk management systems, unsafe trajectories predominate where risks are understood only as evidence of personal failure—which would call into question the principle of individualization and real possibilities of autonomy—while in societies that supplement imperatives of equality with individual freedoms, more secure life courses prevail, because security is a shared societal value reflected in normative principles of the state. In this area, the life course and contractualist schools coincide where both maintain that there are no possibilities for true sociability under generalized conditions of risk. According to these perspectives, the development of capitalism has allowed 'usual risks' to be socially controlled. Under those terms, instead of new risks there would be traditional ones, whose distribution criteria will have been modified by the rupture of national social pacts. Although for these authors, risk is the result of a breakdown of the social pact, in the reflexive school, risk in and of itself is a new, high-level contingency agreement that enables the differentiation between present and possibility.[15] Finally, the main point of convergence between the three theories is, perhaps, that the old ways of regulating social risk have been exhausted.

## WHAT HAS CHANGED

If the welfare society idea takes 40 years to carry out, if the figure of the nation-state is unavoidably identified with the twentieth century (Mayer and Schoepflin 1989), if, ultimately, risk has been more historical norm than exceptionality, what is new about this phenomenon that has been positioned in the center of sociological discussions? The most recent debates about social change that represent each of the perspectives presented here indicate that a powerful sense of uncertainty envelops contemporary societies and social life today (Taylor-Gooby 2005). A certain cloud of doubt, fear and risk purportedly falls upon individuals who, daily and without much success, struggle with the avatars of their existence. In turn, two imposing processes seemingly refer to this pervasive increase in uncertainty: the growth of social complexity and individualization, on one hand, and transformations stemming from globalization, the internationalization of the economy and patterns in the model of accumulation, on the other. Without margins for the nuances, all of this has led to changes in lifestyles, family relations, labor markets and, generally speaking, an opening for possibilities and options (individual and social) capable of enabling a more critical, reflexive and self-responsible agency far removed from tradition, state paternalism and confidence in traditional social service institutions. Whether seen from the functional structuralist or the critical structuralist perspective, structural sediments have been modified and a new social context (structurally different) explains the resurgence of risk in current societies.

Apparently, for the reflexive perspective, the temporary aid of risk expansion is a specific phase of reflexive modernity that departs from the theory of individualization and supposes a social transition that occurs not through a crisis of the previous stage but in terms of what Beck refers to as a radicalization of modernity. The crux of this radicalization is the familiarity of social transformation. The change happens but is unperceived; risk is not desired but becomes natural. Ultimately, uncertainty occurs without historic disaster (Sennet 2000). The institutionalization of risk—its normalization (Bauman 2009) in daily life—generates a sense of facing 'something natural' or routine, whose legitimacy comes from its established, preconfigured nature (Mora Salas 2003a).

For this perspective, the expansion of risk happens in a determined stage of modernity in which there is an escape from institutional control.[16] At the same time that a contraction of the capacities of traditional institutions occurs, an expansion of social alternatives unleashes—alternatives that are ultimately configured by modes of social influence that no one controls directly (Giddens 1996). For the reflexive perspective, this class of analytical endogamy between risk and individualization generally implies an increase in options (and, therefore, in decisions) in a historical moment when social action no longer requires a nation-state for its concretion or an instrumental rationale to sustain it. In this context, action must be restructured in sensible new ways that lead to the restoration of basic trust (Giddens 1996) and a permanent, revised criticism of systems of knowledge (Beck 1997).[17] In the realm of subjectivity, all of the above is associated with heightened critical (self)awareness of these transformations, along with a questioning of traditional institutional structures of modernity (authority, science, the state, the nuclear family, etc.) and the vindication of agency as a breathing, subjective cog of change. The latter, in turn, implies rationality, deliberation, compromise and extremely high confidence in oneself (Mancini 2015).

In this context, primary social change is understood in the context of the emergence of new risks relatively detached from class structure, which, among other things, would yield to more dynamic and individual inequalities. These structural alterations of the social, which profoundly impact subjectivities, lead to an observation of the biographical distribution of dynamic inequalities as inabilities and deficiencies that are not only individual but also primarily personal (Beck and Beck- Gernesheim 2002). The organizational force of new social risks arises from the same place: a structural search for biographical solutions to systemic contradictions (Beck and Beck- Gernesheim 2002, Bauman 2009).

According to the contractualist school, the fundamental social transformation that entails pervasive risk is the social breakdown of a moral order linked to the state that assumed not only an expectation of life that could be controlled through instrumental rationality but that also produced fictions of security that facilitated action based on patterns of institutionally established roles (Rosanvallon 1995, Castel 2004). In contrast to the reflexive school, the basic assumption of this premise is that social action is not possible without security, order and a narrative coherence that is externally induced.

In this theory, the figure of the state has acted, historically, as a mechanism of individualization through collective protections (Gauchet 2003). The roots of this concept can be traced relatively easily in traditional contractualist theory. The Hobbesian individual in the natural state was one who experienced total insecurity and for whom security would become a categorical imperative once the possibility of a pact was established. In either case, security here is understood as: a device, a political technique (Rosanvallon 1995), the result of agreements based on values and moral principles and a legitimate convention with responsibilities and possibilities for socialization. This is the theoretical platform upon which the modern concept of the industrial or salaried society was constructed as differentiated, segmented, stratified and unequal yet protective. This is why, for Castel (2010), the primary difference with the past lies in the excess of inequality in the emphasized present due to an increase in insecurity that exposes not only economic and social crisis but also those that are civilizing (Rosanvallon 1995) (to the extent that they have eroded guiding principles that once upheld basic social pacts based on solidarity and class compromise).

There are at least three major reasons that can explain the deterioration of these principles: the diversification of social categories, the loss of centrality of the nation-state and the qualitative transformation of collective representation (Pérez Sáinz and Mora Salas 2004). The solidification and preservation of the welfare state's prototypical social pacts was possible thanks to the following factors: the homogeneity of social categories based on the social division of labor (including for the identification of marginalized, informal or excluded workers); by the centrality of the state, in order to demarcate the relationship between capital and labor and act as a symbolic referent of social integration; and by the compression of these principles into uniform collectivities with relative ability to exert pressure. In the first case, social risks can no longer be compensated for in their totality, because they are incalculable based on the rise of heterogeneity, complexity and social differentiation. In the second instance, the new spatiotemporal limitation of risks transcends national spheres.[18] Finally, in the third instance, the collective representation that once demanded protection from risks no longer has referents for its interlocution, because risk is transfigured—deliberately—from political power into knowledge.

The life course perspective has emphasized systematizing these transformations in the management of risks based on the classic distinction between traditional, industrial, Fordist and post-industrial types of societies (Leisering 2003, Mayer 2004). In contrast to the reflexive school, this distinction is based exclusively on changes associated with historical models of economic accumulation in terms of the relationship between capital and labor. This theory's conclusions are unmistakable: although in the early stages of development, risks are distributed among individuals and families, upon the intensification of industrialization and financing of the welfare state, we witness an assurance of risks via rights associated with labor and the so-called de-commercialization of the same (Esping Anderson 2001), which implies a degree of individual autonomy vis à vis the market. This is why different studies from this school tend to assimilate this historical period with standardized, regulated, continuous, coherent and stable life courses, whereas, currently, we face the presence of de-temporalized individual and social trajectories.

If there is, indeed, a relative consensus that current societies distribute risks more than they protect them, for the reflexive school, this redistribution occurs more democratically than in the past (Giddens 1997, Beck 1998); while for the life course school, risks become crystallized in individuals through traditional criteria for the use of power (Mayer 1997, Leisering 2003), and this deepens rather than reduces class differences (Breen 1997).

In spite of this polemic, the three perspectives agree that major transformation is related to the complexity of defining exhaustive and exclusive social categories based on the extension of risks. The interpretation of social situations becomes more ambiguous because individualization involves new inclusive distinctions through the creation of individual forms of social inequality that superimpose the structural ones. Social typologies become temporary when, in reality, the categories are different phases in a single life (Lash and Urry 1998). Risk, then, would reveal not social, but temporary segments in biographical trajectories that denote their own plurality. In other words, the possibilities for diverse experiences with social risks widen, but at the same their totalizing or immeasurable nature is compressed into a single life. Therefore, as Rosanvallon (1995) indicates, it would not make a lot of sense to identify those 'at risk' as a social category, considering the latter is not a categorical concept but rather a temporal process that entails ruptures and discontinuities, the disintegration of some social characteristics and the conglomeration of new individualities.[19]

## FINAL CONSIDERATIONS

Throughout this chapter, I have attempted to identify and systematize the basic guiding principle of different theoretical perspectives offered by contemporary sociology in order to demonstrate the genesis, distribution and management of social risks in complex societies. Following this examination, it's beneficial to ponder the theoretical and methodological challenges that a sociologically explanatory model of risk should consider.

To organize the debate around what we consider their common points of departure, we first ought to evaluate the advantages and limitations inherent in binding theoretical perspectives that are more a selection than sociological schools of thought in the strictest sense of the term. This, however, does not justify an undifferentiated treatment of the authors of each school (who, at times, have substantial theoretical divergences), nor a fusion of the different theories to the extent that they lose their specificity.

Second, when doing an analytic work that attempts to explain or interpret positions held by others, one runs the risk of substantially or immanently expanding the problem instead of problematizing the phenomenon and turning it into a working hypothesis. From the present examination of the three theories of social risk, what relationships need to be problematized as the central hypotheses associated with risk? And what type of analytical connections would allow us to explain them? First of all, it would seem that the vast majority of questions that remain here are more empirical than substantive. The generalization and extension of risks or the overlap of social inequalities are research questions the authors themselves have not always carried out (Taylor-Gooby 2005, Mythen 2007, Zinn 2008a, Lupton 2013), so these questions merit a bit more processing in order to advance and potentially unfetter and lighten the debate about social risks. One interesting observation about the three theories dealt with here is the tendency to overgeneralize premises, which sometimes negates acknowledgment of the very complexity one hopes to expose.

Third, are we introducing schools of thought that compete with each other, that make parallel arguments or that could be complementary for an explanatory model of risks? Finally, what kind of analytical tools are these theories offering us in order to build that model? As an appendix to this essay, I introduce a synthetic chart containing the core theoretical elements of each of the three perspectives that may function as a first step in attempting to answer these questions.

Undoubtedly, the reflexive perspective has been a turning point in contemporary sociology. With scant idealism, the authors of this theory have attempted to uncover those social phenomena that are still *up in the air* but are not easily captured through sociological ingenuity. Highlighting infinite possibilities of social modes is a provocative mandate for the other sociological schools of thought. Explanations about the genesis, constitution and distribution of social risks can be seen as part of said mandate. One considerable limitation of this perspective, however, is associated with imposed expectations of generality. Explaining all risks as if everything were a risk has its risks. If the explanatory point of departure is the ontological condition or the inherency of modernity and capitalism, the point of arrival could hardly be anything but their naturalization, refinement or practical consciousness raising. This not only fences in the interpretive possibilities associated with social compromises, historical responsibilities, inequalities or the distribution of power, it also makes the opportunities for social transformation more rigid. At times, the all-encompassing (and certainly reductionist) lack of differentiation in this theory could create as many sociological risks as it hopes to explain (Martell 2009, Rasborg 2012).

In the case of the contractualist school, the explanation for the social construction of risk based on the moral collapse of national social pacts fails to take into account the complex processes of individualization, as well as the political diversity of the distribution of economic power and capital's mechanisms for determining, internationally and innovatively, new social ways of managing traditional risk. If the reflexive school can be accused of excessive methodological individualism, it is also valid to point out the contractualist school's eminent methodological nationalism (Beck 1998), which prevents it from taking into account the trans-nationalization of certain mechanisms associated with risk, its global impact and how it's filtered spatially by nation-states and politically via institutional agreements (as posed by life course theory).

Taking the above criticisms into account, life course theory becomes relatively weak due to an enormous theoretical simplicity for explaining risk as one of social life's undifferentiated resources, easily replaceable by any other attribute or generalizable characteristic of modernity. Beyond its temporal dimension, what is specific to risk isn't clarified sufficiently enough to be able to distinguish it analytically from other social problems.

In the three theories reviewed here, it is difficult to find the cultural imprint assumed by risk management. The move from tradition to individualization, contractual erosion or the spread of globalization is explained more by psychological, social, political, moral, economic and historical factors than by cultural ones. Obviously, the acknowledgment of one doesn't imply the negation of the others. However, without the specific weight that culture imposes upon differentiated risk management, it's very difficult to understand the specificities of different cases and, especially, of their mechanisms of reproduction and maintenance as an innovation of social systems. In this regard, qualitative studies have demonstrated that the concept of risk in common usage is a mixture of premodern notions associated with faith or destiny and modern notions of self-control (Lupton 2013) that warrants more in-depth research. This requires imagining a more ample concept of reflexivity that would include not only rationality but also the affective, hermeneutic, esthetic and habit-related aspects of risk (Zinn 2008a, Lupton 2013). The inclusion of nonrational knowledge, emotions and the trajectories of risk (Zinn 2008b) could contribute enormously to a more profound understanding of this problem.

Finally, it is quite clear that the three perspectives presented here adopt a certain conservative and normative tone upon judging, almost exclusively, social transformations such as nostalgic loss and the grand structures of modernity as the only possibilities for integration and social protection. They obviously are more concerned with the disruptive effects produced by risk without taking into consideration the infinite social mechanisms that are generated daily and permanently in order to diminish their intensity (Millán 2009).

The process of individualization that accompanies risks in the reflexive school, the break from social pacts that is positioned as the genesis of its extension in the contractualist school, or the temporary subjectification of institutional disaffiliation recognized by life course theory, without a doubt reveal the complexity that the diversification of social categorization implies with regard to the expansion of social risks. Thus the problem of risk imposes a new demand on the social sciences: with what analytical tools and methodologies can one read the social map of complex societies when the individual-social category relationship becomes indeterminate; when the contingency is the logical value to best describe social classifications; when, upon seeing ourselves, we ultimately move; when the principle of uncertainty governs the social world.

## APPENDIX: CONCISE CHART OF THE REFLEXIVE, CONTRACTUALIST AND LIFE COURSE PERSPECTIVES ABOUT SOCIAL RISKS IN COMPLEX SOCIETIES

| Analytical Tool | Reflexive School | Contractualist School | Life Course School |
|---|---|---|---|
| **Operative Rationale** | | | |
| **Attribute** | Individual Condition Internal | Event Social External | Individual Condition Institutionalized |
| **Subject** | Reflexive Creative, Critical | Disaffiliated Beneficiary | Biographical New Insecurities |
| **Rationale** | Individualization Reflexivity | Morality of the Social Pact | Political and Cultural |
| **Action** | Reflexive Decision | Beyond Individual Control | Adaptation Improvisation |
| **Principle** | Organizing | Disintegrating | Deregulating |
| **Context** | Reflexive Modernization | Nation-State | Globalization |
| **Constitution** | Political/Historical | Political/Moral | Political/Institutional |
| **Character** | Structural-Systemic | National | Global Filtered by Institutional Agreements |
| **Temporal Dimension** | | | |
| **Time** | Past-Future Rupture | Past-Future Connection | Past-Present-Future Connection |
| **Central Characteristic** | Temporal Subjectification | Superposition Fragmentation | De-synchronization |
| **Nature and Types of Risks** | | | |
| **Values** | Ontological Security Individual Autonomy | Social Security Independence Solidarity | Equality Social Security |
| **Types of Distinctions** | Temporal, Political and Cognitive | Temporal, Political and Social | Temporal and Institutional |
| **Primary Changes** | | | |
| **Processes** | Individualization Detraditionalization | Disaffiliation Social Dislocation Disconnection | Destandardization Deinstitutionalization |
| **Mechanisms** | Social Transition Without Ruptures | Rupture of the Moral Pact | Change in Historical Model of Consumption |

(*Continued*)

| Analytical Tool | Reflexive School | Contractualist School | Life Course School |
|---|---|---|---|
| **Results** | Generalization and Expansion of Risks | Insecurity and De-Socialization | Temporalized Social Inequality |
| **Limitations** | Naturalization Undifferentiation Social Transformation | Complexity International Power Culture | Risk as Resource Specificities Subject as Trajectory |
| **Sociological Challenge** | **A reading of the social map of complex societies from the standpoint of heterogeneity and a diversification of traditional social categories.** | | |

## NOTES

1. The classification theory proposed here is different from, and at the same time complementary to, the excellent analyses carried out by Zinn (2004, 2006, 2008a, 2008b) and Lupton (2013) in recent years. Generally speaking, these authors evaluate five broad sociological approaches to risk theory: risk society theory (Beck 1996, 1998a, 1998b), sociocultural theory (Douglas 1992, 1996), governmentality theory (Foucault 1991, O'Malley 2008), systemic theory (Luhmann 1996, 1998a, 1998b; Japp and Kusche 2008) and the edgework theory (Lupton and Tulloch 2002, Lyng 2008).
2. Obviously, depending on the discipline, the concept of risk has a different ontological, epistemological, and methodological status (Lupton 2013, Zinn 2008b).
3. Structuring the debate in this way acknowledges shared ideas between the different theories without failing to recognize the considerable heterogeneity within each perspective and the important theoretical differences between the authors presented here.
4. The reflexive nature that gives this theory cohesion is based on the possible active responses to risk, including a continuous monitoring of action and its contexts (Giddens 1990) and a pondering and critical evaluation of social institutions (Beck 1998). In other words, the sensitivity to risk acknowledged by this school of thought is possible thanks to the reflexive ability of individuals to observe the world (Lupton 2013).
5. One of the main criticisms of this position is the perception of the sub-socialized individual that necessitates observing him/her from the perspective of methodological individualism (Lash and Urry 1998).
6. This is what Luhmann (1998) calls the brink of disaster. The results of a calculated risk are accepted based on the size of the brink, which can be determined in diverse ways, especially depending on whether or not one participates in the calculation as a decision maker or one affected by these very decisions.
7. In spite of the commonalities between both schools, the symbolic cultural theory strongly criticizes the individualist gaze of risk proposed by the reflexive theory. According to Douglas (1996), the perception of risk is never private and, in and of itself, risk is more a cultural problem than an individual one (Lupton 2013).
8. Since its inception, sociology has recognized that the individual needs meta-experimental configurations in order to confront indeterminacy. For

Weber, the concept of worldview performed that function; for Durkheim, it was the notion of collective representation; and for Bourdieu, the idea of habitus (see Beriain 1996).

9. This line of argumentation is contrary to Giddens and Beck, who maintain that, in the present, risks have become subjectivized and individualized. For the contractualist school, one can only speak of risks to the degree that the negative consequences of behavior can be mutualized.
10. This distinction implies accepting the conditions of structural subordination in which individuals find themselves (Thompson 1993 in Mora Salas 2003a).
11. In the three perspectives there is, moreover, a normative estimate for the concept of risk, inasmuch as it entails the probability of a harm that should be avoided or abolished (Renn 1992, Rigakos and Law 2009). The theory of voluntary risks and edgework (Lyng 2008) distances itself considerably from this explanation.
12. On this point, the three schools come too close to the governmental approach to risk, which claims risk is a moral device for politically disciplining the future (Ewald 1991).
13. Giddens (1996) defines anguish as a spatiotemporal relationship that arises from basic or primitive distrust among human beings.
14. Here it's important to differentiate the theory of individualization from the individualization of social risk process. The theory of individualization emerges in the 1980s and gains strength during the 1990s, when it is becomes unified in the United States under the concept of rational action, and in Europe under the umbrella of reflexive modernity, on one hand, and in postmodern and social dissolution theorists, such as Braudillard (1998), on the other. For Lash and Urry (1998), it also emerges as a reaction to the structural functionalism of Luhmann. In contrast, the individualization of social risk process assumes a current reassessment of the liberal school that considers social inequalities an expression of an order based on differences in talents, gifts, and abilities and therefore as a more individualist vision of the social (Mora Salas 2003a).
15. In fact, social pacts are part of the reflexivity of modernity (Lupton 2013). By definition, modernity assumes self-reflexivity, whether through conventions, as in the past, or the new processes of individualization in the present (Lash 1997).
16. Giddens's well-known reference to society as a *juggernaut*.
17. Lash and Urry (1998) point out that the primary change that a risk society should contemplate is not cognitive, as in the case of Giddens and Beck, but rather esthetic. Their position is that a risk society should contemplate a new understanding of the subject rather than a new regulation of the subject through trust or criticism.
18. Some authors propose an analysis of social risks from a transnational perspective (Yeates 2001, Zinn 2008b).
19. "The insecure do not constitute a social force that mobilizes resources, they are not a new proletariat, they do not have common interests, and they are not an objective class. The insecure are a non-class; they are un-representable and only signify failure" (Rosanvallon 1995).

## REFERENCES


Alexander, J. (2000) *Sociología cultural: formas de clasificación en las sociedades complejas*, Mexico: Anthropos.

Althaus, C. (2005) A disciplinary perspective on the epistemological status of risk, *Risk analysis,* 25 (3), 567–588.

Baudrillard, J. (1998) *The Consumer Society*, London: Sage.

Bauman, Z. (1996) Modernidad y ambivalencia, in Beriain, J. (ed) *Las consecuencias perversas de la modernidad. Modernidad, contingencia y riesgo* (pp. 73–120), Barcelona: Anthropos.

Bauman, Z. (2009) *Tiempos líquidos. Vivir en una época de incertidumbre*, Mexico: Tusquets Editores.

Beck, U. (1996) Teoría de la sociedad del riesgo, in Beriain, J. (comp.) *Las consecuencias perversas de la modernidad. Modernidad, contingencia y riesgo* (pp. 201–222), Barcelona: Anthropos.

Beck, U. (1998a) *La sociedad del riesgo. Hacia una nueva modernidad*, Barcelona: Paidós.

Beck, U. (1998b) Politics of Risk Society, in Franklin, J. (ed.) *The Politics of Risk Society* (pp. 9–22), Cambridge: Polity and Cambridge University Press.

Beck, U. and Beck-Gernesheim, E. (2002) *Individualization: Institutionalized Individualism and Its Social and Political Consequences*, London and Thousand Oaks, CA: Sage.

Berger, P. and Sopp, P. (1993) Differentiation of life courses? Changing patterns of labormarket sequences in West Germany, *European Sociology Review,* 9 (1), 43–65.

Beriain, J. (1996) *Las consecuencias perversas de la modernidad. Modernidad, contingencia y riesgo*, Barcelona: Anthropos.

Beriain, J. (2008) *Aceleración y tiranía del presente. La metamorfosis en las estructuras temporales de la modernidad*, Barcelona; Anthropos.

Bertaux, D. and Kohli, M. (1984) The life story approach: a continental view, *Annual Reviews Sociology,* 10, 215–237.

Blossfeld, H. (2003) Globalization, social inequality and the role of country specific institutions, in Conceicao, P., Heitor, M. and Lundvall, B. (eds.) *Innovation, competence building and social cohesion in Europe: Towards a learning society* (pp. 303–324), Cheltenham: Edward Elgar Publishing.

Blossfeld, H. and Hofmeister, H. (2005) Globalife: Life Courses in the Globalization Process. 1999–2005, *Final Report,* Bamberg: Otto Friedrich University of Bamberg.

Breen, R. (1997) Risk, recommodification and stratification, *Sociology*, 31(3), 473–489.

Castel, R. (2004) *La inseguridad social*, Buenos Aires: Manantial.

Castel, R. (2010) *El nuevo ascenso de las incertidumbres*, Buenos Aires: FCE.

Castells, M. (1995) *La ciudad informacional. Tecnologías de la información, estructuración económica y el proceso urbano-regional,* Madrid: Alianza Editorial.

Cohen, M. and Méndez, L. (2000) La sociedad de riesgo: amenaza y promesa, *Sociológica*, 15(43), 173–201.

DiPetre, T. (2002) Life course risks, mobility regimes, and mobility consequences: a comparison of Sweden, Germany and the United States, *American Journal of Sociology*, 108(2), 267–309.

Douglas, M. (1992) *Risk and Blame: Essays in Cultural Theory*, London: Routledge.

Douglas, M. (1996) *La aceptabilidad del riesgo según las ciencias sociales*, Barcelona: Editorial Paidós.

Douglas, M. and Wildavsky, A. (1982) *Risk and Culture; An Essay on the Selection of Technological and Environmental Dangers*, Berkeley: University of California Press.

Esping Andersen, G. (2001) *Fundamentos Sociales de las Economías Postindustriales,* Barcelona: Ariel.

Ewald, F. (1993) Two infinities of risk, in Massumi, B., (ed.) *The Politics of Everyday Fear* (pp. 221–228), Minneapolis: University of Minnesota Press.

Ewald, F. (1999) Filosofía de la precaución, *L'année sociloque*, 46(2), 383–412.

Ewald, F. and Kessler, D. (2000) Les noces du risque et de la politique, *Le Debat,* 109, 55–72.

Ferrie, J. (2001) Is job insecurity harmful to health? *Journal of the Royal Society of Medicine*, 94, 71–76.

Fitoussi, J.P. and Rosanvallon, P. (1997) *La nueva era de las desigualdades,* Buenos Aires: Manantial.

Foucault, M. (1991) Governmentality, in Burchell, G., Gordon, C. and Miller, P. (eds.) *The Foucault Effect: Studies in Governmentality* (pp. 84–104). Hemel Hempstead: Harvester Wheatsheaf.

Franklin, J. (1998) *The Politics of Risk Society*, Cambridge: Polity.

Furlong, A. and Cartmel, F. (1997) *Young People and Social Change: Individualization and Risk in Late Modernity*, Buckingham: Open University Press.

Gauchet, M. (2003) *La religión en la democracia*, Barcelona: Editorial del Cobre y Editorial Complutense.

Giddens, A. (1996) Modernidad y autoidentidad, in Beriain, J. (comp.) *Las consecuencias perversas de la modernidad. Modernidad, contingencia y riesgo*, Barcelona: Anthropos.

Giddens, A. (1997) Vivir en una sociedad postradicional, in Beck, U., Giddens, A. and Lash, S. *Modernización Reflexiva. Política, tradición y estética en el orden social*, Madrid: Alianza Universidad.

Heinz, W. (2003) From work trajectories to negotiated careers, in Mortimer, J. and Shanahan, M. (ed.) *Handbook of the Life Course* (pp. 185–204). New York: Kluwer Academic Plenum Publishers.

Heinz, W. and Marshall, V. (2003) *Social Dynamics of the Life Course. Transitions, Institutions and Interrelations,* New York: Aldine de Gruyter.

Japp, K. and Kusche, I. (2008) Systems theory and risk, in Zinn, J. (ed.) *Social Theories of Risk and Uncertainty: An Introduction* (pp. 76–105). Oxford: Blackwell.

Johnson, K. (1997) Shiftwork from a work and family perspective, *Research Paper R-98- 2E,* Ottawa: Applied Research Branch, Strategic Policy Group, Human Resources Development.

Kates, R. and Kasperson, J. (1983) Comparative risk analysis of technological Hazards, *Proceedings of the National Academy of Sciences,* 80(22), 7027–7038.

Lash, S. (1997) La reflexividad y sus dobles: estructura, estética, comunidad, in Beck, U., Giddens, A. and Lash, S. *Modernización Reflexiva. Política, tradición y estética en el orden social modern* (pp. 137–208), Madrid: Alianza Universidad.

Lash, S. and Urry, J. (1998) *Economías de Signos y Espacio. Sobre el Capitalismo de la Posorganización,* Buenos Aires: Amorrortu Editores.

Leisering, L. (2003) Government and the life course, in Mortimer, J. and Shanahan, M. (ed.) *Handbook of the Life Course* (pp. 205–225), New York: Kluwer Academic Plenum Publishers.

Lippert, R. and Stenson, K. (2010) Advancing governmentality studies: lessons from social constructionism, *Theoretical criminology*, 14(4), 473–494.

Luhmann, N. (1996) La contingencia como atributo de la sociedad moderna, in Beriain, J. (ed.) *Las consecuencias perversas de la modernidad. Modernidad, contingencia y riesgo* (pp. 173–198), Barcelona: Anthropos.

Luhmann, N. (1998) *Sociología del Riesgo*, Mexico: Triana Editores.

Lupton, D. (2013) *Risk*, London: Routledge.

Lupton, D. and Tulloch, J. (2002) Life would be pretty dull without risk: voluntary risk-taking and its pleasures, *Health, Risk and Society,* 4(2), 13–24.

Lyng, S. (2008) Edgework, risk and uncertainty, in Zinn, J. (ed.) *Social Theories of Risk and Uncertainty: An Introduction* (pp. 106–137), Oxford: Blackwell.

MacDonald, R. and Marsh, J. (2002) Crossing the Rubicon: Youth transitions, poverty, drugs and social exclusion, *International Journal of Drug Policy*, 13, 27–38.

Mancini, F. (2014) El impacto de la incertidumbre laboral sobre la transición a la adultez in Mora Salas, M. and Oliveira, O. (coords.) *Desafíos y paradojas. Jóvenes y transición a la vida adulta en América Latina* (pp. 147–187), Mexico: El Colegio de México.

Mancini, F. (2015) Riesgos sociales en América Latina: una interpelación al debate sobre desigualdad social, *Revista de Ciencias Políticas y Sociales,* UNAM, 223, 237–264.

Martell, L. (2009) Global inequality, human rights and power: a critique of Ulrich Beck's cosmopolitanism, *Critical sociology* 35(2), 253–272.

Martínez Franzoni, J. (2007) Regímenes de Bienestar en América Latina, *Documento de Trabajo N° 11,* Madrid: Fundación Carolina.

Mayer, K. (1997) Notes of Comparative Political Economies of Life Courses, *Comparative Social Research*, 16, 203–226.

Mayer, K. (2001) The Paradox of global social change and national path dependencies. Life course patterns in advance societies, in Woodward, A. and Kohli, M. (eds.) *Inclusions and Exclusions in European Societies* (pp. 89–110), New York: Routledge.

Mayer, K. (2004a) Life course and life chances in comparative perspective, Working paper for the Symposium in Honor of Robert Erikson "Life Chances and Social Origins", Swedish Council for Working Life and Social Research (FAS), Sigtunahöjden, November 24–25, 2003.

Mayer, K. (2004b) Whose lives? How history, societies and institutions define and shape life courses, *Research in Human Development,* 1(3), 161–187.

Mayer, K. and Schoepflin, U. (1989) The State and the life course, *Annual Reviews. Sociology*, 15, 187–209.

Mayock, P. (2009) Exploring transition and change through qualitative longitudinal research: the case of youth homelessness, *Working Paper*, Dublin: School of Social Work and Social Policy, Trinity College.

Millán, R. (2009) Incertidumbre y miedo: visiones sobre la modernidad, in Pamplona, F. (ed.) *Paradojas del miedo* (pp. 75–126), Mexico: UACM.

Millán, R. and Mancini, F. (2014) Riesgos sociales y bienestar subjetivo: un vínculo indeterminado, *Realidad, datos y espacio. Revista internacional de estadística y geografía*, 5(2), 48–79.

Mills, M. (2004) Demand for flexibility or generation of insecurity? The individualization of risk, irregular work shifts and Canadian youth, *Journal of Youth Studies*, 7(2), 115–139.

Mora Salas, M. (2003a) Desigualdad Social: ¿nuevos enfoques, viejos dilemas?, *Cuadernos de Investigación* 2, Mexico: El Colegio de México.

Mora Salas, M. (2003b) El riesgo laboral en tiempos de globalización, *Estudios Sociológicos,* 21(63), 643–666.

Mythen, G. (2007) Reappraising the risk society thesis: telescopic sight or myopic vision?, *Current Sociology*, 55(6), 793–813.

Nolan, J. (2005) Job insecurity, gender and work orientation: an exploratory study of breadwinning and caregiving identity, *GeNet Working Paper* 6, Cambridge: University of Cambridge.

Pedrelli, L. and Cebulla, A. (2011) Perceptions of labor market risks: shifts and continuities across generations, *Current Sociology,* 59(1), 24–41.

Pérez Sáinz, J.P. and Mora Salas, M. (2004) De la oportunidad del empleo formal al riesgo de exclusión laboral. Desigualdades estructurales y dinámicas en los mercados latinoamericanos de trabajo, *Revista Alteridades*, 14(28), 37–49.

Presser, H. (1998) Toward a 24 hour economy: the US experience and implications for the family, in Vannoy, D. and Dubeck, P. (eds.) *Challenges for Work and Family in the Twenty First Century* (pp. 39–47), New York: Aldine De Gruyter.

O'Malley, P. (2008) Governmentality and risk, in Zinn, J. (ed.) *Social Theories of Risk and Uncertainty: An Introduction* (pp. 52–75), Oxford: Blackwell.
Rasborg, K. (2012) World risk society or new rationalities of risk? A critical discussion of Ulrich Beck's theory of reflexive modernity, *Thesis eleven*, 108(1), 3–25.
Renn, O. (1992) Concepts of risk: a classification, in Krimsky, S. and Golding, D. (eds.) *Social Theories of Risk* (pp. 53–79), London: Praeger.
Rigakos, G. and Law, A. (2009) Risk, realism and the politics of resistance, *Critical Sociology*, 35(1), 79–103.
Rosanvallon, P. (1995) *La nueva cuestión social,* Buenos Aires: Manantial.
Sennett, R. (2000) *La corrosión del carácter. Las consecuencias personales del trabajo en el nuevo capitalismo,* Barcelona: Anagrama.
Shirani, F. and Weller, S. (eds.) (2010) Conducting Qualitative Longitudinal Research: Fieldwork Experiences, *Timescapes Working Paper Series 2,* Swindon: Economic and Social Research Council.
Taylor-Gooby, P. (2005) Pervasive uncertainty in second modernity: an empirical test, *Sociological Research Online*, 10(4), 1–9.
Taylor-Gooby, P. and Zinn, O. (2006) Current directions in risk research: new developments in psychology and sociology, *Risk analysis*, 26(2), 397–411.
Thompson, J. (1993) *Ideología y cultura moderna*, Mexico: UNAM-X.
Tulloch, J. (2008) Culture and risk, in Zinn, J. (ed.) *Social Theories of Risk and Uncertainty: An Introduction* (pp. 138–167), Oxford: Blackwell.
Tulloch, J. and Lupton, D. (2003) *Risk and Everyday Life*, London: Sage.
Wagner, P. (1997) *Sociología de la modernidad. Libertad y disciplina*, Barcelona: Herder.
Wilson, W. (1997) *When Work disappears. The World of the New Urban Poor*, New York: Vintage Books Edition.
Yeates, N. (2001) *Globalization and Social Policy*, London: Sage Press.
Zinn, J. (2004) Literature review: sociology and risk, *Working paper 1, SCARR*, Canterbury: University of Kent.
Zinn, J. (2006) Recent developments in sociological risk theory, *Forum Qualitative Social Research*, 7(1), Art. 30, 275–286.
Zinn, J. (2008a) A comparison of sociological theorizing on risk and uncertainty, in Zinn, J. (ed.) *Social Theories of Risk and Uncertainty: An Introduction* (pp. 168–210), Oxford: Blackwell.
Zinn, J. (2008b) Introduction, in Zinn, J. (ed.) *Social Theories of Risk and Uncertainty: An Introduction* (pp. 1–17), Oxford: Blackwell.
Zinn, J. and Taylor-Gooby, P. (2006) Risk as an interdisciplinary research area, in Taylor-Gooby, P. and Zinn, J. (eds.) *Risk in Social Science* (pp. 20–53). Oxford: Oxford University Press.

# 3 Time, Risk and Health

*Andy Alaszewski and Patrick Brown*

## INTRODUCTION

Time is a key element of social life. As Giddens noted, time forms an important feature of all societies and there "is no society in which individuals do not have a sense of past, present and future" (1991: 16). It is also, as we will show, an important component of risk, even though researchers exploring the nature of risk in health and medicine have not given it the same attention as other key components, such as space. For example, disease epidemics such as the nineteenth century cholera epidemics have both a spatial and temporal dimension, yet it is far easier to make the spatial dimension visible by displaying the distribution of cases on a map. John Snow (1855) mapped the incidence of the 1854 epidemic in the City of London showing that proximity to the Broad Street pump increased the probability of being infected. Such mapping provides a physical tangibility to disease through the spatial dimension and can act as a catalyst for the identification and politicization of a specific risk (see Broer's 2007, analysis of the way the mapping of potential noise pollution at Schipol airport predated the establishment of the flight paths). Time can also be made visible, as we show later in this chapter in our discussion of the use of partograms in childbirth, but it tends to get subsumed within composites of space and time.

In this chapter, we contribute to a redressing of this balance by exploring various ways in which time shapes the ways in which health risks are developed and managed. We start with a discussion of the nature of time and explore the ways in which a specific form of time, abstract time, is embedded in the rational model of risk. We then examine the ways in which in health and health care this abstract time interacts with organizational time and personal time.

## PERSONAL, SOCIAL AND ABSTRACT TIME

### Personal Time

In both premodern and modern societies, individuals have their own personal time or, in Durkheim's terms, *my time* (1915: 10). As Martin noted, this personal time is embedded in the taken-for-granted rhythm of everyday life, and the regular performance of domestic chores creates routines that are:

> the mundane process by which meaning is created and maintained even in the face of the chronic flux and disturbance of experience.
>
> Martin (1984: 23)

Personal time is linked to risk in a number of ways. As Giddens (1991) argued, individuals normally live in a state of ontological security in which they implicitly trust that the world and their lives will continue in much the same way. While there is a risk that things can go wrong, for most practical purposes, individuals disregard or bracket out such uncertainty. Given they are not under threat, they have no reason to invest time and energy in thinking about decisions but can rely on their routines and habits as a basis for everyday activities. This routinization of decisions can be seen in the study which Green and her colleagues (2003) undertook into the ways in which UK consumers discussed making choices about food they ate. Green and her colleagues found that despite various food scares, the consumers they interviewed did not engage in complex and time-consuming assessments of risk but simplified and routinized decision making. These consumers described decision making

> as a routine endeavour, aided by a number of 'short cuts' or rules of thumb for establishing food choices as routine and unremarkable. These short cuts divided safe from risky categories of food, but also divided preferred from despised foodstuffs. Rules of thumb provided . . . a sophisticated bulwark against the uncertainties of food risks when events (such as the media concern over BSE) threaten everyday trust in routine decisions.
>
> (Green, Draper and Dowler 2003: 33)

However, Giddens (1991) has noted that the smooth flow of time can be disrupted by events, such as serious illness, which threaten the individual's continued existence. Such disruptions create fateful moments in which 'business as usual' is no longer possible. Risk, the possibility of an adverse outcome, cannot be bracketed out but has to be explicitly addressed and this may involve accessing, evaluating and making decisions on the basis of expert knowledge. Fateful moments are often marked by the involvement of experts such as doctors.

## Time Embedded in Social Settings

Durkheim argued that for organized social activity to take place, there needs to be some agreement about how time is measured and how interactions and activities can be located within time. Social time provides "an abstract and impersonal frame which surrounds not only our individual existence, but that of all humanity" (Durkheim 1915: 10). If an individual wishes to participate in society and community activities, then they need to align their personal time with that of other members of the community; and this alignment involves some agreement about and standardization of time (Zerubavel 1982: 2). Indeed, if the connection between individuals' personal time and the social time of those they would like to interact with becomes disrupted, then they become marginalized and socially isolated. In a study of individuals with physical and mental ill health, Coventry and his colleagues (2014) found that some individuals do not succeed in realigning their personal time with social time and become stuck in a liminal and isolated present in which they struggle to pass time and are unable to reconnect with their past or plan and think about a future:

> For these participants, especially the house bound, day merged with night and the regular intervals associated with the experience of inter-subjective time were absent.
>
> (Coventry, Dickens, and Todd, 2014: 113)

Indeed, Coventry and his colleagues argued that this inability to synchronise personal with social time was a cause of the mental difficulties, especially depression (Coventry, Dickens and Todd 2014). In his review of early systems for measuring time, Sloley (1931) pointed out that it is intrinsically difficult to measure and standardize time, as time itself is elusive and difficult to define; it does not exist in the same way as space, which can be measured by visible objects, such as a length of wood or metal. It is commonly experienced as essentially arbitrary:

> We cannot take a little 'chunk of time' and use it in the same way [as measurements of space such as a ruler]. Before we could grasp it, it would slip through our fingers, as it were, and be-past. Time is not repeatable, not recoverable, not usable again.
>
> (Sloley, 1931: 166)

In premodern societies the measurement and standardization of time were embedded in specific localized social settings. Durkheim (1915) argued that in most premodern societies, the standardization and measurement of time centred on cycles of religious rituals linked to observable natural phenomena such as the daily and seasonal cycle of the sun or the monthly cycle of the moon. In small-scale, face-to-face, premodern societies where coordination is relatively straightforward and simple, the use of natural cycles are adequate. In more large-scale societies, such as dynastic Egypt, more precise systems were needed to predict key events, such as the flooding of the Nile. Sloley (1931) documented the development of Egyptian instruments to measure natural phenomena such as the precise movements of stars and the ways in which these were combined with a religious system of ideas to develop the calendar, an annual cycle of time:

> The Calendar was brought into use by the Egyptians at a very early date, at least 3000 B.C., when New Year's Day 1 (The Opening of the Year; first month of inundation [flooding of the Nile followed by sowing of crops], day 1) coincided with the heliacal rising of Sirius (The Going up of the Goddess Sothis). When Sirius, after a period of invisibility, was first again observed in the sky just before sunrise in the latitude of Memphis, the Egyptians knew that the Nile should begin to rise again.
>
> (Sloley 1931: 168)

While the Egyptian system of measuring time enabled them to predict the key events and undertake appropriate ritual and practical activities to ensure the continued order of the universe and goodwill of the gods, it was limited. For example, both day and night were divided into 12 hours, but the length of an hour varied in accordance with the changing times of sunrise and sunset.

## The Changing Nature of Social Time: From Group Time to Abstract Time

Social and technological changes have altered the nature and use of time, disembedding it from specific localized groups with their religious practices and moving it towards an abstract secularized global universal system (Giddens 1991). In Britain at the start of the nineteenth century social time was based on the local time of sunrise, midday and sunset. Thus midday was approximately 20 minutes earlier in eastern than in western Britain. The development of transport systems, especially the development of the British network of railways in the 1840s, made such variations problematic and potentially dangerous. In the 1840s, the railway companies agreed that all railways clocks should be synchronized with time at the Greenwich observatory in London using the new electric telegraph system and that all train timetables should be based on Greenwich time (Zerubavel 1982, Harrington 2003). As railway companies expanded in the USA, they also developed railway time and agreed a system of four time zones based on Greenwich Meantime (GMT). In 1884, an international conference, despite protests from the French who wanted Paris to be the prime meridian, created an international time zone system with Greenwich as the prime meridian (Zerubavel 1982).

In some settings, local time systems still exist, most notably in Muslim countries where the Islamic calendar remains important and key social and religious events such as the start and ending of fasting during Ramadhan are synchronized with local sunrise and sunset. However, there has been a global movement towards a "*standard system of units of time,* which enables different people to measure the passage of time in an identical manner, and a standard time-reckoning and dating framework" using the 24-hour clock, the Gregorian calendar and dating from the start of the Christian Era (Emphasis in the original Zerubavel 1982: 3).

This standardization is based on an abstract categorization of time with precisely defined measureable units of time each of equal value and quality. Time progresses with a steady and regular linearity, in contrast to some systems such as Hindu religious texts in which time is cyclical and can make bends and loops and move backward on itself. As Brown and his colleagues (2013) noted, modern abstract time units are based on arbitrary but agreed criteria and are central to the development of scientific knowledge about the nature of the world. Past events, such as incidence of specific diseases or deaths can be recorded within time frames, making predictions of future events and incidents possible:

> This universalizing tendency, capturing information and events in their relation to time while these are also 'lifted out' of distinct local contexts, is fundamental to the development of abstract systems of technical knowledge which define experiences of modernity.
>
> (Brown et al. 2013: 480)

## THE IMPACT OF UNIVERSAL TIME AND A MODERN CONCEPTION OF RISK

### Personal Time

The development of abstract time has changed personal time and the ways in which individuals experience time. This can be seen in the development of time-based accounts of the everyday life in diaries and autobiographies. As Alaszewski (2006) has noted, diary keeping, making a personal contemporary record of everyday activities and thoughts, can be traced back to sixteenth century Protestants and was stimulated by the publication of almanacs; "annual calendars of events, which had spaces for individual annotations and facilitated diary keeping" (2006: 6). The production of printed almanacs provided the framework for individual record keeping and for autobiography in which abstract time provides the key anchor points for the personal narrative; key personal events, such as births, are recorded as taking place at specific calendar times.

The development of abstract timing also created the possibility for individuals to view their own lives through the lens of risk. The systematic collection and analysis of information about personal events such as births and deaths during specified time periods is fundamental for the generation of knowledge, such as life expectancies, which can shape how individuals think about time and shape their personal time. This knowledge about the structuring of personal events over time effectively creates a generalized life timetable in which there are designated time periods for particular life activities or events, and individuals are considered to be at risk, or exposed to harm, if they do not undertake normal activities in these periods.

Such processes can be seen in high-income countries in relationship to childbirth. Epidemiological data indicates that the safest time to have a baby is when the mother is aged between 20 and 30 years so that teenage mothers and older mothers are 'at risk'—that is categorized as exposing themselves and their babies to higher risk. Thus for women who are over 30, the 'biological clock' is said to be ticking and, as Locke and Budds (2013) found, not only do these women have to deal with the challenge of becoming pregnant when the risks are higher, but they also have to deal with the increasing possibility of infertility. These women find it difficult to balance personal with social time; there is no 'right time' to become pregnant. Many feel 'panicked' into pregnancy, unable to have a baby in their 'own time'. Locke and Budds described the tension between abstract and personal time in the following way:

> the women in our study claimed to have made decisions about the timing of pregnancy that they inferred possibly warranted justification, owing to the fact that their decisions conflicted with the society's norms regarding the 'right' situation and time to have a baby. Therefore, they were forced to make the decision to either become parents at the 'wrong' time—when they weren't necessarily 'ready' or, alternatively, facing possible childlessness owing to concerns over fertility problems associated with increasing maternal age.
>
> (Locke and Budds 2013: 538)

This tension between the abstract time imposed by organizations and institutions and personal timings is thus an important locus of power relations, as will be explored further in a later section. Personal time will often tend to become colonized by those in more powerful positions and by organizations. Klingemann (2000) denotes the challenging of personal time which is inherent to addiction services, especially those services run within new public management forms of governance. In these contexts, service-users are required to restructure their time or be labelled as at higher risk of relapse. Former drugs users must not only adapt and conform their timetables but are also required to anticipate risk of relapse in the future as a means of managing their time in the present. In this sense, both the quantitative structuring and qualitative living of personal time are imposed through a framework of risk management.

## Abstract and Group Time

As noted in the earlier example (Klingemann 2000), although time has been universalized and abstracted from specific social communities, it is re-embedded in specific organizations and used to control and coordinate activities and minimize risk through organizational timetables or routines. In his description of the ideal type of modern 'rational' organization, the bureaucracy, Weber emphasized order was created though rational rule-based decision making. He did acknowledge some aspects of time, for example the role of paid officials or bureaucrats in being present at specified times in order to make decisions, as well as the role of records or files enabling past decisions to be scrutinized. But since he based his analysis on public administration, Weber effectively disregarded the nature and role of uncertainty about the future and the need to control it. If he had looked more closely at organizations such as nineteenth century railway companies, then the importance of future time would have become clearer. These companies needed abstract time to create train timetables so passengers could plan their journeys. Moreover, the train companies would manage their networks by ensuring rolling stock and suitably trained staff were in the right place at the right time and accordingly managed risk by minimizing the possibility of train collisions (Zerubavel 1982).

The significance of time was also evident in the organizations built in the nineteenth century to manage the social problems such as workhouses, prisons and asylums. The visible architecture of these institutions physically and symbolically divided the normal from the abnormal and internal structures further subdivided the abnormal (Foucault 1967). These institutions used time to manage and control activities. As Foucault noted, the reformers of the early nineteenth century saw therapeutic potential in the orderly management of time, so that

> The pressures of the healthiest needs, the rhythm of the days and the seasons, the calm necessity to feed and shelter oneself, constrain the disorder of the madman to a regular observance.
>
> (Foucault 1967: 194)

In the small-scale asylums of the early nineteenth century, such as the Retreat established by the Quakers in York, there was an attempt to reproduce an orderly household in which the insane were occupied by a regime of activities and participated in social events, such as meals and tea parties (Tuke 1813). As the number and size of institutions and the therapeutic optimism of 'moral treatment' was replaced by the pessimism of the late nineteenth century, so the therapeutic and flexible routines of the early asylums were replaced by more rigid controlling and processing routines. When Goffman (1961) wrote his highly influential essays on asylums drawing on his research in a mega-institution, the seven thousand patient St Elizabeth Hospital in Washington DC, USA, he drew on Weber's theory of bureaucracy. For example he argued that rules and the hierarchy of officials played a role in "the bureaucratic organization of whole blocks of people" (Goffman

1967: 6). However, Goffman added time to Weber's specification, noting that the institutional routine was one of the defining features of the bureaucratic 'total institution' in which

> All phases of the day's activities are tightly scheduled, with one activity leading at a prearranged time into the next, the whole sequence of activities being imposed from above by a system of formal rules and a body of officials.
>
> (Goffman1961: 6)

Given the size and complexity of institutions, such 'prearranged time' could only be based on abstract clock time. This use of time to manage and judge patients was not restricted to mental hospitals but was evident in general hospitals (Sellerberg 1991). As Lorber (1975) noted, surgical patients were categorized and managed through staff routines:

> For the sake of the smooth and efficient running of the institution, patients are categorized so they can be worked on with routines established as proper for their category.
>
> (Lorber 1975: 213)

Patients who disrupted these time structures were judged to be difficult or bad patients and experienced moral opprobrium, even punitive treatment:

> The doctors and nurses tended to term patients who interrupted well-established routines and made extra work for them "problem patients" . . . Possible consequences of being labeled a problem patient are premature discharge, neglect, and referral to a psychiatrist.
>
> (Lorber 1975: 213)

The disruption of routines is not limited to patients; in a study of the thrombolysis for stroke survivors, Cluckie (2014) showed that stroke doctors are aware that the clock is ticking when they first admit a patient. They need to rapidly access services from other departments, such as medical images of the patient's brain, so they do not miss the narrow window of opportunity for the treatment and at the same time minimize the risk of a harmful outcome, such as a brain bleed. However, the disruption of the routines of other departments creates tension or conflict which Cluckie described as 'turf wars' between departments:

> These turf wars illustrate an unexpected consequence of the sudden and unpredictable nature of stroke. Whilst there were disruptions to the usual activities of the stroke team, these turf wars again illustrate the disruption to usual clinical routines that are experienced beyond

> the stroke unit into the ED [emergency department] and the radiology department.
>
> (Cluckie 2014: 131)

Managing the complex routines of a hospital is a defining skill of a competent practitioner. Yoels and Clair described how junior hospital doctors in the USA learn to deal with the problem of 'never enough time' by learning to save time and manage "the *conveyor belt* of scheduled patient appointments" (emphasis in the original, 1999: 142).

## Comment

Although time is a key element of social life, it is one that is frequently overlooked. To some extent, this relates to its taken-for-grantedness; but partly this relates to the difficulty of defining and making time visible and tangible. Thus Weber, who developed his ideal type of bureaucracy from public bodies using rules to make decisions in stable predictable conditions—that is, ones of low risk—did not treat time as a key phenomenon, whereas Goffman, in developing his ideal type of bureaucratic total institution from mental hospitals operating in a higher-risk environment dealing with large numbers of unpredictable people, did include time as a defining feature.

Heightened sensitivities towards risk can thus be seen as rendering time more explicit both within everyday lived experiences and social scientific analysis. Knowledge of risks have been noted in this section as disrupting the experiential passage of time in the present as well as demanding an increasing attentiveness to the future (Giddens 1991). Risk as a social phenomenon can thus be associated with more intense experiences of personal time (as we will show later). The notion of women's 'ticking body clock' and the association of age and fertility are by no means modern—as various Old and New Testament Bible stories make evident. What is distinctively modern, however, is a much more precise and increasingly compressed understanding of 'normal' or safe periods of time and, correspondingly, a widened problematization of abnormality and of being 'at risk'.

Modern standardization and measurement of time therefore is not only vital as a basis for the construction of knowledge regarding which risks are salient, but in structuring the social contexts in which the 'doing' (Montelius and Nygren 2014) or managing of risk is more or less successfully accomplished. We have noted that abstract time is imposed upon actors' personal time and becomes a locus of power relations through which actors are expected or required to align themselves and be held accountable for their success in doing so. These different processes connecting time to risk and risk to time denote the socially constructed format of modern abstract time and attempt to rationalize the world through this standardized medium. This tendency towards rationalization is a defining hallmark of risk, and yet risk also involves the resistance of nature and technology to time management, as becomes clear in contexts where complex technological processes are 'tightly coupled' to one another to the extent that human thinking and planning struggles to keep up (Perrow 1984). It is to such relations between time, risk and rationality which we now turn.

## RISK AND INSTITUTIONAL ATTEMPTS TO RATIONALIZE TIME

As Perrow (1984) has noted, the growth in size, complexity and interconnectivity of organizations in modern society means that major failures or, in his terms 'normal accidents', have become common. In our study of health policy (Alaszewski and Brown 2012), we note a similar trend in health care in the UK. Partially in response to such dysfunctions in the second half of the twentieth century, Power (2004) described how risk and its management became pervasive in all types of organizations:

> Risk management and risk 'talk' are all around us. The risk-based description of organizational life is conspicuous. [All organizations including hospitals and the central government have] been invaded to varying degrees by ideas about risk and its management.
>
> (Power 2004: 9)

Organizations, especially those which are publicly funded and/or overtly concerned with human well-being, such as hospitals, have to demonstrate that they do not harm their staff or patients and therefore claim to use rational approaches to risk. However, closer examination of how these organizations manage uncertainty and particularly of the ways in which time shapes identification and management of risk indicates that underlying risk is a discourse of power which is difficult to resist because of the apparent benevolence and objectivity of risk.

In the 1950s, before medical power and autonomy had been challenged by policies such as clinical governance, the American sociologist, Roth (1957), undertook a study of hospitals treating patients with tuberculosis. Roth observed that while tuberculosis is a contagious or infectious disease, there was uncertainty over how contagious, how it was transmitted between individuals and the most effective way of preventing its transmission. He argued that while the hospital had measures which it claimed were based on rational risk management, in reality the failure to apply these measures consistently meant that they were in practice irrational, even magical:

> These uncertainties leave the way open for ritualized procedures that often depend more on convenience and ease of administration than on rationally deduced probabilities. They also leave the way open for irrational practices that can properly be called "magic".
>
> (Roth, 1957: 310)

Roth reached this conclusion by examining the ways in which protective devices such as masks, gloves and gowns were used. He found that their use was shaped by social not biological factors, including: power, the most powerful groups, doctors, tended to avoid such protection; spatial, interactions in non-clinical spaces tended not to include protective barriers; and temporal, the 'rules suggest that the tubercle bacillus works only during business hours' (Roth 1957: 313–314). The influence of time was evident in its categorization, with hospital staff 'protecting' themselves during working time but not when they were off duty:

> The ward employee tends to wear protective clothing when carrying out her duties, but not when 'socializing' with the patients . . . Apparently, these nurses believe they need protection only when working.
>
> (Roth 1957: 314)

Thus for Roth, the different ways in which time influenced the use of protective measures reflected the role of power and symbolism in managing uncertainty, not rational evidence-based risk management. The role of time in organizational creation and management of uncertainty is also evident in the temporal structuring of childbirth. The continuities and changes in this field can be seen by comparing two studies separated by 50 years: a US study of an obstetrical hospital (Rosengren and DeVault 1963) and a UK study of midwifery (Scamell and Alaszewski 2012 and Scamell and Stewart 2014). These two studies found that while most births were routine and did not require any intervention, uncertainty about the birthing process meant that the possibility of things going wrong was ever present. Rosengren and DeVault found that:

> Pregnancy does not necessarily entail abnormal complications, but the possibility always exists. Because of this the demeanor of the doctors and nurses takes on a studied casualness about childbirth—but always with a watchful eye towards unforeseen difficulties.
>
> (1963: 280)

Scamell and her colleagues described similar findings. They noted that in high-income countries, childbirth is typically considered a fateful moment with a lot at stake for both mothers and midwives. In a culture of blame with limited tolerance for accidents (Green 1999), if things go wrong, then all actions will be scrutinized and blame allocated. In such a context, all births are potentially abnormal and only some become defined as normal in hindsight:

> Within a linguistic context where normality and unassisted safety could only be envisaged as the non-occurrence of unwanted futures, imagined futures where things go wrong took on a very real existence in the

> present, thereby impacting upon how birth could be conceptualised and managed. As such, midwifery activity functions not to preserve normality, but to introduce a pathologisation process where birth can never be imagined to be normal until it is over.
>
> (Scamell and Alaszewski 2012: 219)

They argued that this pathologisation is based on a precautionary approach to risk management which disregards the probabilities of events, in this case, the low probability of adverse outcomes, and "casts the future principally in negative, potentially catastrophic terms" (Alaszewski and Burgess 2007: 349). In both studies, time is a key element in the management of uncertainty, but time was used in different ways in the two studies. In the doctor-dominated context of the early 1960s, women giving birth were expected to fit in with medical expectations of time. Thus women who asked for pain relief when staff did not think it was the right time were categorized as difficult patients as they were "upsetting the rhythmic expectations to which the team members have become accustomed" (Rosengren and DeVault 1963: 281). The routine of childbirth was symbolically represented by the spatial structure of the unit, and all women had to go through the same circuit of rooms, even if it did not fit the timing of their birth:

> The normal circuit . . . is adhered to scrupulously. The physiological rhythm [of a woman's birthing] would often indicate that at least one or more rooms might better be forgotten, but the patient must adhere to this timing of movements from region to region, even if it means at a fast trot.
>
> (Rosengren and DeVault 1963: 283).

Medical power was evident in the delivery room. In this space there were medical norms of time based on custom and practice and routine practices to keep deliveries to time. Doctors were expected to deliver babies within 40 to 50 minutes and to use interventions such as forceps to meet these deadlines:

> The use of forceps is also a means by which the tempo is maintained in the delivery room, and they are so often used that the procedure is regarded as normal.
>
> (Rosengren and DeVault 1963: 283)

In the 50 years between Rosengren and DeVault's study and Scamell's, there have been major changes in practice. The paternalism of unfettered medical power in which professional judgments defined norms and facilitated moral judgments about patients who disrupted time rhythms has, in many countries (though by no means all), been replaced by a system based on the rhetoric of patient choice and informed consent in which professional actions are justified in terms of encoded knowledge, such as national guidelines and protocols. As Scamell and her colleagues show in this context, midwives' practice is highly controlled through a system of rules and procedures justified in terms of scientific knowledge. Central to this system is the partogram, a visual timetable on which midwives have to record the progress of the labour in terms of the dilation of the labouring woman's cervix. The partogram is an ongoing record of their surveillance of the labour and is also a record that can be used to scrutinize a midwife's actions if the labour does not go to plan and timetable. They noted that:

> Individual midwives are required to use an agreed timetable embodied in the partogram to manage labour so that they identify labours that are too slow and take action to minimise potential risk to mother and baby. To maintain their surveillance of the cervix, midwives are expected to undertake regular and intrusive internal vaginal examinations.
>
> (Scamell and Stewart 2014: 87)

Most of the midwives and mothers in Scamell and Stewart's study accepted the use of the partogram timetable and saw it as beneficial, as a way of using scientific knowledge to manage the uncertainty of the future and minimize the possibility of harmful outcomes. However, Scamell and Stewart did observe occasional acts of defiance in which midwives sought to 'stop the clock' and replace the abstract time encoded in the partogram with labouring women's own embodied time. In these circumstances, midwives used their own intuitive knowledge to justify disregarding the institutional timetable but, given the surveillance built into the partogram timetable, they had to do this covertly, for example by not recording the start of labour:

> Midwives indicated that they wanted to minimise risks to the pregnant women and at times saw the prescribed pathways and timetables as potentially hazardous. This meant that at crucial points in the process when the clock started ticking, start of established labour and onset of birth, midwives created 'grey areas' [by delaying appropriate recordings] that enabled them to delay the start of the clock.
>
> (Scamell and Stewart 2014: 92)

## Comment

As Power (2004) has argued, risk has become a central issue for organizations which seek to manage the uncertainties they face. Their explicit risk management strategies use time to pace and control activities. In health-care organizations, the rationale for such time structuring has changed over time. In the 1950s and 1960s, risk management was embedded in medical practice. The medical profession dominated the specification of time norms, the routine of activities and sanctions against individuals, including patients who disrupted the rhythm of activities. By the end of the twentieth century, the autonomy of the individual practitioner was itself considered a risk and subjected to new formal systems of risk management, such as clinical governance with the externalization of norms in formal 'evidence-based' guidelines and protocols. While these systems are justified as rational, based on evidence, various studies have depicted risk management as an illusion, whereby organizations can claim that they can provide protection, but in reality it is impossible to predict every outcome:

> Can we know the risks we face, now or in the future? No, we cannot: but yes, we must act as if we do.
>
> (Power 2004: 9)

This gap between aspirations and practices accounts for the more irrational dimensions of organizational time: in Roth's study as the symbolic or magical use of protective clothing, in Rosengren and DeVault as the ritualist movement of birthing women through the sequence of rooms even when this meant doing it at a brisk trot and in Scamell's study where the rigidity of the partogram timetable meant that midwives had to conceal information and actions if they wanted to create time for a woman to birth in her own time.

## RISK, ILLNESS AND LIVED EXPERIENCES OF TIME

### The Disruption of Personal Time Amidst the Illness Experience

When individuals are ill, the nature of personal time and the relationship between personal and other forms of time changes. Illness fosters a heightened awareness of uncertainty where, as Bury (1982) has explored, the onset of chronic illness changes the lived experience of personal time, creating a biographical disruption in which the anticipated relationship between past, present and future can become undermined. In her analysis of narratives of chronic illness, Charmaz (1991) similarly noted that illness experiences were marked by crises and threats to the individual's usual patterns of daily life. Amidst such crises, individuals tended to focus on the immediate present. Charmaz argued that the extent to which such a crisis "engulfs everyone in the present", while "the fear of death clouds the future", meant that "images of the future remain vague and elusive". (Charmaz 1991: 35).

In Alaszewski and his colleagues' studies of stroke survivors,[1] survivors used time as a way of telling their story and as a way of attempting to piece back together a chronology decimated by the disruption and uncertainties of their post-stroke lives (Alaszewski 2006).The survivors experienced stroke as an unexpected and unforeseen disruption of the smooth and regular flow of life and time, undermining their sense of ontological security:

> The lack of warning meant that survivors experienced their stroke as a traumatic event, one which undermined the confidence which they had in the "taken-for-grantedness" of everyday life. Stroke survivors could no longer take-for-granted every day activities and perceptions of dangers that had previously been 'bracketed out' now needed to be explicitly considered and managed.

Stroke survivors' accounts represented their stroke "as a terrifying and violent intrusion upon the normal flow of day-to-day life" (Alaszewski and Wilkinson 2014: 8). In telling their stories, survivors contrasted the normality of everyday life pre-stroke with post-stroke abnormality. For example one of the survivors in our stroke study, a 34-year-old woman, described normality in terms of the regular routine of events when managing a household with young children:

> Up until that point [the stroke], I was driving my son to school every morning, then driving my daughter to hers, both are out of walking reach, they are too far to walk. Coming home, doing my normal thing of the shopping and the cooking and the ironing and the cleaning and all the things you take for granted.
>
> (Alaszewski and Wilkinson 2014: 8)

A survivor who was 58 years old when he had his stroke described pre-stroke normality in terms of leisure, improving his personal best time by running against the clock:

> I was determined [before the stroke] that I was going to be super fit and the only way you can do that is to push out the standards so that every time I [went] for a run I was looking at the time and trying to get it a little bit better.

Stroke survivors contrasted these descriptions of pre-stroke normality against descriptions of abnormality of life and time after stroke. Since most of the survivors in our study were admitted to hospital following their stroke, images of the abnormality of hospital life and routine—and of the colonization of their personal time by institutional time—dominated their accounts. A survivor who was 45 when she had her stroke had experienced various health problems before her stroke, including chronic fatigue. She described the ways in which the hospital routine disrupted her normal routine and made it difficult to get the rest she needed:

> I've got tiredness anyway, so I don't know [if the stroke made any difference]. I can't say I felt any more tired. Only from the fact that because

> they made us get up so early in hospital in the morning I was very tired. But I'm tired anyway. And my mornings are like 10 o'clock time usually I surface and in the hospital it was something like 5.45 they were getting me up. And then they wouldn't let you back into your bed.

Clearly apparent in this account was the intrusion into personal time of the timetable of the institution by which the rhythm of the individual patient becomes colonized and interfered with by the organizational rhythm of the hospital. Indeed the tension between these two formats of time were important in shaping the physical difficulties of tiredness she encountered.

Stroke survivors' accounts of stroke also highlighted the ways in which the stroke itself disrupted their experience of personal time, particularly the relationship between past, present and future. Their pre-stroke past was no longer a reliable indicator of a newly destabilized and uncertain future. Indeed stroke survivors found it difficult to talk about the future, one in which the possibility of another stroke was an ever-present reality. For example one survivor, a 59 year-old-man, who kept a research diary wrote:

> Again very tired this afternoon—still trying to maintain a positive attitude although am scared that another more serious stroke may occur—trying to prevent this by doing everything I am told by doctor and community stroke team.
>
> (Alaszewski 2006: 53)

Meanwhile, another survivor, in this case a 34-year-old woman, described in her diary the way in which she could no longer take her life for granted as she was "living on borrowed time" (Alaszewski 2006: 54).

## Working With Time to Generate Meaning and to Recast Futures

Survivors used time to account for what had happened and what was happening to them. Over time, survivors developed ways of making sense of and describing their situations. Some survivors sought to reconnect with their pre-stroke lives by emphasizing their personal resilience and the continuity of their biography and life (Ezzy 2000). Other survivors accepted that the stroke had created a disruption; some of these survivors described the ways in which they were creating a new normality with its own past, present and future, whereas others described the ways in which they had become stuck in the abnormality with neither a past or future just a present.

The survivors who reconnected with their pre-stroke past minimized the disruption of their stroke and recalled the continuity and normality of their life, for example by recounting the ways they rapidly returned to pre-stroke activities and routines. For example a survivor who was 49 when he had his stroke and who ran his own business described in his final interview his rapid resumption of everyday activities and return to work:

> I had the stroke on the Thursday and I went into work on the [following] Wednesday. I mean I was sort of going down and having a chat with the lads . . . But I think about three weeks later I actually went back to work full-time. (Fourth Interview)

He emphasized his personal resilience and the continuity of his biography by comparing his response to his stroke with the ways he had overcome pre-stroke adversity:

> I smashed it [his leg] in about twenty places [in a motor cycle accident] and he [the consultant] said, 'you probably won't walk without a stick', and that was like a red rag to a bull, I mean particularly because after the operation I was driving our transit camper up to London every day which wasn't the brightest thing I could have done but it was the bloody-minded part of it that, you know, it's not going to stop me.

A survivor who was 45 when she had her stroke also distanced herself from her stroke: "So I count myself very lucky and it's [the stroke] in the past now" (Second Interview). In her interviews, she recalled and reconnected with her pre-stroke life and biography, which in her case had been one of chronic illness:

> I got chicken pox when I was 30 and the bank didn't believe my doctor that I had chicken pox. They got really nasty so I was so glad to leave in the end . . . I had shingles and it left me with this fibromyalgia and chronic fatigue syndrome and it kind of all goes hand in hand and I think that's far worse than ever having that stroke. (Fourth Interview)

Other survivors found it more difficult to bracket stroke out of their life stories and continued to describe it as a key defining event in their lives and biography. Some of these survivors were able to tell a new story in which they had created a new form of more restricted normality with a more limited relationship between their past (post-stroke), present (recovery) and future (adjusted expectations). A survivor who was 58 years old when he had his stroke described his stroke as a significant one-off event whose consequences he could manage through hard work and rational effective planning. Within such a 'linear-restitution' narrative (Ezzy 2000), he accounted for his stroke as a mechanical failure of his body and described how he could control the future and prevent a reoccurrence by being more careful:

> I see it as a plumbing problem in the sense that there was a weak pipe in there [my body] which was waiting to burst really and I'd put it

> under a lot of strain with my exercise regime and I think it's significant that it burst when I was really, really pushing hard on my bicycle and it burst . . . so the risk of it happening again is very low although they would say you are damaged goods, so don't [overdo] it . . . don't tempt fate . . . (Third Interview)

This participant described his approach to life as a form of rational planning, one grounded in realism but oriented to the future, to achieving targets. In his final interview, he responded to a question about what advice he would give to other stroke survivors in the following way:

> To work at it I think. Don't give into it . . . it may be the way I deal with things but you have to put some effort in but to accept that you've got limits. So you've got to make targets to aim at but if you don't achieve them then don't get too disappointed, move the target and think well I got that bit wrong, I'll have another go. So get some method into it. (Third Interview)

However, for one group of survivors, stroke remained an ever-present reality, an event they could not forget or get away from; so it left them stuck in the present in an abnormal and/or chaotic narrative (Ezzy 2000). In his final interview 18 months after his stroke, a survivor who was 44 years old at the time of his stroke described how he had rapidly recovered his physical ability and made a quick return to work, albeit one which he later regretted:

> I was probably too eager to be trying to portray to people I think that I hadn't had a stroke. Against the stroke nurses advice I went back to work on the third week . . . I wish that I had taken a couple of months and just sat quietly and got myself back into it gently rather than bang, off you go, I'm alright, nothing's happened to me . . . I would like to turn the clock back a few years to when I could do it [work] for fun. (Fourth Interview)

He described how he could not move on from his stroke and was experiencing continuing anxiety. He could not rid himself of the memory of being admitted via the Accident and Emergency department (A&E) to hospital, returning to this experience repeatedly in this final interview:

> That period when you're in A&E for you personally is very traumatic, no matter what you've got wrong with you, and when you're just left there and nobody seems to be taking any notice of you, and when they do it's are you alright love? You know, it's terrifying . . . I mean I was crying most of the time I was there and I just wish somebody had come over and said look this is probably what's happened to you, what we're gonna do is this and in a minute you'll be taken to a ward and

> you'll be assessed. But no, to be lying there for 4 hours thinking I can't move, something has occurred to me or happened to me, was terrifying. (Fourth Interview)

Even though he was making an excellent physical recovery from his stroke, since the past was ever present, he described how this shaped his inability to think of and plan for the future:

> I tend not to think of the long term future for myself personally. I mean I am frightened to death that it will happen again . . . I don't make any great plans for the future. [Fourth Interview]

A survivor who was 43 when she had her stroke described how her initial post-stroke recovery was undermined by a series of major health problems, and she was unable to reconnect with her hectic pre-stroke life:

> Yeah. You could say that [the stroke has changed things]. It's had a huge impact on my life. Whereas 18 months ago, when I first had my stroke I was well on the road to recovery and I was almost cocky with my attitude and what have you I soon . . . the epilepsy and the ensuing medical problems that I've had has brought me back down to earth with a bump, you know? And it's just been a nightmare. That's all I can say. [Fourth Interview]

Her sense of being stuck in the present was exacerbated by the feeling that professionals were unwilling or unable to give her a recovery timetable, to tell her if and when she would regain use of parts of her body. In response to a question about whether she was recovering she said:

> Not really and nobody seems to give me straight answers because I still haven't regained full use of my right arm and when I approached the physio[therapist]s, whether it be at the hospital or home visits and what have you, no-one can give me a straight answer as to whether I will ever regain or regain a certain amount of use, albeit limited or restricted in any way. They just don't tell you. They just say well everybody's different and they brush it under the carpet. But a stupid thing like regaining my right arm means all the world to the individual. You know . . . because I can't even type 2-handed. So looking at my job prospects for the future I can't do anything. (Fourth Interview)

At the time of her final interview, 18 months after her stroke, this participant could see no way forward. She was trapped in an abnormal situation in which even day-to-day survival was difficult. She summarized her sense of hopelessness in her final interview and diary entry:

> I can't walk any distance anymore. It's just . . . It's simply just a question of confidence, a) in the tablets to control my epilepsy and in myself. And

> until I've built that up it's just been a nightmare. My whole world consists of this room, literally. (Fourth Interview) I'm beginning to wonder if I'll ever be well again. (Final Diary Entry)

In the accounts of the stroke survivors, we have explored the deeply problematic disruption of time through uncertainty as an important feature of lived experiences of illness. Such disruption could be countered by attempts to restore a linear narrative of progress and recovery in order to bring about a less unpredictable and more normal future. However, we have also noted various examples where this attempt to return to a normal format of personal time was not possible, and in some instances, personal time was further disrupted by organizational time.

Individuals may also work with time in various ways in order to manage uncertainty, as is also evident in the literature. In Brown and de Graaf's study of the ways in which individuals responded to uncertainty following a diagnosis of terminal cancer, individuals had to deal with the information that they had a limited time left to live—a personalized life expectancy based on diagnostic data and probabilistic inferences drawn from these. Brown and de Graaf found that individuals incorporated this information into their own lives while also personalizing such considerations of future-time, both in terms of its quality and quantity. In some instances, individuals with a terminal diagnosis intensively reflected upon such future-time, endowing it with heightened personal meaning. For example in their interviews they discussed:

> The significance of time spent with family, grandchildren in particular, and the imagined loss of this future is experienced as significantly problematic. As time spent living with the prognosis continues, so does future-time become more deeply considered, appreciated and thus its potential loss becomes all the more palpable.
>
> (Brown and de Graaf 2013: 550)

In their interviews, terminally-ill individuals reflected on their futures and found a variety of ways of reworking the information that they had a limited quantity of time left. For example some argued that there might be a cure or that their cancer would respond to an experimental treatment so they would gain more time. As Brown and de Graaf explored, in these situations, time was not made up of a fixed quantity of abstract time but was (re-)constructed by:

> various human and non-human actors involved in the cancer experience. Subjective experiences of perceived or embodied time are more obviously shaped by social and illness context . . . but clock time (quantity of time) in the future is also constructed through the probabilistic inferences of professionals, the reinterpretation by the patient within a specific social setting and illness experience, and is in various cases

> extended or 'fed' by hope in certain surgical or pharmaceutical interventions. The impact of how these two aspects of future-time—quality and quantity—are constructed and experienced was vividly apparent within the illness narratives of the participants.
>
> (Brown and de Graaf 2013: 558)

The nature of risk information and its provision to individuals is important here in understanding the agency of individual patients to rework futures in the midst of uncertainty. Probabilistic information about futures is helpful in predicting tendencies across groups but much less useful for any one individual in understanding whether he or she will be a typical patient or an outlier. The residual uncertainty can then be reworked through hope by which the future is made malleable and extended in light of new possibilities provided by medical technologies.

## Comment

Serious ill health brings time into sharp focus. As the illness undermines individuals' sense of ontological security, it means that they can no longer bracket out risk but need to directly confront it. As the routines of everyday life are fragmented and replaced by alien even hostile time structures, such as hospital routines, so the relationship between past, present and future is fragmented. Reconstructing this relationship is a challenge. To reconnect with the normality of pre-illness life requires the use of selective memory, some of the shock and disruption of the illness have to be forgotten, remembering earlier successful overcoming of adversity facilitates this. However, such selective remembering may be difficult to achieve as Tullock, a sociologist who survived the 9/9 bombings in London noted in his struggle to overcome post-traumatic stress:

> The emotional consequences stemming from the frightening lack of warning of a catastrophic invasion of one's personal health; the anxiety about recurrence of the attack; the breakdown of everyday confidence or sense of ontological security; and, in reaction to all this anxiety, the painstaking and minutely detailed planning of everyday activities like crossing a road or making a cup of tea which hitherto had been taken for granted.
>
> (Tulloch 2008: 452)

Those who cannot reconnect with the past seek to create a new normality, a new relationship between their post-illness past, the present and the future. Hope in this context becomes an invaluable tool for working with and reworking future time. Those who are unable to create a new normality become stuck, in the present, in an intolerable situation which has to be endured.

## CONCLUSION

Risk and uncertainty are both concepts that are time oriented, particularly towards future-time; uncertainty concerns the essential unpredictability of the future, while risk is grounded in a faith in its predictability and control. Thus in response to the question 'What will happen?' the answer in terms of uncertainty is 'anything' whereas in terms of risk it is 'the probability or likelihood of specific definable outcomes'. Serious illness is disruptive of everyday life, normality and time. It creates uncertainty by disrupting the relationship between past, present and future and the taken-for-grantedness that the future will somehow be like the past. As stroke survivors make clear in their accounts, after their stroke, nothing is ever quite the same. There is for example the ever-present possibility of another and fatal stroke.

Experts and the organizations they work within use routines based on abstract time to attempt to attain control amidst uncertainty, though we noted how such routines can be difficult to maintain in the context of unpredictable workloads and differences between cases, for example with the speed of birthing in an birthing unit. These routines are justified as ones which are based on a rational management of risk, but this tends to overlook the various ways in which they may become warped manifestations of professional and organizational power.

Patients and professionals thus experience time in different ways. What for a professional is a routine event is for the patient a unique event that has the potential to change his or her relationship with him or herself and with time. Serious illness is associated with the loss of control over personal time and routines; and if patients are admitted to hospital, they then have to make sense of a new and alien form of time embedded in organizational routines. However, in most high-income countries, this hospital stay is usually only a short and temporary interlude before they return to everyday places and life. Yet memories of what they have been through and ongoing difficulties may leave them needing to make sense of the relationship between past, present and future either by reconnecting with past biography or, if possible, by creating a new albeit more restricted relationship between past, present and future.

## NOTE

1. In this chapter, we draw on two studies of stroke survivors undertaken by Alaszewski and his colleagues in the early 2000s. The first study was a one-off interview survey of stroke survivors (Alaszewski, Alaszewski and Potter 2006), the second was a longitudinal study post-stroke and included a series of four interviews over 18 month and diaries (Alaszewski and Wilkinson 2014). We use data from published articles and the original data set.

## REFERENCES


Alaszewski, A. (2006). Diaries as a source of suffering narratives: A critical commentary, *Health, Risk & Society*, 8: 43–58.

Alaszewski, A., Alaszewski, H. and Potter, J. (2006). Risk, uncertainty and life threatening trauma: Analysing stroke survivor's accounts of life after stroke, *Forum: Qualitative Social Research* [On-line Journal], 7(1), Art. 18. http://www.qualitative-research.net/fqs-texte/1–06/06–1–18-e.htm

Alaszewski, A. and Brown, P. (2012). *Making Health Policy: A Critical Introduction*. Cambridge: Polity.

Alaszewski, A. and Burgess, A. (2007). Risk, time and reason, *Health, Risk & Society*, 9: 349–358.

Alaszewski, A. and Wilkinson, I. (2014). The paradox of hope for working age adults recovering from stroke *Health (London)*, 19(2): 172–187.

Bröer, C. (2007). Aircraft noise and risk politics, *Health, Risk & Society*, 9(1): 37–52.

Brown, P., Heyman, B. and Alaszewski, A. (2013). Time-framing and health risks, *Health, Risk & Society*, 15: 479–488.

Brown, P. and de Graaf, S. (2013). Considering a future which may not exist: The construction of time and expectations amidst advanced-stage cancer, *Health, Risk & Society*, 15(6–7): 543–560.

Bury, M. (1982). Chronic illness as biographical disruption. *Sociology of Health and Illness*, 4: 167–182.

Charmaz, K. (1991). *Good Days, Bad Days: The Self in Chronic Illness and Time*. New Brunswick, NJ: Rutgers University Press.

Cluckie, G. (2014). *An ethnographic study of risk in thrombolysis treatment for acute stroke*, unpublished PhD, King's College, London.

Coventry, P.A., Dickens, C. and Todd, C. (2014). How does mental-physical multimorbidity express itself in lived time and space? A phenomenological analysis of encounters with depression and chronic physical illness, *Social Science & Medicine*, 118: 108–118.

Durkheim, E. (1915). *The Elementary Forms of the Religious Life*. London: George Allen and Unwin.

Ezzy, D. (2000). Illness narratives: Time, hope and HIV. *Social Science & Medicine* 50: 605–617.

Foucault, M. (1967). *Madness and Civilisation: A History of Insanity in the Age of Reason*. London: Tavistock.

Giddens, A. (1991). *Modernity and Self-Identity: Self and Society in the Late Modern Age*, Cambridge: Polity Press.

Goffman, E. (1961). *Asylums: Essays on the Social Situation of Mental Patients and Other Inmates*, republished 2007, New Brunswick, USA: Aldine Transaction.

Goffman, E. (1967). *Interaction Ritual: Essays on Face-to-Face Behaviour*. New York: Anchor Books.

Green, J. (1999). From accidents to risk: Public health and preventable injury, *Health, Risk & Society*, 1: 25–39.

Green, J., Draper, A. and Dowler, E. (2003). Short cuts to safety: Risk and 'rules of thumb' in accounts of food choice, *Health, Risk & Society*, 5: 33–52.

Harrington, R. (2003). *Trains, Technology and Time-travellers: How the Victorians Re-invented Time*. http://www.greycat.org/papers/timetrav.html, accessed 24 September 2014.

Heyman, B., Alaszewski, A. and Brown, P. (2013). Probabilistic thinking and health risks: An editorial, *Health, Risk and Society* 15:1–11.

Klingemann, H. (2000). 'To everything there is a season'—social time and clock time in addiction treatment. *Social Science and Medicine* 51: 1231–1240.

Lorber, J. (1975). Good patients and problem patients: Conformity and deviance in a general hospital, *Journal of Health and Social Behavior*, 16: 213–225.

Locke, A. and Budds, K. (2013). 'We thought if it's going to take two years then we need to start that now': Age, infertility risk and the timing of pregnancy in older first-time mothers, *Health, Risk & Society*, 15(6–7): 525–542.

Martin, B. (1984). Mother wouldn't like it: Housework as magic, *Theory Culture Society*, 2: 19–36.

Montelius, E. and Nygren, K. G. (2014). 'Doing' risk, 'doing' difference: Towards an understanding of the intersections of risk, morality and taste, *Health, Risk and Society*, 16: 431–443.

Perrow, C. (1984). *Normal Accidents: Living with High-Risk Technologies*, New York: Basic Books.

Power, M. (2004). *The Risk Management of Everything: Rethinking the Politics of Uncertainty*, London: Demos.

Rosengren, W. R. and DeVault, S. (1963). The Sociology of Time and Space in an Obstetrical Hospital. In: E. Freidson (ed.) *The Hospital in Modern Society*. New York: The Free Press of Glencoe, pp. 266–292.

Roth, J. A. (1957). Ritual and magic in the control of Contagion, *American Sociological Review*, 22: 310–314.

Scamell, M. and Alaszewski, A. (2012). Fateful moments and the categorisation of risk: Midwifery practice and the ever-narrowing window of normality during childbirth, *Health, Risk & Society*, 14: 207–222.

Scamell, M. and Stewart, M. (2014). Time, risk and midwife practice: The vaginal examination, *Health, Risk & Society*, 16: 84–100.

Sellerberg, A. M. (1991). Expressivity within a time schedule: Subordinated interaction on geriatric wards, *Sociology of Health and Illness* 13: 68–81.

Sloley, R. W. (1931). Primitive methods of measuring time: With special reference to Egypt. *The Journal of Egyptian Archaeology*, 17(3/4) (November): 166–178.

Snow, J. (1855). *On the Mode of Communication of Cholera*. London: John Churchill.

Tuke, S. (1813). *Description of the Retreat and Institution near York for Insane Persons of the Society of Friends*. York: W. Alexander.

Tulloch, J. (2008). Risk and subjectivity: Experiencing terror, *Health, Risk & Society*, 10: 451–465.

Yoels, W. C. and Clair, J. M. (1999). Never enough time: How medical residents manage a scarce resource, In: K. Charmaz and D.A. Paterniti (eds.) *Health, Illness and Healing: Society, Social Context and Self, An Anthology*, Los Angeles, California: Roxbury, pp.131–144.

Zerubavel, E. (1982). The standardization of time: A sociohistorical perspective, *American Journal of Sociology*, 88: 1–23.

# 4 Using Medicines in the Face of Uncertainty

## Developing a Habermasian Understanding of Medicines' Lifeworlds

*Patrick Brown*

## INTRODUCTION

> What are Americans afraid of? Nothing much except the food they eat, the water they drink, the air they breathe, the land they live on and the energy they consume. In the amazing short space of fifteen to twenty years, confidence about the physical world has been turned to doubt. Once the source of safety, science and technology has become the source of risk.
>
> (Douglas and Wildavsky 1983: 10)

This familiar quotation, from a classic study of the cultural functioning of risk, points towards a sea-change in Americans' interaction with technology. An earlier position of confidence and hope had seemingly been replaced by one of doubt and risk. As a central feature of the presence of science and technology within everyday life, biomedicine and medicinal products in particular might well have been added to this list of fears—'the drugs they consume'. Indeed it would be tempting to write a similar sweeping narrative describing a concurrent shift in late-modern discourses regarding growing doubt in medicine and medicines, yet this would be far too neat and schematic for a range of reasons.

First, as Douglas and Wildavsky are very well attuned to, this shift towards seeing the world as 'risky' is not as new as it might first appear (c.f. Beck 1992). Indeed we can understand much of the professionalization processes around medicine in northern Europe in the mid-nineteenth century as bound up with a politicisation of fears and concerns regarding the dangers of what came to be labelled as 'quackery' and 'quack medicines', with various power struggles and claims-makers shaping these concerns (Burney 2007).

Second, it becomes increasingly difficult to substantiate an argument for increased risk perceptions amongst late-moderns when looking at data regarding medicines usage. Angell (2005: 3) observes that the amount spent on prescription drugs in the United States during the period referred to by Douglas and Wildavsky remained stable before tripling in the two decades after 1980. If risks were perceived, then this did not appear to compel Americans to use medicines less (even when taking pricing shifts into account). It is possible, however, that patients were prescribed more medicines but did not then ingest them, but over-the-counter sales have expanded greatly.

Third, it is problematic to use 'Americans' as a proxy for all 'late-moderns'. Both of these wide categories belie highly intricate variations in medicines usage and forms of 'consumerism' across different national and local social contexts (Abraham 2010). Each context furthermore varies in terms of its cultural formations and the related 'strengths' and 'directions' of social and moral critiques (Douglas and Wildavsky 1983: 7).

Political and institutional infrastructures and practices also differ, and this in turn may shape lived experiences, cultural memory and ongoing medicines usage (van der Geest et al. 1996: 156; Abraham 2010). In 1960, the American Food and Drug Administration refused approval for the drug thalidomide, which had been successfully marketed across Germany, the United Kingdom, Canada and many other countries. In contrast to thousands of foetuses/infants which died or suffered deformities as a result of pregnant mothers being prescribed the drug for morning sickness and other symptoms elsewhere, a much smaller number of babies (impacted through trial usage of the drug) were affected in the United States.

Varying social histories and related sociocultural processes may create rather locally specific ways of *seeing* and *knowing* medicines and attributing to them particular 'cultural-symbolic logics' (van der Geest et al. 1996: 155). Yet as has already been glimpsed, these cognitive horizons—or lifeworlds—of medicines use may be importantly shaped by political institutions and interests (Britten 2008; Krumholz et al. 2007; Abraham 2010). Within such lifeworlds, risks never merely *exist* and indeed within critical social science accounts, it has become fairly standard practice to emphasise the extent to which risks are socioculturally contingent. The emergence of *risk* amidst contexts of modernity has been deemed to indicate the centrality of particular configurations of objects, knowledge and attribution—although these relationships have been considered via a highly contrasting array of analytical perspectives (Beck 1992; Douglas 1992; Luhmann 1993; Dean 1999; van Loon 2014). Such social theories of risk, however diverse (see Zinn 2008b for a useful overview), nevertheless possess various aspects of common ground, including a basic notion that 'the type of society generates the type of accountability and focuses concern on particular dangers' (Douglas and Wildavsky 1983: 7).

Implicit within this latter, ostensibly simple, quotation are at least two key social phenomena which are highly salient for analysing how and why medicines come to be deemed risky—as 'particular dangers' being focused upon—or not: a) a concern with the 'type of society' points us towards the importance of identifying the structural properties and dynamics of a society through which particular perceptions of risks are generated and structured and b) meanwhile, the 'type of accountability' implies that risk is very much political, a means of allocating blame and, in doing so, a basis of shaping how we think about (or disregard) linkages of cause and effect (Douglas 1992; Szmukler 2003).

In analysing how the structure of the social world shapes perceptions and experiences of risk and uncertainty around medicines, this chapter will follow Britten (2008) in exploring various considerations of medicine-users' (MUs) lifeworlds (Schutz 1967; Habermas 1987). As a cognitive horizon for sense-making in the present, or as a lens of possibilities for framing the future, the concept of lifeworld will be employed in considering how various features of cultural, social and identity-related processes (Habermas 1987) shape the ways in which MUs perceive and expect—either more explicitly or 'take-for-grantedly'—various properties of the medicines they are prescribed or which they otherwise come to use. In particular, different mechanisms will be considered in terms of: how cultural properties of common-lived experiences lead MUs to assume *truths*, or question uncertainties, around medicines; how MUs' particular membership and relative location within social groups and communities shape the perceived *legitimacy* of using particular medicines or, in contrast, the legitimacy of particular risks attributed to medicines; and how an individual MU's biographically acquired sense of self (identity) may become bound up with practices of medicines (non-) use in relation to experiences of *authenticity* (Habermas 1987).

These different layers of MUs' lifeworlds—culture, society, identity[1]—can be seen as shaping their *knowing* of, or uncertainty towards, medicines in respective relation to these notions of truth, legitimacy and authenticity. Wider cultural sense-making, social position and narrative identity interweave to form cognitive horizons through which the knowing of medicines functions but which may be refined or reworked through critical communication with others and related processes of reflexivity. Yet Habermas (1987) warns that the possibility for the effective ongoing refinement of norms and understandings, which structure how we construe and use medicines, are impeded by the (systemic) functioning of power and money.

From a Habermasian (1987: 118) perspective, all social contexts (macro to micro) involve structures of meaning-making and belonging (lifeworlds), as well as structures of demands and achievement (systems). Processes of meaning-making and questioning amidst lifeworlds become distorted and warped, however, by the financial and other interests of the system. So although there has been an ongoing rationalisation of medicines lifeworlds whereby, for example, medicines are less seen as 'magic bullets' and more as manufactured products which may heal or harm (Britten 2008: 46), such disenchantment and reflexivity remain incomplete and distorted due to the insidious influence of various configurations of power and money—not least that of the pharmaceutical industry. The apparent 'boomerang effects' (Beck 1992: 205) of thalidomide, tranquilisers (Gabe and Bury 1996) or

Vioxx (Krumholz et al. 2007)—whereby sophisticated technologies come to be seen as creating harm rather than treating/reducing it—have indeed led to a growing politics and reflexivity around risk (Beck 1992; Gabe and Bury 1996). Nevertheless, the influence of this politics and the development of reflexivity within the public sphere and across MUs' lifeworlds is a disjointed one.

The goal of this chapter is to develop the application of Habermasian theory in exploring how structures of societies—as lifeworlds and systemic influences upon lifeworlds—come to lead MUs to certain attributions and related concerns with, or the overlooking of, the uncertainties bound up with using or not using various medicines. This analytical framework will be developed in relation to a number of key considerations:

- First, a deeper exploration of the properties and rationalisation of the lifeworld, as proposed by Schutz (1967) and reworked and refined by Habermas (1987), will be sketched in greater detail.
- By emphasising the distinct layers/functions of the lifeworld in relation to culture, society and identity, a more nuanced awareness of how these contrasting but related functional dynamics of society shape MUs' horizons will then be facilitated.
- It is important though not to depict MUs as lacking agency by externally shaped/imposed lifeworlds, thus attention will also be given to how MUs actively construct and bracket off their lifeworlds through processes of risk, trust and hope in relation to medicines (Zinn 2008a; Brown et al. 2014a). The experience of vulnerability and the felt need to cope with this is one mechanism which drives trust and hope around medicines use, leading some to refer to 'coercive trust' (Robb and Greenhalgh 2006) and 'political-economies of hope' (Good 2001).
- This latter warping of cognitive horizons by political and economic interests will be conceptualised further in relation to the colonisation by the system of the lifeworld's potential for continued refinement and rationalisation.
- This colonisation of the lifeworld thesis will itself be held up for critical reflection in light of related theories of reflexive modernity and risk society. Here the contrasting conceptualisations of lifeworld (following either Schutz 1967 or Habermas 1987) lead us towards rather different conclusions. A more 'individualised' lifeworld (Beck 2009: 198) is a political enfeebled one, in its Habermasian (1987) sense, yet lifeworld resistance against colonisation may still be apparent—albeit in far more dispersed and less perceptible forms.

In developing this theoretical framework, I will draw on examples from my own research and that of others by way of illustration and adding empirical nuance.

## DEVELOPING A THEORY OF MEDICINES LIFEWORLD(S)—MOVING BEYOND SCHUTZ AND DOUGLAS

This chapter is by no means the first to develop a Habermasian perspective towards medicine or medicines use more particularly. Scambler's (2001) edited volume surveys an array of health-care contexts where system-lifeworld perspectives offer important analytical purchase and Britten's (2008) excellent text on *Medicines in Society* is very effectively grounded in a system-lifeworld framework. This latter study does touch at various points upon risk and uncertainty—both theoretically (pp.16–18) and more empirically (e.g. pp.160–162)—however, while lifeworld and system are very clearly explicated early on, the empirical emphasis within the book directs the analysis towards using these concepts to draw threads together rather than interrogating these concepts in more detail. In contrast, this chapter will not be able to offer anywhere close to the breadth and depth of Britten's empirical illumination but instead aims to build upon her system-lifeworld perspective on medicines use towards a more detailed understanding of lifeworld processes regarding uncertainty and risk.

In order to develop a more thorough understanding of Habermas's conceptualisation of lifeworld, it is first useful to trace the concept from its more phenomenological roots. For Schutz (1967), the lifeworld[2] is the basic sense-making tool upon which our being in the world and our interactions with others depends. As a 'reality which seems self-evident to men remaining within the natural attitude' of taken-for-granted interactions in everyday life (Schutz and Luckmann 1973:3), Schutz's lifeworld can be considered as a 'horizon of possibilities' or lens through which the meaning of the social world becomes intelligible. It is thus through the structures of this lifeworld that a particular social setting 'appears to me in coherent arrangements of well-circumscribed Objects [such as medicines] having determinate properties' (Schutz and Luckmann 1973: 4). While there was some ambivalence across Schutz's work on whether lifeworlds were person-specific or shared, his later work and the refinement of his ideas, as completed (after Schutz's death) by Luckmann (Schutz and Luckmann 1973), suggest a shared lifeworld which is rooted in common understandings as accumulated over the life course (stocks-of-knowledge). The lifeworld thus has a sense-making function within which the meanings of other actors (such as prescribing professionals) or objects (such as medicines) are imbued but also functions on the basis of common socialisation experiences 'which are presupposed, so to speak, and provide the basis for intersubjective understanding' (Schutz and Luckmann 1973: 261).

Although grounded somewhat differently—within Mead, Durkheim and Weber, in contrast to Schutz's reworking of Weber via Husserl and Bergson—Habermas's concept of lifeworld shares this primary sense-making function. However, whereas Schutz's shared lifeworlds require common socialisation as having occurred already, Habermas's much broader conceptualisation (via Mead and Durkheim) incorporates socialisation and integration as part of the lifeworld mechanism (Habermas 1987: 109; Outhwaite 2009: 83). Habermas's lifeworld does not, therefore, merely facilitate interaction and understanding within the social world but achieves a binding cohesion which is seen by Mead as becoming more encompassing as societies develop (Habermas 1987: 110). Developing this consideration of societal evolution further by rehearsing Durkheim's interactions with Spencer, Habermas (1987: 115) proceeds to explore how the communicative aspects of the lifeworld, in terms of mutual understanding and questioning, can also achieve and maintain consensus. To this end, Spencer is quoted in considering how 'social life, just as all life in general, can naturally organise itself only by an unconscious, spontaneous adaption under the immediate pressure of needs' (Habermas 1987: 115).

At this point in the analysis, our formulation of lifeworld comes to resonate strongly with Douglas's conceptualisation of risk cultures—where both involve a means of making sense of the world through implicit categorisations and as a functionalist tool in binding groups and maintaining social structures (Douglas and Wildavsky 1983; Douglas 1992). For Douglas, how the world is perceived in relation to risk is significantly shaped by an individual's or group's position within broader social formations, as well as the social structure of these formations. Being positioned either more centrally or on the edge of a community, as well as how 'tight' this community is, will shape an individual's attentiveness to risk as well as which risks a person is concerned with:

> In a tight community a man has his work cut out to meet his neighbor's standards. This is where he gets the health information which he cannot ignore. When the community bond is weaker, he can relax . . . but unless he is totally isolated, his acquaintances to whom he goes for solace are his sources of risk warning.
>
> (Douglas and Wildavsky 1983: 85)

It is in this sense that a broader cultural basis of sense-making is shaped more specifically by group dynamics and position, whereby the truth or validity of particular knowledge about medicines or risks of medicines becomes interwoven with the possibility and legitimacy of heeding and acting upon such sources (Desmond 2009). This starts to take us beyond the 'culturalistic concept of lifeworld' of Schutz as a sense-making tool (Habermas 1987: 134), towards a more action-oriented formulation of lifeworld—one which is geared towards analysing action itself, rather than analysing how social beings make sense of action (ibid.).

As apparent in the earlier quotation, Douglas and Wildavsky's framework (elaborated more systematically as a 'grid-group' approach—see Douglas 2006) would seem attuned to this combination of cultural and social structural shaping of risk perceptions *and* actions. It is in this sense that Habermas's lifeworld may be deemed more analytically powerful than Schutz's, as a means of analysing not just how MUs perceive or make sense of medicines but moreover how they act and (mis)use medicines or not. Seeing the lifeworld as a socialising force which (de)legitimates action is therefore vital.

The socialising force of the lifeworld which imposes neighbours' standards on individuals is also bound up with the second main analytical feature which Habermas's lifeworld analyses share with Douglas's cultural theory of risk—that of integration. Durkheim's common influence across both frameworks helps explain how communicative action within the lifeworld or risk attributions within Douglas's cultural settings both act to regulate interpersonal relations and bind communities (Habermas 1987: 120, 139; Douglas 2006:1–2). Habermas (1987: 140) is keen to avoid the interpretations of Durkheim by some functionalists, by which analyses of culture and identity are reduced to their integrating functions. Douglas (2006) seems similarly sensitive to the importance of avoiding functionalist reductionism. Therefore although she affirms her 'Durkheimian thesis' whereby 'classification underwrites all attempts to co-ordinate activities, any thing that challenges the habitual classifications is rejected' (Douglas 2006: 2), so much of her work pursues processes of classification and risk as of interest in their own right and which are seldom reduced to their functionalist roles.

Where Habermas departs from Douglas however is by way of his concern to describe and explain late-modern processes as distinctive, in contrast to Douglas who through her more historical and anthropological framing tends more towards emphasising recurring themes (Wilkinson 2010). Habermas (1987:169) argues that in more traditional societies, the reproduction of the political and that of the social were fully interwoven, with the dominion of royal courts, the influence of religious 'ideologies' (more than mere theologies) and the generation of cultural tendencies upholding one another amidst their relation to various economic underpinnings. Similarly in various traditional societies it has been seen that the economic 'exchange of women in marriage is both social and system integration' (Outhwaite 2009: 87). By contrast, modernity witnesses the increasing disaggregation of power from theology and later on 'the economic system does tend to operate according to its own principles, and administrative systems too, tend to be differentiated, and relatively independent of direct state control' (Outhwaite 2009: 87).

It is this uncoupling of the sociocultural lifeworld from the political-economic system which, for Habermas, renders more functionalist analyses of unitary social systems decreasingly satisfactory. For as modernity progresses, it becomes increasingly apparent that 'social consensus (via social integration) and political consensus (regarding the orientation of economy and administration)—are no longer two sides of the same coin but each come to develop increasingly independently of one another' (Brown 2014: 398). It is at this stage that the value of a Habermasian lifeworld analysis of medicines use amidst uncertainty becomes clearer, in that Douglas's approach has less purchase on this unmooring of the political-economic and its consequences for cultural processes through which uncertainty and risk are experienced. This section has already noted the limitations of a Schutzian lifeworld in analysing *action* beyond cultural understandings of action.

## THE DEVELOPMENT OF MULTIDIMENSIONAL MEDICINES LIFEWORLDS

Habermas sees the lifeworld as reproduced through communicative action, between individuals and across a broader public sphere, as constituted by three layers or dimensions—culture, society and identity. In this three dimensional conceptualisation, communicative action refers to or implies: interpretations of an objective world, which can be considered true or not (in relation to a common cultural stock of knowledge); the ordering of a social world, which can be deemed legitimate or not (in relation to a membership of a particular community); and the expression of experiences of a subjective world, which can be deemed authentic or not (in relation to a particular narrative identity) (Habermas, 1987: 120, 138, 139). The salience of all three lifeworld components was considered in the preceding section, thus rendering communicative action as involving 'not only processes of cultural interpretation in which "cultural knowledge" is tested against the world; they are at the same time processes of integration and socialisation' (Habermas 1987: 139).

### Cultural Rationalisation in Relation to Truth

In the reproducing of the lifeworld, effectively functioning communicative action moreover comes to refine these three components in terms of a rationalisation of knowledge, a maintaining or enhancing of solidarity of citizens and a commitment of identity (Habermas 1987: 141). The rationalisation of cultural meanings around medicines is thus one such product of lifeworld refinement. A critical public sphere, within a broader social context of modernity, has led to a greater questioning of medicines, their properties and the validity of various truth claims made about medicines' effectiveness and safety. The more magical properties attributed to medicines have increasingly been questioned within a form of Weberian disenchantment. This reduced valuing of the mystical aspects of medicines can be seen as resulting from, while simultaneously contributing to, the proliferation of medical knowledge which has come to form a discursive basis upon which the relative effectiveness and risks of medicine use can be considered.

As Britten (2008) acknowledges, the lifeworld consideration of truth claims regarding efficacy may partly take place within the public sphere, as well as within smaller group and more micro-interactional contexts, and furthermore in light of personal experiences with medicines. Rather than seeing all social contexts as 'simultaneously' systems and lifeworlds (Habermas 1987:118) however, Britten's (2008: 43, 85,171) analysis tends to posit 'lay' experiences, non-biomedical activities and associations as 'part of the lifeworld' in contrast to the realms of professionals, pharmaceutical manufacturing and regulation which form the 'system'. This leads to an underplaying of the extent to which regulatory decision making, for example, may offer possibilities for communicative action. Conceptualising such contexts as both systems *and* lifeworlds in turn enables more nuanced analyses of how rationalisations of understanding within institutional contexts create manifold possibilities for more 'strategic' (system-based) action to parasitically excerpt influence and distort (Outhwaite 2009:44).

In seeking to develop effective criteria for considering truth claims over the effectiveness of medicines, the National Institute for Health and Care Excellence (NICE) in England can be seen as one basis through which communicative action exposes various claims about effective health care (within development of NICE guidelines), alongside manufacturers' claims about medicines' effectiveness (within NICE technological appraisals), to discursive scrutiny as a means of testing the validity of these truth claims. Various ways in which system-influences impede communicative action in these context will be returned to (see later section), but these processes of guideline formulation and technological appraisals are very much oriented towards testing and challenging interpretations of an objective world, which can be considered true or not, in relation to a common cultural stock of knowledge. Although it is very much biomedical knowledge which is privileged (Milewa and Barry 2005; Britten 2008), the gradual adjustment of NICE processes has in various ways sought to include a broader range of voices and experiences and to take these into account (Moreira 2011).

Alongside more official regulatory organisations, the broader public sphere can be seen as facilitating reflexive considerations of interpretations of an objective world. Habermas (1991) bemoans the loss of a bygone (eighteenth century) print media and coffee house culture which facilitated relatively free and undistorted communication within a rather select public. Nevertheless, the mainstream mass media and a whole host of Internet-based critical journalism and pressure group publications and sites can be seen as modestly successful in a) holding pharmaceutical manufacturers more accountable for the processes of drug development and b) enabling the growth of public discussions and movements which critically evaluate the effectiveness and side-effects of medicines, at least in some cases.

Gardner and Dew (2011), adopting an actor-network-theory approach, explore how radio, newspaper and parliamentary discussion, amongst other platforms, facilitated a discussion and greater awareness of the potentially damaging effects to changes in the manufacturing of Eltroxin, used to treat hypothyroidism. Local radio in particular was seen to be a basis of critical reflection on medicine effectiveness and side effects but also enabled the forming of public associations (cohesion and collective consciousness) and the reworking of identities. As with the eighteenth century public sphere, Internet usage in relation to medicines knowledge is limited to certain groups within society (Seale 2005) but may furthermore offer 'new spaces or forums for challenging or reworking prevailing understandings and practices' of medicines use (Williams et al. 2011: 716).

## Legitimacy of Medicines and Group Membership

The differential access to and participation within certain media, and the public sphere in general, makes evident the limitations of lifeworld reduced to culture, as already noted. In an earlier section we quoted Douglas and Wildavsky (1983: 85) in noting how different social networks and 'neighbours' played important roles in exposing actors to varying types of knowledge, risk awareness and concerns. Moreover, membership of social groups and communities leads to social actors being held accountable for their presentation-of-self, with this rendering certain beliefs and actions as legitimate and others illegitimate or even unimaginable. These insights enable a 'thicker' grasp of social action around medicines and risks in that, far from a mere intellectual exercise of reflexivity towards knowledge and various truth claims therein, this action is profoundly structured by location within particular social spaces, within particular communities.

This perspective points towards the need, for example, for an intersectional consideration of how accomplishing gender, class and ethnicity within specific communities places demands and facilitates certain practices towards medicines while precluding others. Montelius and Giritli-Nygren (2014) have explored how consuming healthy food is complexly interwoven with implicit demands of class, gender and a performing of taste; a similar interrogation of medicines usage would be very illuminating. Norms of *healthy* consumption could accordingly demand certain types of legitimate use of medicines from some actors more than others, with relative status within a social context and community being affected as a result. Broader demands to combine intensive study with a busy student lifestyle were thus relevant in understanding the prescription and non-prescription use of Ritalin amongst university students in Amsterdam (Hupli 2013).

Membership and relative position within social contexts generate specific demands, for example, for concentrated academic-study or performing 'health', but these social locations also breed sensibilities towards uncertainty and risk. Guillaume's (2014) study in southern France of young women's practices involving 'fourth generation' contraceptive pills found these to be shaped by discussions and problematization of this type of pill within the broader French media but also within small networks of female friends. This new questioning of the interpretation of an objective world, in relation to truth claims about the relative efficacy and safety of the pill, in turn uncovered a whole array of assumptions about the 'naturalness' of taking the pill when one reached the 'appropriate' age, as normalised within peer groups and education-system settings. Broader media debates, alongside the personal-embodied experiences with the pill amongst acquaintances, therefore shaped the legitimacy of questioning these taken-for-granted assumptions about the appropriateness of the pill. Whereas before a more legitimate risk concern was about getting pregnant, concerns with pill safety and hormone-associated risk to one's body became increasingly legitimised (Guillaume 2014).

### Authenticity of Medicines Usage and Risks in Relation to Identity

A new questioning of the values and legitimacy of medicines use, as seen in Guillaume's study, makes evident the mechanisms of 'switching stations' where processes *within* either culture, society or identity come to impact on each other (Habermas 1987: 216–217). In this case study, a rationalising questioning of various interpretations of evidence around the pill led to it becoming demystified—shifting from a relatively unproblematic cultural trope ('the pill') of women's empowerment towards a hormone-shifting medicine of a particular 'generation' which impacts significantly, and sometimes problematically, on the 'normal' functioning of women's bodies (Guillaume 2014: 45). This renewed questioning of normality within the cultural dimension comes to impact the legitimacy of various demands and ordering within the social sphere, with Guillaume's young French women's position and membership of various friendship circles reworked in the process.

Further switching stations are, in turn, observable where the 'doing' of health and risk (Montelius and Giritli-Nygren 2014) bear upon and must be compatible with identity in order for actions to feel authentic. Use and non-use of particular technologies, in relation to cultural perceptions and membership or exclusion of groups, can come to bear importantly on experiences of selfhood (Guillaume 2014: 38). The ordering and framing of actions as 'everyday', or as unusual and risky, drawing upon narratives within broader culture, either legitimated or undermined particular actions and frames within social circles and communities, bearing significantly upon narrative identity (Ezzy 1998; Guillaume 2014). Habermas's stress upon the socialisation of identity suggests the imposing of selves upon subjects so as to be 'in harmony with collective forms of life' (Habermas 1987: 141). This Mead-oriented understanding limits agency for self-narration of identity (see Ezzy 1998). Yet, as will be examined in the next section, lifeworlds do not just impose lived experiences but are also able to be actively reworked by MUs.

## EMPHASISING AGENCY: REWORKING LIFEWORLDS THROUGH BRACKETING UNCERTAINTY AND COLLAGING RISK, HOPE AND TRUST

For Habermas, the lifeworld is an encompassing totality which cannot be stepped outside of. In a similar manner by which we cannot think outside of language: 'In a situation of action, the lifeworld forms a horizon behind which we cannot go' (Habermas 1987: 149). So whereas agency and critical reflection may function within the lifeworld, which can lead to a gradual refining of a shared lifeworld, individual actors' experiences of this lifeworld itself are not amenable to reworking. This argument can be seen as similar to that of Schutz and Luckmann (1973) who posit that the structures of the lifeworld are open to examination through social scientific investigation but not within the 'natural attitude' of everyday, taken-for-granted existence.

This section will progress to re-examine these understandings of the lifeworld in the light of various recent research into how actors consider medicines (and drugs), including our own recent work into cancer patients' use of trial medicines (Brown et al. 2014a, 2014b). In particular, we will proceed to conceptualise various processes through which uncertainty regarding the future is framed in a particular way or 'looked past', focused upon or bracketed off (Kierkegaard 1957). While these processes do not give MUs full insight into or complete control over their lifeworlds, they do enable a reworking of their cognitive horizons, which grants agency over what aspects of their illness experience and medicines use are confronted. This reconfiguring of lifeworlds will be explored under two main processes: the re-categorising of risk and the bracketing off and reworking of uncertainty through processes of risk, trust and hope.

## Re-categorising Risk

As has already been stressed, risks never simply exist and come to be perceived through social processes of attribution and framing (Douglas and Wildavsky 1983: 7). Heyman and colleagues (2013) suggest that implicit within any reference to risk are notions of valuing (regarding what might be lost), categorisation (by which inferences regarding the probability of 'an event' assume a homogeneity across observations of occurrences of this 'type' of event in the past), as well as particular modes of construing probability and framing time. In particular, processes of categorising the 'type of event' which is more or less likely to occur have been stressed as defining the social construction of risk (Douglas and Wildavsky 1983), for example, whereby objects or events considered as abnormal or which defy neat categories are more likely to be deemed as 'other' and thus risky.

The cultural categorising of 'medicines' used within the domain of 'health care' as 'normal' and regulated by various trusted networks of actors (Brown and Calnan 2012), in contrast to 'illicit drugs' associated with 'deviant' networks of actors, can be considered one basic example of such a process. Ongoing use of the former accordingly tends to be assumed to be far less risky than that of the latter, although these neatly categorised interpretations of an objective world have recently been subjected to modest contestation within the UK public sphere (Collins 2011). Evidence of individual propensities to challenge and subvert these cultural categories is apparent within Caita-Zufferey's (2012) research with Swiss men who combined working lifestyles with recreational use of heroin and/or cocaine. These men categorised their use of these products as normal, drawing upon comparisons with more socially legitimate practices. They 'erased any distinction between substances (cognac, heroin), activities (drinking a cognac, having a cup of tea, taking a bath, smoking heroin) and experiences (celebrating the pleasure of living, experiencing a good moment, using drugs)' (Caita-Zufferey 2012: 436).

Mainstream cultural interpretations of the objective world in terms of risk are thus open to critical reflection, partly facilitated through Swiss drug laws, the way truth claims about the effects of 'illicit drugs' are challenged by some scientists and other voices in the public sphere (Caita-Zufferey 2012). Moreover, because the development of knowledge about probabilistic relationships between behaviours and outcomes for groups has little predictive value for any one individual (Heyman et al. 2011), the meaning of probabilities is readily open to reinterpretation by individual MUs in line with their identity and status (Montelius and Giritli-Nygren 2014).

Yet as pliable as these cognitive lenses for considering risk may appear, the three-dimensionality of Habermas's lifeworld nevertheless points towards certain limitations for this 'freedom' to categorise drug use and riskiness. By drawing on other accessible (albeit marginalised) cultural scripts, Caita-Zufferey's participants could subvert mainstream understandings in ways which created new truths about heroin and cocaine use, which in turn facilitated a more authentic and responsible identity, yet these views and related actions were not necessarily legitimated within their wider communities and social networks. This undermining of the integration within actors' lifeworlds may lead to experiences of alienation for such individuals (Habermas 1987: 143). Hence prevailing lifeworld interpretations, norms and beliefs around medicines can be challenged via risk categorisations but at a cost. In Gardner and Dew's (2011) study, initial challenges to positive cultural interpretations of Eltroxin's safety by individual hypothyroid patients based on personal experiences were not legitimated. However, as time passed, communicative action through radio and other media enabled a reinterpretation of understandings of these patients' medicines which was legitimated through membership of a collective and which, in turn, enabled the authenticating of personal negative lived experiences involving these medicines.

## Trust and Hope as a Means of Attempting to Bracket Off Uncertainty

Risk is one way of illuminating uncertainty as a means of coping with vulnerability in social contexts (Zinn 2008a). However, as noted in the preceding subsection, risk information may be of limited utility for individual actors—due to the difficulty in interpreting probabilistic information in a manner which resolves problems of uncertain futures. For example, the advanced-cancer patients in our study were often given probabilistic prognoses of their likelihood of surviving one year or of being eligible for an operation to remove a tumour, but being told they had a 10 per cent chance of an outcome happening nevertheless left them unsure as to whether they were one of the lucky 10 or less fortunate 90. Risk therefore illuminates objects (medicines) and potential futures (outcomes from medicines) in a particular light, but it does overcome the lingering problem of induction by which the future is never knowable (Möllering 2001; Heyman et al. 2011).

Zinn (2008a) and others (e.g. Möllering 2001) therefore suggest that, for individuals seeking to cope with vulnerability amidst uncertainty, other tools for working with uncertainty are drawn upon. One such approach already briefly referred to is trust. The greater safety attributed to medicines used within health-care contexts (in contrast to heroine bought through a drug dealer) is importantly understood through the network of trust relations involved (Brown and Calnan 2012). The esteem of the expertise and motivations of the prescribing doctor or recommending pharmacist are important here, but broader systems-related assumptions about the training and professional commitments of the doctor, alongside systems of medicines regulation, may also exist as taken-for-granted assumptions which further undergird such trust (Möllering 2005).

Möllering (2001) describes trust as involving a 'leap of faith' in overcoming the unknowable to reach positive expectations about the future. Uncertainty continues to linger, therefore, but is looked past—enabling individuals to act 'as if' (Lewis and Weigert 1985) the future was known. Thus lifeworlds characterised by trust may well contain uncertainty but trust enables this uncertainty to be 'bracketed off' (Möllering 2001). Brown (2009) emphasises that this bracketing or leaping is, as these terms suggest, active: 'Trust in this phenomenological sense results from actively "putting the world in brackets" (Sartre 1962: 25) rather than from a passive consequence of external attributes' (Brown 2009:402) of the context or trustee.

In contrast to managing uncertainty in terms of probability (risk), or bracketing off uncertainty (trust), hope represents one further example of coping amidst vulnerability where uncertainty remains more palpable. This was certainly the case for the advanced-cancer patients involved in our study who hoped for, and sometimes focused upon, brighter futures (at least in the shorter term). Yet as one participant explained, 'at the back of my mind . . . I have an illness which can't be cured' (Brown and de Graaf 2013: 555). Hope in medicines could enable a more positive horizon of possibilities, yet 'darker' futures nevertheless lingered on that same horizon—sometimes towards the margins but in a number of cases looming more explicitly.

Hope and trust—as with risk—therefore enable the reworking of experiences and perceptions within the cognitive horizons of lifeworlds—albeit in different ways and with different costs. Trusting incorporates actors looking past uncertainty but in trusting they also create new possibilities for being let down by trustees (Barbalet 2009). Hoping meanwhile involves focusing on positive possibilities *alongside* an awareness of more negative futures, with the tensions that exist between these different futures coming to characterise the difficulties of hoping (Brown et al. 2014b).

A pertinent analytical avenue emerging from Zinn's (2008a) framework relates to the combining of risk, trust, hope and other means of managing vulnerability amidst uncertainty—and thus of reworking lifeworlds. Trust may be combined with risk in various ways as a basis of dealing with uncertainty—for example, the cancer patients in our study trusted professionals to interpret probabilistic information for them, heeding their recommendations in light of this (Brown et al. 2014b). Although their trust in these doctors led the patients to take these numbers seriously, these probabilities still required interpretation. Hope could become relevant here, for example, where patients focused upon rather small probabilities as possibilities nonetheless (Brown et al. 2014b). The advanced-cancer patients taking part in our study were (or had recently been) involved in medicines trials. Smaller possibilities of surviving longer with the existing treatment were sometimes then attached to hope in further possibilities, such as new medicines becoming accessible via future trials. These different hopes, partly facilitated by trust in doctors, could lead to the reworking of low survival probabilities and the extension of possible futures—thus rendering future horizons far more malleable for these patients (Brown et al. 2014b).

## SYSTEM COLONISATIONS OF MEDICINES LIFEWORLDS

The processes of reworking the presence and recognition of uncertainty around medicines, as experienced by individuals within particular lifeworlds, was explored in the preceding section where an emphasis was placed upon the agency of MUs within their lifeworld. This analysis, involving the active recasting of uncertain futures through processes of risk, trust and hope, owes much to phenomenology (Brown 2009) and, accordingly, to analyses of the lifeworld which begin with the individual. In working with Schutz and Mead, Habermas (1987) is aware of this person-centred analytical basis—which can then be expanded out into broader processes of shared meaning-making (culture). Yet he also emphasises the need for analyses which are more rooted in societal level phenomena, such as collective consciousness and solidarity—following Durkheim and, as we have noted, echoing Douglas. The Habermasian conceptualisation of lifeworld thus tries to bridge this dualism between individual and societal analytical orientations. However, this working between the individual and the collective is not straightforward.

### Colonisation of Culture: Hope Which Limits a Questioning Truth and Uncertainty

In stressing the agency of MUs within lifeworlds, the previous section could be critiqued for a relative blindness to deeper layers of collective consciousness.

Hence, for example, hope was considered as a process through which MUs *actively* reworked their lifeworld horizons of possibilities, yet patients' narratives of hope and of being hopeful need to be considered as expressions of cultural 'vocabularies' (Mills 1940) available to individuals when coping. In turn, these cultural vocabularies are underpinned by yet deeper assumptions regarding the need to cope. As we reflected upon within our own data analysis of cancer patients' accounts of trust and hope amidst conditions of uncertainty, 'narratives of hope, for example, should be read in light of broader cultures (Good et al. 1990) or 'regimes' of hope (Brown 2005) rather than simply 'reified and imputed to human nature as underlying principles of . . . action' (Mills 1940: 913) (Brown et al. 2014b). In continuing to explore the lifeworld in greater detail, therefore, we come across more and more layers (Schutz 1967: 7) or 'depths' of assumptions which can be seen as bearing upon how medicines are perceived and thus used (Brown et al. 2014b). In doing this we also uncover more and more processes by which communicative action—which would lead to the reproduction and rationalisation of the lifeworld—is impeded by systemic tendencies relating to power. Habermas (1987) refers to this as the colonisation of the lifeworld by the system.

There are manifold ways in which communicative action around medicines use is impeded by system processes, a number of which are reflected in Britten's (2008) analysis albeit less explicitly in relation to each of the three dimensions of the lifeworld. For the purposes of this chapter, the analysis will be restricted to a small number of colonisation tendencies, emphasising those which involve the disregarding of uncertainty. Deeper assumptions limit what is thinkable and therefore questionable as uncertain, especially where system-related tendencies of demands and achievement (instrumentality) come to perpetuate these assumptions.

One example of such instrumentality, in the sphere of medicines, is what has been referred to as a 'culture of hope' or 'political economy of hope' (Good et al. 1990; Good 2001). Hope can be seen as profoundly 'communicative', in encouraging the questioning of the *status quo*, binding solidarity amongst those sharing a common hope and affirming committed identities (Brown et al. 2014b). Yet Good (2001) and colleagues (1990) describe various ways in which hope can also develop potent instrumental properties. The interests of biomedical science, pharmaceutical manufacturers, health-care professionals and individual patients can all be seen as being furthered by cultures of hope (Good 2001): promoting hopes of new breakthroughs in what science could achieve leads to the elevated status of science and greater income and investment in order to 'bring technology into being' (Hedgecoe 2004: 16); by emphasising hopes, pharmaceutical manufacturers similarly attract investment, foster a demand for their products and challenge regulators who could be construed as threatening patients' hopes (Brown 2011); in our study some of the advanced-cancer patients referred to being less likely to raise concerns with their doctors due to the position of these medical professionals as gatekeepers of hope, with patients' fearful of jeopardising access to hope-giving medicines (Brown et al. 2014b); outside of trial contexts, van Dantzig and de Swaan (1978) furthermore describe a 'system of hope' within a cancer hospital by which positive aspirations are falsely maintained in order to limit the difficult emotional labour of dealing with death; this system delegated the tasks of dealing with bad news and despair to less senior professionals, while patients were also complicit in this system due to their need to hope.

Through such system-related properties, everyone has something to gain from maintaining hope and hence it can be seen to develop a function which shuts down communication action while also reproducing power relations (van Dantzig and de Swaan 1978). Good (2001) shows how the cultural, in terms of imagination around novel technologies; the social, in terms of relational commitments and obligations; and identity-related aspects of patients' individual 'clinical narratives' help sustain one another, whereby 'affective and imaginative dimensions of biotechnology envelope patients within a 'biotechnical embrace' (Brown et al. 2014b: 2).

Through Good's (2001) analysis, the instrumentality of hope can be seen to impact upon all three dimensions of the lifeworld, whereby affective aspects of hope—those relating to desire (Simpson 2004)—shape cultural, social and personal sensibilities which stifle questions regarding the uncertainty around the development, trialling, prescribing and use of medicines. Focusing upon the cultural dimension, a questioning of interpretations of an objective world in relation to truth (Habermas 1987:120) becomes severely inhibited by the increasing intertwining of 'regimes of truth' with 'regimes of hope' (Brown 2005: 333). Correspondingly, effects of hope render the confronting of present uncertainties increasingly difficult and unlikely:

> This [merging of facts and values] is also parasitical in that the uncertainties of present doubt and the potential for future certainty or truths are in dynamic relationship with one another; that is, the present absence of certainty is itself constitutive of the hope for, and drive toward, future truths.
>
> (Brown 2005: 333)

Hope has been the focus of this subsection, although in considering how system demands involving power and money limit the challenging of truth, it would have been equally pertinent to consider the negative effects of blind trust placed in systems of medical knowledge (Calnan and Rowe 2008). Moreover, dominant understandings of the risk presented by medicines, as publicised within the scientific and mass media or as shaped by medicines regulators, can also be seen as being warped by regimes of truth driven by the financial and political might of large pharmaceutical manufacturers and their ability to distort the publication of findings (Smith 2005) and to 'capture' regulatory organisations (Abraham 1995).

## Colonisation of 'Society': Trust and Its Impact on Legitimacy of Medicines Use

Communicative action and a related successful reproduction of the lifeworld within the societal dimension involves integration and, in particular, the 'coordination of actions via intersubjectively recognised validity claims' (Habermas 1987: 144). Trust can be seen as an important component within this dimension in enabling the reproduction of social commitments, as well as facilitating the kind of communication which enables the development of a mutually beneficial (rather than obliged) consensus (Brown 2009). Where medicines decisions are discussed within doctor-patient encounters, the potential exists for various forms of instrumentality to emerge whereby both patient and professional pursue strategic action to attain something, thus inhibiting effective mutual understanding and recognition (Greenhalgh et al. 2006; Britten 2008). Moreover, the biomedical context of this interaction also has the potential to undermine real consensus building:

> When a doctor, wittingly or otherwise, dominates or controls an encounter with a patient this typically has the effect of absorbing and dissolving the patients' self-understanding into . . . the framework of technical biomedicine.
>
> (Scambler and Britten 2001: 55)

As with hope, trust has the potential to be vitally communicative or, when warped by power, to become strategic (Greenhalgh et al. 2006). Blind trust on the part of the patient, rooted in asymmetric knowledge, may facilitate more superficial and unequal clinical interactions. Alternatively, where patients feel they have little option but to trust, then a 'coercive trust' (Robb and Greenhalgh 2006) may lead to interactions where concerns and worries, information about patients' (non)cooperation with medicines emerges and/or other aspects of uncertainty are unable to be openly discussed. In stark contrast to more communicative and critical trust whereby uncertainties can be openly expressed and addressed in reaching consensus on medicines use (Calnan and Rowe 2008), these instrumentalised forms of trust may result in unreported non-cooperation with medication plans, continued use of medicines amidst anxiety or various forms of ineffective treatment plans due to a lack of information exchange. In short, consensus is unable to be generated or maintained.

## Colonisation of Identity: Authentic Medicines Use Inhibited by Risks

In contexts where consensus is unable to be achieved due to a dearth of communicative trust, the legitimacy of medicines use is thus unable to be generated in that 'newly arising situations' are not being 'connected up with existing conditions . . . in the dimension of social space' (Habermas 1987: 140). These limitations within the social dimension have knock-on ('switching point') implications for the identity dimension of the lifeworld, were MUs' use or non-use of medicines remain unchallenged and where individual MUs are not put 'in a position to take part in processes of reaching understanding and thereby to assert [their] own identity' (Habermas 1987: 138).

By its stimulating of reflexivity or 'self-confrontation' (Elliott 2002), risk can be seen as a potential enabler of communicative action in the lifeworld dimension of identity. However, related analyses also emphasise how risk processes also foster an individualisation, which could be seen as antithetical to the lifeworld (as will be returned to in the conclusion). Hence risk, as a way of illuminating the world and various uncertainties therein can—once more—be seen as possessing both communicative and more instrumental tendencies. That risk appears to be a neutral mode of considering probable outcomes, thus belying an inherently and staunchly political character (Douglas 1992) suggests the potential for significant strategic influence to function parasitically within ostensibly communicative action (Habermas 1987).

One further setting where such colonisation of the lifeworld may take place around medicines use is within regulatory decision making. While it may be neater to consider regulation solely as a 'system' function (Britten 2008), significant communicative action regarding truth testing, membership of 'working groups' and the identity of individual decision makers are vital to considering how regulatory committees make decisions on new medicines. Here I refer to our recent research into cost-effectiveness appraisals of expensive new medicines as carried out by the NICE.[3] These decisions, which regulate which expensive new medicines are to be made available in the English National Health Service, bear importantly upon medicines use and can be seen as being shaped by various ways the members of the decision-making committee deal with risk and uncertainty.

Within the Single Technological Appraisals we researched, the considering of hypothetical patient outcomes, based on evidence from the past as expressed through probabilistic inference and confidence intervals regarding uncertainty, can be understood through a lens of 'risk'. Different decision makers on the committee dealt with and interpreted this probabilistic modelling in different ways, in consonance with their background—as an expert clinician, as a lay member or as a researcher working for a pharmaceutical manufacturer. Identity was implicitly very influential over how models (developed by the medicine manufacturer) were scrutinised and accepted (or not), which forms of uncertainty were queried and which were overlooked and how manifold complexity was overcome: through focusing on those aspects with which the decision makers were familiar, by trusting particular colleagues and some expert outsiders and mistrusting other outsiders and in deferring to colleagues within the decision-making process. This structuring of what was questioned inevitably led to some uncertainties being taken-for-granted or dismissed and not subject to examination.

## CONCLUSION: THE INCOMPLETE AND DISJOINTED RATIONALISATION OF MEDICINES LIFEWORLDS

Late-modern discourses around medicines use are nothing if not convoluted. On the one hand, narratives regarding the damaging effects of medicines and self-interested profiteering of pharmaceutical manufacturers would seem more visible in the public sphere than in some earlier phases of modernity (Brown and Calnan 2012). Such discourses are seemingly part of a broader sensitivity towards risks attributed to science and technology (Douglas and Wildavsky 1983), one where medicines lifeworlds are more reflexive and critical. On the other hand, many academic accounts describe tendencies towards a pharmaceuticalisation of society whereby heightened experiences of vulnerabilities within a medicalized late-modernity extend the scope of medicines-based solutions (Williams et al. 2011) and the hopes invested in these (Brown 2005).

The cultural dimension of medicines lifeworlds can be said to be becoming more rationalised in some senses via a disenchantment with the magic of medicines and a growing public awareness of uncertainty of medicines use and the fallibility of manufacturers and prescribers. However, this shift away from a more mystical meaning attached to medicines use is far from complete, and the hopes invested in chemotherapy drugs, for example, can be seen as partial re-enchantments which encourage individual MUs to look past uncertainty within their illness-shaped lifeworlds. Political-economies of hope (Good 2001), as well as warped understandings of risk and ongoing systems-trust in biomedicine, therefore stifle the questioning of powerful truth regimes which assert or imply the effectiveness and relative safety of medicines (Habermas 1987; Brown 2005).

The societal dimensions of medicines lifeworlds need to be understood within a public sphere which is increasingly heterogeneous and individualised (Beck 2009:198). This means that even where truth regimes involving medicines may be questioned within the public sphere, reflexivity typically remains more individual rather than coordinated, rendering a broader reshaping of collective consciousness around medicines less likely. More particularly, the bracketing of uncertainty through personal strategies of risk, trust and hope means that concerns and misgivings regarding medicines' efficacy and safety are less likely to be collectively recognised, politicised and legitimated—especially when media accounts of uncertainty are warped within narratives of risk, hope and trust which serve biomedical and pharmaceutical interests.

The legitimation and commonality of particular patterns of medicines use, alongside the relative lack of legitimacy of alternative accounts, within public contexts render individual narratives of reflexivity and questioning more precarious. Medicines use practices need to be made compatible with personal identities but also legitimised by social networks and neighbours. Individual analytical approaches to lifeworlds (Schutz 1967) which focus only on cultural 'sense-making' tend to underplay the influence of authenticity and social legitimacy for particular meanings and uses of medicines.

The advantages of the Habermasian (1987) framework outlined in this chapter is this recognition of legitimacy of action (c.f. Schutz 1967) and its attentiveness towards divergent logics of system and lifeworld (c.f. Douglas 1992). This divergence may, as has been explored, often lead to an impinging upon the refinement of social consensus and meanings around medicine. Yet this same system-lifeworld uncoupling may also lead to an instrumentality of medicines development and manufacture which is so glaringly out of touch with social consensus (Outhwaite 2009: 91) that a more radical and collective re-evaluation of medicines remains possible within certain settings.

## NOTES

1. Thomas McCarthy directly translates Persönlichkeit as 'personality', however I use 'identity' here as common conceptualisations of the latter term offer a better reflection of Habermas's (1987: 129) conceptualisation.
2. Schutz's spelling of life-world is different to that of Habermas's lifeworld and indeed these differences will be maintained throughout the chapter to clarify when Schutzian conceptualisations are being referred to.
3. I conducted this research with Mike Calnan and Ferhana Hashem at the University of Kent. The research was funded by the UK Economic and Social Research Council.

## REFERENCES


Abraham, J. (1995) *Science, Politics and the Pharmaceutical Industry: Controversy and Bias in Drug Regulation.* London: UCL Press.

Abraham, J. (2010) Pharmaceuticalisation of society in context: Theoretical and empirical dimensions *Sociology* 44(4):603–622.

Angell, M. (2005) *The Truth about the Drug Companies: How They Deceive Us and What to Do about Us* New York: Random House.

Barbalet, J. (2009) A characterisation of trust and its consequences *Theory & Society* 38(4):367–382.

Beck, U. (1992) Modern society as a risk society, in Stehr, N. and Ericson, R. (editors) *The Culture and Power of Knowledge* Berlin: Walter de Gruyter.

Beck, U. (2009) *World at Risk* Cambridge: Polity.

Britten, N. (2008) *Medicines and Society: Patients, Professionals and the Dominance of Pharmaceuticals* Basingstoke: Palgrave.

Brown, N. (2005) Shifting tenses: reconnecting regimes of truth and hope *Configurations* 13(3):331–335.

Brown, P. (2009) The phenomenology of trust: a Schutzian analysis of the social construction of knowledge by gynae-oncology patients *Health Risk & Society* 11(5):391–407.

Brown, P. (2011) The dark side of hope and trust: constructed expectations and the value-for-money regulation of new medicines *Health Sociology Review* 20(4):407–419.

Brown, P. (2014) Risk and social theory: the legitimacy of risks and risk as a tool of legitimation *Health Risk & Society* 16(5):391–397.

Brown, P. and Calnan, M. (2012) Braving a faceless new world? Conceptualising trust in the pharmaceutical industry and its products *Health* 16(1):57–75.

Brown, P. and de Graaf, S. (2013) Considering a future which may not exist: the construction of time and expectations amidst advanced-stage cancer *Health, Risk & Society* 15(6):543–560.

Brown, P., de Graaf, S. and Hillen, M. (2014) The inherent tensions and ambiguities of hope: towards a post-formal analysis of experiences of advanced-cancer patients. *Health* 19:207–225.

Brown, P., de Graaf, S., Hillen, M., Smets, E. and Laarhoven, H. W. (2014a) The interweaving of pharmaceutical and medical expectations as dynamics of micro-pharmaceuticalisation: advanced-stage cancer patients' hope in medicines alongside trust in professionals. *Social Science & Medicine* 131(1):313–321.

Burney, I. (2007) The politics of particularism: medicalisation and medical reform in 19th century Britain, in Bivins, R. and Pickstone, J. (editors) *Medicine, Madness and Social History: Essays in honour of Roy Porter*. Basingstoke: Palgrave.

Caita-Zufferey, M. (2012) From danger to risk: categorising and valuing recreational heroin and cocaine use *Health Risk & Society* 14(5):427–443.

Calnan, M. and Rowe, R. (2008) *Trust Matters in Healthcare* Basingstoke: Palgrave.

Collins, J. (2011) Sending a message: Ecstasy, equasy and the media politics of drug classification *Health Risk & Society* 13(3):221–237.

Dean, M. (1999) *Governmentality: Power and Rule in Modern Society* London: Sage.

Desmond, N. (2009) *Ni kubahatisha tu!' It's just a game of chance: adaptation and resignation to socially constructed perceptions of risk in rural Tanzania* PhD Thesis, University of Glasgow.

Douglas, M. (1992) *Risk and Blame: Essays in Cultural Theory* London: Routledge.

Douglas, M. (2006) *A history of grid and group cultural theory*. http://projects.chass.utoronto.ca/semiotics/cyber/douglas1.pdf (accessed 29 January 2012).

Douglas, M. and Wildavsky, A. (1983) *Risk and Culture: An Essay on the Selection of Technological and Environmental Dangers* Berkeley, CA: University of California Press.

Elliott, A. (2002) Beck's sociology of risk: a critical assessment *Sociology* 36(2): 293–315.

Ezzy, D. (1998) Theorising narrative identity. *Sociological Quarterly* 39(2):239–252.

Gabe, J. and Bury, M. (1996) Risking tranquiliser use: cultural and lay dimensions, in Williams, S. and Calnan, M. (editors) *Modern Medicine: Lay Perspectives and Experiences* London: UCL Press.

Gardner, K. and Dew, K. (2011) The eltroxin controversy: risk and how actors construct their world *Health, Risk & Society* 13(5):397–411.

Guillaume, H. (2014) *Daughters of the Pill—Getting off? Women's Stories of Contraceptive Use in France* Unpublished MSc Thesis, University of Amsterdam.

Good, M.J.D. (2001) The biotechnical embrace *Culture, Medicine & Psychiatry* 25(4):395–410.

Good, M.J.D., Good, B., Schaffer, C. and Lind, S. (1990) American oncology and the discourse on hope *Culture, Medicine & Psychiatry* 14:59–79.

Greenhalgh, T., Robb, N. and Scambler, G. (2006) Communicative and strategic action in interpreted consultations in primary care: a Habermasian perspective *Social Science & Medicine* 63(5):1170–1187.

Habermas, J. (1987) *Theory of Communicative Action: Vol II. Lifeworld and System: A Critique of Functionalist Reason* Cambridge: Polity.

Habermas, J. (1991) *The Structural Transformation of the Public Sphere* Cambridge: Polity.
Hedgecoe, A. (2004) *The Politics of Personalised Medicine* Cambridge: Cambridge University Press.
Heyman, B., Alaszewski, A. and Brown, P. (2013) Probabalistic thinking and health risks *Health, Risk & Society* 15(1):1–11.
Heyman, B., Alaszewski, A., Shaw, M., and Titterton, M. (2011) *Risk, Safety and Clinical Practice*. Oxford: Oxford University Press.
Hupli, A. (2013) *Perceptions, practices and ethics of cognitive enhancement drugs. A case study among academic youth in Amsterdam*. Unpublished MSc thesis, University of Amsterdam.
Kierkegaard, S. (1957) *Concept of Dread* Princeton: Princeton University Press.
Krumholz, H., Ross, J., Pressler, A., and Egilman, D. (2007) What have we learnt from Vioxx? *British Medical Journal* 334:120–123.
Lewis, J. and Weigert, A. (1985) Trust as a social reality. *Social Forces* 63:967–985.
Luhmann, N. (1993) *Risk: A Sociological Theory*. New York: Aldine de Gruyter.
Milewa, T. and Barry, C. (2005) Health and the politics of evidence *Social Policy & Administration* 39(5):498–512.
Mills, C. W. (1940) Situated actions and vocabularies of motive *American Sociological Review* 5(6):904–913.
Möllering, G. (2001) The nature of trust: From Georg Simmel to a theory of expectation, interpretation and suspension. *Sociology* 35:403–420.
Möllering, G. (2005) The trust control duality: an integrative perspective on positive expectations of others. *International Sociology* 20(3):283–305.
Montelius, E. and Giritli-Nygren, K. (2014) Doing risk, doing difference: towards an understanding of intersections of risk, morality and taste *Health, Risk & Society* 16(5):431–443.
Moreira, T. (2011) Health care rationing in an age of uncertainty: A conceptual model. *Social Science and Medicine* 72(8):1333–1341.
Outhwaite, W. (2009) *Habermas: A Critical Introduction* Cambridge: Polity.
Robb, N. and Greenhalgh, T. (2006) 'You have to cover up the words of the doctor': the mediation of trust in interpreted consultations in primary care *Journal of Health Organisation Management* 20(5):434–455.
Sartre, J. P. (1962) *A Sketch for a Theory of the Emotions* London: Methuen.
Scambler, G. (2001) *Habermas, Critical Theory and Health* London: Routledge.
Scambler, G. and Britten, N. (2001) System, lifeworld and doctor-patient interaction: issues of trust in a changing world, in Scambler, G. (editor) *Habermas, Critical Theory and Health*. London: Routledge.
Schutz, A. (1967) *The Phenomenology of the Social World* Evanston: Northwestern University Press.
Schutz, A. and Luckmann, T. (1973) *The Structures of the Lifeworld* Evanston: Northwestern University Press.
Seale, C. (2005) New directions for critical internet health studies: representing cancer experience on the web. *Sociology of Health and Illness* 27(4):515–540.
Simpson, C. (2004) When hope makes us vulnerable: a discussion of patient—healthcare provider interactions in the context of hope. *Bioethics* 18(5):428–447.
Smith, R. (2005) Medical journals are an extension of the marketing arm of pharmaceutical companies *PLOS Medicine* 2(5): e138.
Szmukler, G. (2003) Risk assessment: numbers and values *Psychiatric Bulletin* 27:205–207.
van Dantzig, A. and de Swaan, A. (1978) *Omgaan met angst in een kankerziekenhuis* Amsterdam: Aula.

van der Geest, S., Whyte, S. and Hardon, A. (1996) The anthropology of pharmaceuticals: a biographical approach *Annual Review of Anthropology* 25:153–178.
van Loon, J. (2014) Remediating risk as matter-energy-information flows of avian influenza and BSE *Health, Risk & Society* 16(5):44–458.
Wilkinson, I. (2010) *Risk and Vulnerability in Everyday Life* London: Routledge.
Williams, S., Martin, P. and Gabe, J. (2011) The pharmaceuticalisation of society? A framework for analysis. *Sociology of Health & Illness* 33(5):710–725.
Zinn, J. (2008a) Heading into the unknown: everyday strategies for managing risk and uncertainty *Health Risk & Society* 10(5):439–450.
Zinn, J. (2008b) *Social Theories of Risk and Uncertainty* Oxford: Blackwell.

# 5 Performing Risk and Power

## Predictive Technologies in Personalized Medicine

*Nadav Even Chorev*

## INTRODUCTION

> Disease is no longer the object of anguish for the healthy man; it has become instead the object of study for the theorist of health.
>
> (Canguilhem, 1989: 43)

The emerging medical practice termed 'personalized medicine' is founded on the assumption that personal health risks can be predicted and mitigated before they materialize. It is an attempt to change medicine's central paradigm, no less, from one which is retrospective and evidence-based to one which is prospective and molecular-driven (Mendelsohn, 2013: 17). Medicine, according to this perspective, will remain evidence-based, yet the nature of the evidence will change. Personalized medicine has many strands, yet in all of them the characterization of an individual patient's molecular make-up forms the starting point for prediction upon which subsequent action is taken.

In this chapter, I will discuss how quantified predictions of risk and efficacy, produced and used by artifacts and humans in the field of personalized medicine, reflect forms of power. For this purpose, I will review a case study of a specific cancer clinical trial in which a personalized method to tailor treatment is applied. The WINTHER (Worldwide Innovative Network THERapeutic) trial, about which I will elaborate in the following sections, does not test a new therapy but a personalized method by which to choose between various possible therapies. In order to achieve this goal, the trial makes use of computerized matches between the molecular characteristics of the participating patients and information on drugs. As part of this trial, an algorithm was developed to rank drugs according to their projected effectiveness for a specific patient, based on analysis comparing his or her gene expression in the tumor to that in the normal tissue. The investigators factor these results into their decision-making process on suitable treatment for the specific patient (WIN Consortium Press Release, 28/06/2012, 03/09/2013. Presentation by Dr. Fabrice Andre, 28/06/2012, www.gustaveroussy.fr, downloaded 15/10/2013).

The method developed for the trial is formulated in a patent. In a critique of current cancer treatment practices, the authors of the patent state that: "These approaches tend to enrich the patient cohort for a given chemotherapy rather than to select a targeted individual therapy for a given patient on the basis of the intrinsic tumoral characteristics" (Lazar, Soria, Ducreux & Tursz, 2011: 4). This approach, I argue, attests to a new development that has implications for the governmental understanding of risk. Risk, according to this approach, is not only attached to the body by the application of epidemiological assessments (Weir, 1996: 381). Estimations of risk and uncertainty are also reached from within the individual body. This partly reverses the rationality of risk as conceptualized by governmental studies. Indeed, as I will show, epidemiological and large statistical distributions still play a role in personalized medicine. The connection between a disease and a therapy and states of molecular mechanisms cannot be established without them. Yet in this developing medical trend, they are embedded in the background of the process by which individual risk assessment or therapeutic decisions are reached. A course of actions is chosen on the basis of the patient's personal characteristics, not by fitting the patient into known, existing standards of care based on such large distributions. Thus, I claim, in this sense, individual patients and their attributes are not completely "submerged or stripped away and only certain recurring characteristics attended to" (O'Malley: 57).

My aim here is to demonstrate how this shift in the understanding of risk and uncertainty occurs in actuality. Starting from Foucault's concept of power, I will show that information artifacts enact their performative capacity in the context of the trial while interacting with human actors and other discursive and nondiscursive elements. By producing predictive and probabilistic estimations of an uncertain future (in this case, the projected efficacy of therapeutic drugs for a specific patient), they exert what is termed 'power to': the capacity to carry out actions (Lukes, 2005: 34). However, I claim that when examined in the framework of the trial, this form of power gains a relational quality, usually ascribed to the domination of one actor over another or 'power over'. This comes about through 'naming' the immediate future with numerical probabilistic estimations that characterize risk as a technology of government. Thus estimations of risk and efficacy produced by artifacts and engaged by humans designate a field of intervention through the new field of biomedicine.

Though at first sight the analysis offered here may seem narrow, its importance may be found in the fact that medicine is a central site through which to examine changes in risk and uncertainty in late-modern liberal societies. If the vision of personalized medicine is to act before health risks materialize—that is, to prevent disease—its focus on the individual can be understood beyond the context of scientific developments. The spread of personalized medicine can have far-reaching effects on health-care systems at large (Davis, Ma &Sutaria, 2010), while the solution it offers will always remain at the individual level, in the individual's molecular details. Thus individual answers are still suggested as a way to deal with increasing risk and uncertainty, which may be propelled by forces well beyond individual reach (Beck, 1992, 2006, 2009).

In what follows, I will describe the scope and methodology of the research in brief. I will then discuss how risk and power are related analytically, focusing on the conceptualization of risk in governmentality studies which draw on Foucault's formulation of power. I will also explore how this formulation of risk relates to performativity as an aspect of 'power to'. As implied by Langdon Winner (1980), a detailed understanding of the technological artifact in its social setting is necessary for uncovering its inner political mechanisms. Accordingly, I will describe the WINTHER trial in its context and describe the process of reaching a therapeutic decision in the case of a specific patient. Finally, I will discuss the actual ways in which power and risk are expressed in the trial.

## METHODOLOGY

The analysis offered here of a case study research explores the ways in which risk is configured in the field of personalized medicine, focusing particularly on the role played by information technologies in this process. The case study strategy enables a clear delineation of the scope of the research, which becomes useful when engaging with current phenomena in real contexts (Yin, 2009: 18). In the case of the WINTHER trial, the context consists of institutional, clinical, scientific, technological and social dimensions. Risk and uncertainty are examined, in this case, through their numerical manifestations and articulations in trial documents. They are also considered through the discourse of professionals formulating clinical decisions based on these same numerical assessments. Both these of aspects comprise the process of tailoring personalized treatment. The WINTHER trial can be considered to exemplify what Flyvbjerg (2011: 307–308) terms a 'paradigmatic case' through which one can achieve an understanding of a new research domain and thus highlight its general societal characteristics.

The empirical material collected for this study consists of texts including patents, newspaper articles, textbooks and professional articles on personalized medicine; computerized outputs, records and the software codes, databases and algorithms on which they are founded; semi-structured, in-depth interviews with specialists and physicians; and recordings of their online consultations. In this chapter, I rely specifically on publicly available material as well as on trial documents and specific clinical data, results of molecular analysis and discussions pertaining to a specific patient. All references to participants were anonymized.

The main analysis of empirical material was carried out employing a 'Membership Categorization Analysis' (MCA) technique, which is suitable for identifying the uses of various categories in real situations. This methodology is used to identify the 'categorization devices' participants of a conversation employ and evoke, which, in turn, consist of categories, their attributes and rules for application. By locating these devices in the analysis of a conversation, in this case clinical discussions, MCA seeks to pinpoint the knowledge on which participants draw. Furthermore, the order in which categories appear during a discussion is important as well as the specific actors who use them, as they attest to the hierarchies and assumptions implicit in the conversation. Such hierarchies and assumptions, in turn, can be related to an external context (King, 2010; Lepper, 2000).The analysis was performed using the ATLAS.ti version 7 Qualitative Data Analysis software package (Friese, 2014).

## RISK, POWER AND TECHNOLOGICAL PERFORMATIVITY

Ongoing debates about the definition of power, its origins, modes of legitimation and the conditions under which it materializes can be traced throughout the history of Western social and political thought. The convergence of thinking about risk and power took shape in recent years following Ulricih Beck's positioning of risk in the late 1980s as a central stratifying variable, essential for the sociological understanding of late-modern society (Beck, 1992). Within the vast literature dealing with risk (see Zinn, 2008 for a comprehensive review), governmentality studies have taken on an analytical engagement with risk as a form of power. This perspective and line of research draws upon Foucault's conception of power and applies it to various facets of social and political life. Thus risk has been studied as an example of technologies of security central to the governmental form of power and has been examined both as a rationality and as a practical apparatus for deploying such a rationality. As I will try to show here, governmental studies of risk, though concerned with risk as a concept governing human conduct, give rise to a concept of power which is ambivalent in that it suggests both domination and capacity.

Although the Foucauldian conception of power resides on the side of 'power over', it cannot be understood exclusively in terms of one actor subordinating another actor to its will. For Foucault, power is not an all-encompassing "mode of subjugation" or a "general system of domination" (Foucault, 1978: 92) but rather a set of multiple forces that constitute their field of operation. Power should not be viewed as a unity emanating from a single omnipotent source but as an aggregate network or process in which power relations are produced by every point in the field at any given minute:

> power is not an institution, and not a structure; neither is it a certain strength we are endowed with; it is the name that one attributes to a complex strategical situation in a particular society.
>
> (Foucault, 1978: 93)

As is well known, governmentality according to Foucault is a historically specific instance of the exercise of power, appearing in Europe in the 18th century(Foucault, 1991). It is an ensemble of strategies that rose in connection with the increasing salience of 'population' as a social and political subject. Governmentality functions to maintain the security of the population by developing and employing forms of knowledge relating to this population such as statistics, economics, criminology, public health and more. Foucault stresses that the governmental form of power does not point to linear historical development and does not displace sovereignty or disciplinary power. It is specific, however, in its constitution of 'population' as a new field of intervention. Thus viewing risk as a form of government, and following from Foucault's concept of power, Francois Ewald made the now famous assertion that:

> Nothing is a risk in itself; there is no risk in reality. But on the other hand, anything *can* be a risk; it all depends on how one analyzes the danger, considers the event. As Kant might have put it, the category of risk is a category of the understanding; it cannot be given in sensibility or intuition.
>
> (Ewald, 1991: 199)

Risk, then, is both a feature of government and a way of thinking about government (O'Malley, 2008: 56). In this sense, it is not a unique mechanism of power. Risk does, however, have specific attributes that set it apart from other practices of government. According to Pat O'Malley, risk

> is a statistical and probabilistic technique, whereby large numbers of events are sorted into a distribution, and the distribution in turn is used as a means of making probabilistic predictions. In this process, the particular details of each individual case which have been the focus of disciplinary technologies are submerged or stripped away and only certain recurring characteristics attended to.
>
> (O'Malley: 57)

As I will show, this rationality of risk is partly reversed in personalized medicine in that the calculations of risk and attempts to reduce uncertainty in this field begin with individual characteristics and, moreover, cannot be undertaken without them.

Risk as a governmental rationality of ordering reality in calculative terms is, according to Mitchell Dean, not significant in itself. Its significance lies with what it "gets attached to": the moral and political programs in which it is developed and used (Dean, 2010: 206). This view of risk is compatible with Foucault's perspective on power. Power is not an institution but a 'name' given to a set of complex forces (to use Foucault's terms) under particular historical conditions. In this view, 'risk' is a 'name' given to a set of practices that are meant to render certain aspects of an uncertain present-day and future reality legible by calculative means and make them governable.

The ambiguity contained in the concept of power, implied by the capacity to give a 'name' and thus open up a field of intervention has been debated in current discussions of the concept. For example, Pamela Pansardi, discussing the distinction between 'power over' and 'power to', claims that these two perceptions of power are not mutually exclusive. They characterize a unified social power. In this view, both notions of power have relational aspects and refer to the same class of social facts across many research domains (Pansardi, 2012). A governmental perspective would consider this stance as attributing a constant essence to power. Governmentality, as represented by Dean, approaches the concept of power by tracing it through a series of antinomies, such as 'power to' versus 'power over', which appear in debates on the subject. Thus power itself, according to Dean, is no different from the concept of power. It is a meta-concept, a 'signature':

> What is distinctive about the concept of power is the way the notion refers us to an opposition that in turn can become a unity in another opposition. What the discussions of the concept of power thereby reveal is that there is an 'excess' in the concept of power beyond what it might signify, which marks it and forces this movement towards oppositions, their unification and further opposition.
>
> (Dean, 2012: 107)

The development of concepts of power is dialectic but has no deterministic direction. Power should be analyzed while suspending the dichotomies related to it. It should be viewed as both "being and action". It follows, according to Dean, that power should be examined through its substantive, concrete instances (Dean, 108).

Risk, therefore, is power to the extent that it gives a 'name', phrased in calculative terms, to a field of intervention (Butler, 1997: 34–36). It thus invents the field, the ways of intervention, of governing conduct and the subjects to be governed (Hacking, 1996). In this sense, risk can be viewed as performing and designating a domain of action in specific discursive ways. Dean sees in "performation" one aspect of a signature of power. It is not only the post hoc result of a network of 'actants', as in Latour's formulation, but part and parcel of assemblages of human and nonhuman actors (Dean, 2012: 106). I argue that, following Dean's rationale, the performativity of artifacts as an expression of power can be used to understand power in a certain area of governmental practices. Power as performed by these objects resides in the naming of a set of practices as 'risk'. This 'name' refers to calculations pertaining to future uncertainty that can be employed on any analytical level. The performance of such objects allows uncertainty to be perceived as reduced and controlled.

The performativity of information artifacts is a recurrent theme in writings on information systems, algorithms and program codes, specifically in medicine, biomedicine and molecular biology (Berg and Bowker, 1997; Mackenzie, 2005; 2006; Orlikowski, 2005). Drawing on Butler, Adrian Mackenzie asserts that the performativity of an algorithm, a section of code or a system lies in the set of practices which allows them to do things. These things, deeds or actions, are not entirely discursive, and since they are embedded within a set of practices, they are not entirely material either (Mackenzie, 2005: 76). In other words, they cannot be entirely reduced into either discourse or materiality. Objects and discourses can be simultaneously located in an existing set of practices and viewed as performing a calculative action. It is here that the performativity of artifacts is associated with power. As I will demonstrate, this association is a form of exercising power, in this case as risk, within a concrete setting. Performativity thus becomes a part of an actual process of governing the future and can be useful for understanding the exercising of power in new emerging domains. Power, according to this perspective, still carries analytical utility.

## DELIBERATING A PERSONALIZED MEDICAL DECISION

The process of reaching a therapeutic decision in the WINTHER trial exemplifies the application of a personalized medical approach. I will present this process in the form of a narrative beginning with the underlying assumptions informing the trial and ending with the moment of reaching a clinical decision. Although I outline this narrative chronologically, it is far from linear. As this case demonstrates, the course of events in the trial are subject to contingencies and does not necessarily follow the formal 'standard operating procedure' (SOP). The case I follow is representative of other decisions made in the trial in that on the one hand it is unique and presents investigators with its distinct challenges, and, on the other hand, the specific decision is made with regard to a patient who has passed the inclusion threshold and thus has commonalities with other patients in the trial. Put differently, all the cases in the trial are similar in that they are exceptional. This case demonstrates the dynamic relations between artifacts and human actors characterizing all decisions in the trial.

### The Case Study in and as Context: A Brief Description

The WINTHER trial was initiated and is managed by the WIN Consortium (Worldwide Innovative Networking in personalized cancer medicine, http://www.winconsortium.org/), a nonprofit based in Paris. The actual trial began in April 2013. Currently it takes place in four medical centers: in Israel, France, Spain and recently in Canada, with the intention of launching in a center in the United States as well. The trial is scheduled to include 200 patients. The WINTHER trial should first and foremost be placed in the general context of personalized medicine. As indicated in the introduction, personalized medicine embodies an ethical principle according to which it is necessary to act in the present in order to mitigate future risks. Dealing with such health risks can be accomplished by behavioral as well as by medical interventions. This principle can be discerned in the vision of personalized medicine, as stated, for example, by the American nonprofit Personalized Medicine Coalition:

> Personalized medicine introduces the ability to use molecular markers that signal the risk of disease or its presence before clinical signs and symptoms appear. This information underlies a healthcare strategy focused on prevention and early intervention, rather than a reaction to advanced stages of disease.
>
> (Feinstein Kean Healthcare & Silver, 2009: 6)

The goals of the WINTHER clinical trial should thus be understood against the backdrop of the attempt to overhaul medical practice. Indeed there is a temporal gap here. Action in the present to mitigate future health risk is different from formulating a personalized cancer treatment in the here and now of a clinical trial. Nelson, Keating & Cambrosio (2013) describe this gap as the difference between 'long term personalized risk management' and 'actionability', yet both practices fall under the category of 'personalized'. As I will demonstrate in the current section, 'actionability' coalesces with personalized risk management through "a predictive efficacy score for all existing drugs for each individual patient" (WIN Consortium Press Release, 03/09/2013). In other words, in this case at least, personalized predictions are made in the present.

The vision of personalized medicine as described earlier is integrated into the trial's goals. The trial, as the protocol clearly states, does not test some new therapy but explicitly examines the effectiveness of a method for the personalized treatment of cancer: "The aim is to provide a rational personalized therapeutic choice to all (100%) patients enrolled in the study, harboring oncogenic events (mutations/translocations/amplifications, etc.) or not" (http://clinicaltrials.gov/ct2/show/study/NCT01856296). The overarching goal is to overcome the deadlock which cancer treatment has reached in recent years, in which even DNA targeted therapy provides a solution to only about 30 percent of advanced cancer patients (Lazar, Soria, Ducreux and Tursz, 2011, 1–2; WIN Consortium Press Release, 03/09/2013). In this way, the trial, its goals and the predictive tools it employs serve personalized medicine's aspiration to replace current standardized medical practices with future-oriented, patient-focused, biologically based practices (Mendelsohn, 2013). To use the trial's terms, they reflect an attempt to reduce uncertainty by rational therapeutic choice. Rational choice here means a therapeutic decision reached on the basis of molecular information of the patient and on second-order predictions resulting from this same information.

The patients admitted to the trial are cancer patients in advanced stages, who have exhausted all conventional therapeutic options, a state described as "therapeutic failure" (Lazar, Soria, Ducreux & Tursz, 2011: 32). They entered this trial since they are still considered to have sufficient life expectancy for the results of the treatment by the trial's method to be meaningful. Such results are measured in the trial by an indicator called Progression Free Survival (PFS). The trial will be considered successful if this indicator will be significantly larger than the one measured before entering the trial. That is, whether the patients' period in which the disease does not progress is significantly longer, in statistical terms, after applying the method than the period measured for the last line of treatment before entering the trial (http://clinicaltrials.gov/ct2/show/study/NCT01856296). Designating PFS as the outcome by which to measure success in the trial is significant for two main reasons. First, it can be statistically validated though the sample of the trial is not large. Second and more importantly, this indicator measures the state of the tumor numerically. Unlike other cancer treatment indicators, it does not necessarily attest to the overall benefit for the patient (Booth and Eisenhauer, 2012). It is thus in line with the calculative rationality of risk and serves as a relatively stable measurement of the effect of the method employed in the trial for patients who are in 'therapeutic failure'.

According to the trial's procedure (presentation by Dr. Fabrice Andre, 28/06/2012, 7), two biopsies are performed for each patient: one from normal tissue of the organ in which the cancer originated and the other from the tumor or from a metastasis. The tumor tissue is sent for DNA analysis at an American biotech company (testing for about 230 genes, termed Arm A in the trial) to locate DNA alterations (also referred to as oncogenic events) in the tumor. The result is a report for each patient that matches the identified DNA alterations with known and approved targeted drugs or with clinical trials testing treatments targeting these alterations.

For about half the patients in the trial (Interview with Bioinformatician, 12/05/2013), no such DNA alteration is identified. So, in parallel, both the normal and cancerous samples are sent for a differential, comparative gene expression analysis (termed Arm B). They are run against a much wider collection of genes, approximately 1400. The genes for this test were compiled from a public database of drugs and chemicals known to be related with gene expression (http://ctdbase.org/, expression measured here in the amount of RNA produced). This analysis is meant to identify the genes which are deregulated in the tumor in comparison with the normal tissue, either over- or under-expressed, (Lazar, Soria, Ducreux & Tursz, 2011).An algorithm developed specifically for the trial produces a score for each drug drawn from the filtered public database. It calculates the number of genes found to be deregulated in the tumor in comparison with the normal tissue (based on the Arm B analysis) together with the extent of 'deviation' of each deregulated gene. The result is a score produced for each drug for a given patient (Lazar, Soria, Ducreux & Tursz 2011).

The Clinical Management Committee (termed CMC) of the trial convenes biweekly to discuss the results for each patient and decide on the appropriate treatment. The committee consists of the principle investigators who are high-profile oncologists, a bioinformatician, a representative of the company performing the DNA analysis and administrators from the WIN Consortium. This is not an unusual composition for trials of this kind (Nelson et al., 2013). The committee uses an online portal that includes the data available for each patient: clinical information, the DNA report and a dynamically produced table that orders and ranks the drugs according to the calculated score. According to the protocol, the committee members first discuss the results of the Arm A analysis (Presentation by Dr. Fabrice Andre, 28/06/2012, 7). At this stage, the specialists decide which alteration from those identified in the patient tumor DNA analysis is an 'actionable' one, i.e., an alteration worth acting upon, on which to target the therapy (Nelson et al., 2013). If no approved drug is matched with the alterations identified, or in a case where drugs are not available in the treating center or there are no suitable clinical trials, the specialists move to consider the drug-ranking table of Arm B. They can then probe deeper into the results of gene expression for each drug. The decision reached is then recorded in the portal. Later the patient's progress is recorded as well.

## Decision Making in Practice

In order to demonstrate how personalized medicine is put into practice in the trial, I will focus on the process of reaching a clinical decision for a particular patient. Again it should be remembered that although described in the order of events, this process is somewhat iterative and does not necessarily follow the formal framework of the protocol. Each patient's treating physician presents his or her case. The patient in this example is a middle-aged person who suffers from 'squamous cell carcinoma', a type of soft-tissue cancer. The disease originated in the tongue and oral cavity, and metastases were found in the lungs. The patient had already undergone four lines of treatment with partial success (Clinical data sheet, WINTHER Portal, downloaded 11/05/2014). After reviewing the patient's treatment history, the specialists examined the DNA analysis report, which identified four DNA alterations of different kinds. These alterations were not matched with any drugs, meaning there are no approved drugs specifically targeting the molecular mechanisms in which these genes are involved. However, the report mentions eight clinical trials testing drugs that do target these alterations (Genomic alterations report, WINTHER Portal, downloaded 11/05/2014).

After consulting the representative of the company performing the genomic analysis, the doctors decided to act upon one of the identified DNA changes, the amplification of the MDM2 gene:

| | |
|---|---|
| Oncologist 1 | Well, I mean, we have a clinical trial that is going to open very soon, with [pharmaceutical company] MDM2 inhibitor, hopefully by next month, that could be an option . . . 2, you have an opinion? |
| Oncologist 2 | Sorry. But I think that the best one would be the clinical trial for sure. I wonder if the gene expression profiling, I don't think we have any drugs in the database, I don't have the ranking, so I don't think we will find a MDM3 inhibitor there. But it would be nice to go to the raw data and see if we see a high expression of MDM2. |
| Bioinformatician | But you do realize that SOP do not. . . |
| Oncologist 1 | We do realize, we are evaluating the SOP. (Clinical online consultation, 25/06/2013) |

Based on this information, the treating physician suggests putting the patient on a clinical trial available at his center. The decision is based on the genomic characteristics of the patient's tumor (an Arm A decision). He consults his colleague who agrees but asks whether they can review the results of the RNA analysis for the MDM2 gene for supporting evidence. The treating physician dismisses the bioinformatician's concerns that this deviates from the designated standard operation procedure. The problem here, from the bioinformatician's point of view, is that an Arm A decision is made based on information from both analyses, while it should have been made on the basis of the genomic analysis alone.

The gene expression data (referred to by oncologist 2 as 'the raw data') includes an analysis (termed 'probe') for each version (isoform) of RNA produced from each gene included in the aforementioned filtered CTD database. Thus, in this case, the MDM2 gene identified in this patient's tumor DNA analysis produced 14 versions of RNA (that is, 14 isoforms). These versions are examined in the pathological cancer tissue and compared to the normal tissue. The raw data, a long table, consists of an analysis serial number, gene symbol (MDM2 in this example), the amount of RNA found for each of the versions of the genes in the cancer tissue, the RNA amount found for each of the versions (isoforms) of these genes in the normal tissue and a simple ratio between these two amounts (Comparative RNA data table, WINTHER Portal, downloaded 11/05/201).The physicians ask the bioinformatics lab assistant to describe the results of this analysis for this patient: the analyses (probes) of 13 out of the 14 versions (isoforms) indicate that, as measured by the amount of the RNA produced, the MDM2 gene is overexpressed in the cancer tissue as compared to the normal tissue

(Comparative RNA data table, WINTHER Portal, downloaded 11/05/2014. Clinical online consultation, 25/06/2013). Overexpression here means that the cancer tissue produces significantly more RNA for the MDM2 gene, as compared with the results for this same gene in the normal tissue. The MDM2 gene is therefore deregulated in the cancer tissue of this patient. Thus by referring to the raw data of the expression report, the physicians gain confidence in their Arm A decision.

The treating physician (an oncologist) is more or less content with this decision. Then the plot thickens. One of the oncologists taking part in the consultation recalls one of the other genes identified as altered in the patient's DNA analysis, the TP53 gene, and raises a question:

| | |
|---|---|
| Oncologist 3 | What is the significance of the TP53 mutation, because MDM2 targets TP53 and if we like the target of MDM2, it's like having a resistance to MDM2 inhibitor. |
| Oncologist 1 | Ok, Dr. 3 has just destroyed our whole decision, because he thinks that . . . [?] MDM amplified because it's TP53 mutant and might not work. So he's probably. . . So can you tell us what is this P53 mutant? Is it [a] pathogenic mutant? What is this? . . . but the point of Dr. 3 is quite clear, is that the mechanism of resistance to the drug is already imprinted in the genetic background of the tumor. So, do we still go for MDM2? Is that something that still makes sense or . . . so we are assessing the patient file, so the patient file, patient is currently perform in status one, so he is doing ok, so probably he can wait. (Clinical online consultation, 25/06/2013) |

The first decision, the Arm A decision to enter the patient into a clinical trial testing an MDM2 targeting therapy, is scrapped. The reason is that the MDM2 and TP53 gene products are involved in the same molecular mechanism in which they cancel each other's effect, and thus targeting one of them will not yield any results. This is not implied in any of the outputs the physicians viewed so far and is derived from their own knowledge and experience. This information takes them back to the trial's formal procedure. At this stage, the physicians move to the processed results of the analysis of Arm B. These are presented in a dynamically produced table. The table is generated by a code running of the predictive algorithm. The algorithm runs on the table of raw data containing the patient's results of the comparative gene expression analysis and matches the genes in this table with an additional drug table. It produces a third table that ranks drugs according to the extent of discrepancy between the normal and the pathological expression of genes. Each drug receives a score based on this discrepancy, which is intended to predict its efficacy for the specific patient. This table is presented on the trial's Internet portal. After reviewing the ranking of drugs presented in the table and again examining the details of the raw data, the physicians decide on the drug to be administered to the patient:

| | |
|---|---|
| Oncologist 2 | Yes. What you are saying here is that any met inhibitor could work. |
| Oncologist 1 | In that case, how come [Drug A] or [Drug B] do not appear in the list? Can you check that, Bioinformatician? |
| Bioinformatician | Yes, just a second. |
| . . . | |
| Oncologist 1 | Ok, so [Drug B] could be a choice. So either we put the patient in the phase one trial of the met inhibitor from [pharmaceutical company], if he is met positive. And if not, we treat him with [Drug B], but this is by decision of Arm B. Are we in agreement with that? (Clinical online consultation, 25/06/2013). |

The oncologists do not readily accept the first drug on the list. They choose a drug according to their understanding and according to the treatment options available to them (either administering a drug or directing the patient to a suitable clinical trial). Yet their choice is based on the same molecular mechanism targeted by the drug ranked first on the list. In other words, the drug chosen (which belongs to a relatively new class of therapies) is predicted to be effective since the genes it is associated with are involved in a certain cellular process (connected with the cell's energy production cycle) and have been found to be deregulated in the results of the RNA analysis of this patient.

In the process described here, it can be seen that the physicians exercise their discretion regarding the decision to be made. No automated system makes that decision for them. However, the decision is taken in relation to information provided by various computerized outputs. These outputs translate the molecular characteristics of the patient into higher-order information, upon which action can be taken. This is the way in which personalization is interpreted in the trial. It comes down to the very molecular mechanisms of the individual patient. Details are important to describe in this context, since they comprise the foundations for a personalized clinical decision. This process demonstrates the interplay between the framework of the trial (including its goals and procedures), biological matter translated into information, systems that present this information and human actors. This process, to the extent that it can be seen as representative of personalized medicine, reverses the rationality of risk described by O'Malley (2008: 57). The decision relies on statistical and probabilistic information and the numbers are independent from the subject from whom they are produced. However, the large distributions are implicit in the background of the trial, and as shown in the earlier example, the decision starts from the specific individual and cannot be reached without taking the patient's particularities into account. In this the trial's personalized medical decisions differ also from Lorna Weir's characterization of clinical risks (1996). The physicians can exercise discretion and draw on prior knowledge in understanding these particularities and in choosing whether to locate them in larger distributions and if so where.

## DISCUSSION

As I suggested earlier, the role of information artifacts in the case of personalized clinical decision making can be better understood by employing a perspective of risk as a governmental practice of power. I argued that risk can be viewed as power through the performativity of various artifacts when these are placed in the context of practices which enable them to 'perform'. I claimed furthermore that this performativity of objects, which produces risk as power, lies in the capacity of objects to 'name' the future. That is, objects reduce uncertainty by calculative means and thus open up a field of intervention. In this case, the field constituted is that of personalized medicine where action in the present is mandated by the endeavor to mitigate future health risks.

According to this perspective, the predictive algorithm and the databases matching biological information with drugs produce a dual effect which carries implications for the ethics of personalized medicine: it simultaneously sets the future in fixed numerical terms and opens up the potential for undetermined deliberation and negotiation. In other words, the effect is that of reducing uncertainty in one sense and increasing it in another. In the first instance, in both arms of the trial, the results of the patients' biological molecular analyses are run against databases of matching drugs. The drugs are found to be suitable in varying degrees of confidence. In the case of the Arm A DNA analysis, it is a simple matching between mutations and known drugs. In the case of Arm B, the score produced by the predictive algorithm cannot be regarded with the same level of confidence. Thus, for example, the algorithm produces higher scores for drugs interacting with a single gene than for those interacting with multiple genes (biased upward, Interview with bioinformatician, 12/05/2013). Yet the score itself generally goes undisputed when discussed by the physicians. They accept the statistical assumptions on which it is founded. More importantly, the score is accepted as an indication of the expected efficacy of the drug, and, subsequently, is viewed as a route to reducing uncertainty. In both cases, the process of translating biological material into information is manifested by the couplings of drugs with molecular information, and is presented in a standardized manner.

However, as clearly demonstrated in the example I provided earlier, in the second instance, the database matches and scores are only the starting point for an open discussion. The physicians are compelled to accept the results of database matches of mutations and drugs only in the case of Arm

A. This is mainly for ethical reasons: if a known and approved therapy exists, it has to be offered to the patient (Interview with WIN Consortium staff, 15/1/2014). Yet even in Arm A, drugs are matched according to identified DNA mutations, not according to the type of cancer. They can thus be recommended off-label and deviate from standard regimens. In the case of Arm B, the physicians are not obliged to accept the highest scoring drug, though the goal of the trial is to guide the therapeutic choice according to these scores. In the example I brought here, neither arms contribute to a decisive reduction of uncertainty. In addition, the therapy that is eventually selected is not determined in advance. The score produced by the predictive algorithm serves as a starting point for a nonlinear discussion. The therapy selected can be said to be partly an unintended consequence of this process. The drug is selected in a process that deviates from accepted standards and protocols. This is exactly the intention of the so-called paradigmatic shift, which personalized medicine aims to achieve, yet uncertainty has not been eliminated from the process.

How does this dual effect come about? The performativity of technological artifacts, to recall, is enabled by the context in which they are located. The trial moves between discursive and material components which engage with one another. Discursive elements include wider contexts and existing forms of knowledge in which the trial itself is situated and which provide the background for the various assumptions on which it relies. These consist, for example, of vision statements for personalized medicine, such as the one offered above by the Personalized Medicine Coalition (Feinstein Kean Healthcare & Silver, 2009). More specifically, the trial's goal to rationally choose a therapy based on the comparison, in Arm B, of normal and pathological gene expression stems from this broader context. The threshold for the discrepancy between the normal and the pathological tissue is another example of such an assumption (Lazar, Soria, Ducreux & Tursz, 2011: 11). It was determined based on existing biological scientific knowledge on what is considered a meaningful result versus what is considered 'noise' (Interview with bioinformatics lab manager, 29/09/2014).

The role of information technology artifacts in processing the results of biological material analyses is enabled within these contexts. That is, the operation of nondiscursive components can take place in the discursive context. Thus the trial's procedure stipulates extracting tissue samples, both the normal and the pathological, in a particular manner. The samples are processed to extract DNA and RNA, which are, in turn, translated into legible information of sequence and order (Mackenzie, 2006) by Next Generation Sequencing (NGS) technologies in specialized laboratories. This information is further processed to produce higher-order information. From the point of view of cancer treatment, the main contribution of the trial is the comparative RNA analysis between the normal tissue and the cancer tissue (Interview with WIN Consortium staff, 15/1/2014. Interview with bioinformatics lab manager, 29/09/2014). It is here that the performative capacity of technological artifacts is expressed most clearly. Algorithms, according to Robert Kowalski's classic definition, consist of 'logic': a problem which they are meant to solve and the knowledge used to solve it. They also include 'control': the ways and means by which the problem will be solved(Kowalski, 1979). The algorithm can thus be understood as the coupling of knowledge and action (Totaro and Ninno, 2014: 30). The algorithm developed and used in Arm B of the trial is intended to interpret gene deregulation between normal and pathological tissues. It employs existing knowledge extracted from the CTD database and the products of the patient's RNA analysis. Its action consists of the production of a score per drug, which will serve as an indication of the drug's projected efficacy. By this action, it 'does something'—that is, creates a new piece of information, a new statement. The algorithm thus exercises its "hierarchizing power" of reordering information (Goffey, 2008: 19). In the trial, the algorithm runs on structured data, which originated from the patients' unstructured, contingent, biological matter to produce a second-order structured piece of information. The latter serves to inform further action designed eventually to reintegrate the contingent body. The predictive algorithm, born as a logical abstraction of existing knowledge applied to the problem domain of cancer treatment, acts upon the interpretation of actual biological matter and then feeds back into the therapeutic choice. It is embedded into the setting of the trial, which enables it to operate. It 'performs' by giving a 'name' in the form of a numerical score to the molecular state of the patient. Otherwise, it would "only ever have a paper reality as the artifacts of a formal language" (Goffey:17).

Decision making in the trial can thus be viewed as a discursive move based on the products of nondiscursive components. Decision making itself, as exemplified in the case brought here, is not a standardized process. Each decision is tailored to a specific patient. In the trial, personalization is achieved not only through matching molecular alterations with drugs but also through the drugs' predicted efficacy for the specific patient. The patients participating in the trial are, to recall, in 'therapeutic failure'. They are all 'borderline' cases. The trial does not seek to cure them. In this sense, clinical decisions in the trial are by definition not carried out by seeking commonalities. This is what Wood, Prior and Gray characterize as "recurrent pattern recognition"(2003) or, to come back to risk and governmentality, what O'Malley describes as "certain recurring characteristics attended to" (O'Malley, 2008: 57). Patterns are not sought after, only as the end result of the trial (for example, a statistically significant increase in PFS). The products of the information artifacts serve as input for the decisions taken in an uncertain context, occasionally augmented, as shown in the case study, by sometimes indeterminate knowledge. As Pascale Bourret and her colleagues put it, "the ascription of diagnostic, and in particular predictive agency to genomic tests turns them into key non-human intermediaries between medical oncologists, pathologists, medical biologists, and their patients" (Bourret, Keating & Cambrosio, 2011: 822). That is, as demonstrated in the trial, in certain circumstances agency is not a zero-sum game, and the performative role played by 'non-human intermediaries' does not lessen human agency and discretion.

What is at stake here? The rationale of the trial contends that if the personalized method for selecting therapy for a patient proves successful (as measured in a statistically significant increase in PFS), it could be applied in earlier lines of treatment (Lazar, Soria, Ducreux & Tursz, 2011: 31–32). This is accomplished in the trial by making therapeutic decisions for actual patients. These decisions will most likely not save their lives. The aggregate effect of the trial is the accumulation of new knowledge on how to act in states of advanced metastatic cancer and offer new ways to help patients (Interview with bioinformatician, 12/05/2013). Thus the decisions are taken for patients facing imminent death, yet are made in an attempt to find ways to prolong life by fighting disease. Physicians in the trial are concerned more by the risk of missing an opportunity for therapy and less by risks of toxicity (Interview with bioinformatician, 12/05/2013).

As demonstrated here, pathology is interpreted in the trial through molecular abnormality. According to the bioinformatics lab manager, dealing with cancer in these terms is not new, nor is there any bioinformatic innovation in the trial. The novelty lies in the fact that physicians have to take the analyses of such abnormalities into account when deciding on therapeutic options. However, continues the lab manager, the predictive algorithm employed in Arm B does give an indication of efficacy of drugs (Interview with bioinformatics lab manager, 29/09/2014). In the case of Arm B, the gene expression (the amount of RNA produced) is compared between the normal and the pathological tissues. In this sense, pathological gene deregulation (over- or under-expression) in the cancerous tissue is simply what Georges Canguilhem describes as a quantitative extension of the normal state (1989: 38–46). However, the therapeutic choice is based on a manipulation of this understanding of pathology processed by databases and algorithms. As I argue, the process of finding a therapy for participating patients can be seen as an exercise of power expressed as risk leading to actions based on calculations. The predictive algorithm of Arm B of the trial, for example, expresses 'power to': through its performative capacity it gives a 'name' to the discrepancy between a pathological and normal molecular state. As shown in the example discussed here, this 'name' given in calculative terms both reduces risk and uncertainty and increases them at the same time. This 'name' is designed to be used as input in clinical decision making and in practice is used as such. Thus information technology artifacts are deeply implicated in the process through the predictive indications they provide.

## CONCLUSION

The case I surveyed here is relatively well delimited and deals mainly with the role of professionals. It shows that despite the interaction with technologies, the role of discretion by the experts increases. Through exercising a kind of power, technological artifacts play an ambiguous role. In this sense, the rather specific phenomenon dealt with can point to the place these artifacts occupy in a society where the logic of risk, or at least that of risk management (Power, 2004), gains salience. The analysis of the performative role of technologies offered here sheds light on aspects of the collective and individual need to deal with uncertainty brought about by the "Janus-faced consequences of human decisions" (Beck, 2006: 333) and, hopefully, demonstrates the continuing importance of posing questions concerning the changing character of risk and uncertainty and the strategies devised to deal with this dynamic development.

## ACKNOWLEDGMENTS

I wish to thank the specialists and clinicians, especially the WIN Consortium operational team, who kindly agreed to be interviewed for this research and review drafts of this paper. I also thank my instructor, Prof. DaniFilc. Thanks also to Rony Blank from McGill University, Dr. Katrin Amelang from Goethe University Frankfurt, the participants of the panel on quantification at the EASST conference, Torun, Poland, September 2014, and the participants of the PhD workshops in the Department of Politics and Government, Ben-Gurion University of the Negev, Israel, for commenting on earlier versions of the text. My gratitude to Talya Ezrahi for her devoted editing. Transcriptions were funded with the assistance of a grant from the Israel Science Foundation.

## REFERENCES

Beck, U. (1992). *Risk Society: Towards a New Modernity.* London: Sage Publications.

Beck, U. (2006). Living in the world risk society. *Economy and Society,* 35(3), 329–345.

Beck, U. (2009). *World at Risk*. Cambridge: Polity.

Berg, M. and Bowker, G. (1997). The multiple bodies of the medical record: Toward a sociology of an artifact. *The Sociological Quarterly*, 38(3), 513–537.

Booth, C. M. and Eisenhauer, E. A. (2012). Progression-free survival: Meaningful or simply measurable? *Journal of Clinical Oncology*, 30: 1030–1033.

Bourret, P., Keating, P. & Cambrosio, A. (2011). Regulating diagnosis in post-genomic medicine: Re-aligning clinical judgment. *Social Science & Medicine*, 73: 816–824.

Butler, J. (1997). *Excitable Speech: A Politics of the Performative.* New York: Routledge.

Canguilhem, G. (1989). *The Normal and the Pathological.* New York: Zone Books.

Davis, J., Ma, P. & Sutaria, S. (2010). *The Microeconomics of Personalized Medicine.* Palo Alto, CA: McKinsey.

Dean, M. (2010). *Governmentality: Rule and Power in Modern Society.* London: Sage.

Dean, M. (2012). The signature of power. *Journal of Political Power*, 5: 101–117.
Ewald, F. (1991). *Insurance and Risk*. In G. Burchell, C. Gordon & P. Miller (Eds.), *The Foucault Effect: Studies in Governmentality, with Two Lectures by and an Interview with Michel Foucault* (pp. 197–210). Chicago: The University of Chicago Press.
Feinstein Kean Healthcare & Silver, M. (2009). *The Case for Personalized Medicine*. Washington: Personalized Medicine Coalition.
Flyvbjerg, B. (2011). *Case Study*. In N.K. Denzin and Y.S. Lincoln (Eds.), The SAGE *Handbook of Qualitative Research* (4th ed., pp. 301–316). London: Sage Publications.
Foucault, M. (1978). *The History of Sexuality, Volume I: An Introduction* (R. Hurley, Trans.). New York: Pantheon Books.
Foucault, M. (1991). *Governmentality*. In G. Burchell, C. Gordon and P. Miller (Eds.), *The Foucault Effect: Studies in Governmentality, with Two Lectures by and an Interview with Michel Foucault* (pp. 87–104). Chicago: The University of Chicago Press.
Friese, S. (2014). *Qualitative Data Analysis with ATLAS.ti*. London: Sage.
Goffey, A. (2008). *Algorithm*. In M. Fuller (Ed.), *Software Studies: A Lexicon* (pp. 15–20). Cambridge, MA: MIT Press.
Hacking, I. (1996). *The Looping Effects of Human Kinds*. In D. Sperber, D. Premack & A.J. Premack (Eds.), *Causal Cognition: A Multi-Disciplinary Debate* (351–383). Oxford: Clarendon Press.
King, A. (2010). 'Membership matters': Applying Membership Categorisation Analysis (MCA) to qualitative data using Computer-Assisted Qualitative Data Analysis (CAQDAS) Software. *International Journal of Social Research Methodology*, 13(1), 1–16.
Kowalski, R. (1979). Algorithm = Logic + Control. *Communications of the ACM*, 22(7), 424–436.
Lazar, V., Soria, J.-C., Ducreux, M. & Tursz, T. (2011). *Method for Predicting Efficacy of Drugs in a Patient* (WO 2011/003911 A1). France: World Intellectual Property Organization.
Lepper, G. (2000). *Categories in Text and Talk: A Practical Introduction to Categorization Analysis*. London: Sage.
Lukes, S. (2005). *Power: A Radical View*. Houndmills, Basingstoke: Palgrave.
Mackenzie, A. (2005). The performativity of code: Software and cultures of circulation. *Theory, Culture & Society*, 22: 71–92.
Mackenzie, A. (2006). *Cutting Code: Software and Sociality*. New York: Peter Lang.
Mendelsohn, J. (2013). Personalizing oncology: Perspectives and prospects. *Journal of Clinical Oncology*, 31(15), 1904–1911. doi: 10.1200/jco.2012.45.3605
Nelson, N.C., Keating, P., & Cambrosio, A. (2013). On being 'actionable': Clinical sequencing and the emerging contours of a regime of genomic medicine in oncology. *New Genetics and Society*, 32: 405–428.
O'Malley, P. (2008). *Governmentality and Risk*. In J.O. Zinn (Ed.), *Social Theories of Risk and Uncertainty: An Introduction* (pp. 52–75). Oxford: Blackwell.
Orlikowski, W.J. (2005). Material works: Exploring the situated entanglement of technological performativity and human agency. *Scandinavian Journal of Information Systems*, 17: 183–186.
Pansardi, P. (2012). Power to and power over: Two distinct concepts of power? *Journal of Political Power*, 5: 73–89.
Power, M. (2004). *The Risk Management of Everything: Rethinking the Politics of Uncertainty*. London: Demos.
Totaro, P., & Ninno, D. (2014). The concept of algorithm as an interpretative key of modern rationality. *Theory Culture & Society*, 31: 29–49.

Weir, L. (1996). Recent developments in the government of pregnancy. *Economy and Society*, 25(3), 373–392.

Winner, L. (1980). Do artifacts have politics? *Daedalus*, 109(1), 121–136.

Wood, F., Prior, L. & Gray, J. (2003). Translations of risk: Decision making in a cancer genetics service. *Health, Risk & Society*, 5: 185–199.

Worldwide Innovative Networking in personalized cancer medicine Consortium (2012, June 28).*Official launch of the clinical, academic and international trial WINTHER: A bioinformatics scoring system that predicts the response to known treatments for each patient* [Press release]. Paris.

Worldwide Innovative Networking in personalized cancer medicine Consortium (2013, September 3).*WIN Consortium receives 3 Million Euro EU FP7 grant to conduct WINTHER, WIN's first cancer personalized medicine clinical trial* [Press release]. Paris.

Yin, R.K. (2009). *Case Study Research: Design and Methods*. London: Sage Publications.

Zinn, J.O. (2008). *A Comparison of Sociological Theorizing on Risk and Uncertainty*. In J.O. Zinn (Ed.), *Social Theories of Risk and Uncertainty: An Introduction* (pp. 168–210). Oxford: Blackwell.

# 6 Balancing Risk and Recovery in Mental Health

## An Analysis of the Way in Which Policy Objectives Around Risk and Recovery Affect Professional Practice in England

*Jeremy Dixon*

## INTRODUCTION

In this chapter, I explore two dominant themes within mental health care today—risk and recovery. Concern about the risk that people with a mental disorder may pose to themselves or others is not new, although members of the public tend to significantly overestimate how significant this is (Markowitz, 2011). My focus in this chapter is on professional practice in England where evidence-based practices have had a significant influence on policy makers since the 1990s (Flynn, 2002; Harrison, 2009). This has led to an increase in law and policy focused on risk management. The most significant of these was the Mental Health Act 2007 (DH, 2007a), which introduced powers for some patients to receive compulsory treatment in the community. In addition, this mental health policy directed professionals and individuals to assess and manage risk in certain ways. However, a focus on risk only tells half of the story. In line with the US, the UK government has adopted a focus on recovery within mental health policy. The mental health literature is now awash with articles focusing on recovery, although what recovery means remains contested. Common to most definitions is a vision that service users should be enabled to define what recovery means for them. This poses an implicit challenge to mental health professionals seeking to frame and manage risk. It also opens up the question of who is enabled to define concepts of risk and recovery and how conflicts are resolved. Within this chapter, I am concerned to highlight different interpretations of risk and recovery before considering how they have been adopted within mental health law and policy. In outlining these structures, it is recognised that legal and policy frameworks act to provide an ideal by government as to how mental illness should be managed and that they do not in themselves represent a social reality. I seek to balance this through providing examples from the research literature as to how these concepts have been interpreted or resisted by professionals.

Governmentality theory provides a useful means through which to analyse the extent to which professionals are shaped by and respond to mental health law and policy. The theory draws on Foucault's (1991) analysis of the way in which the exercise of power changed in Europe between the sixteenth and seventeenth centuries from one in which compliance was enforced through public displays of punishment to a more complex system of governance formed "by the institutions, procedures, analyses and reflections, the calculations and tactics that allow [for] the exercise of this very specific albeit complex form of power" (1991, 102). In other words, it provides an account of how the mechanisms for exercising power became more diffuse with a greater reliance on organisational and professional knowledge. Foucault notes that this change came about in recognition of beliefs that aspects of society such as 'population' and 'economy' had their own laws (such as patterns of births and deaths within the population). In addition to this, individuals were also seen to be self-regulating. These aspects of everyday life needed to be taken into account if effective governance were to occur. This then led to recognition that effective governance could not be enacted by obedience to the sovereign or to the rule of law alone. This did not mean that governments relinquished all control over individuals or professionals. Governmental power remained important as a means of legitimating professional responses, and governments might act to shape professional responses through law and policy. When considering the effects of governance mechanisms, the question then becomes, "Who governs what? According to what logics? With what techniques? Towards what ends?" (Rose et al., 2006, 85). In thinking about how risk has come to be governed in England we therefore need to focus on the development of professional knowledge on risk before considering how such knowledge has come to be adapted within law and policy and how such policy has been interpreted.

## THE DEVELOPMENT OF RISK THINKING AMONGST MENTAL HEALTH PROFESSIONALS

In his development of Foucault's theory, Castel (1991) identifies how psychiatry developed as an organisational site of power through particular forms of social control. Castel is concerned to chart the centrality that risk practices have come to play in psychiatric thinking. A key part of Castel's argument is the way in which psychiatry had become concerned with managing risk. Castel argued that psychiatry went through significant developments as a discipline between the late eighteenth to early nineteenth centuries in which diagnostic systems to identify mental disorder were developed. These systems were concerned with assessing both symptoms of illness and levels of danger within individuals. Where 'dangerousness' was detected, this was seen to be an intrinsic quality within individuals, meaning that they might pose a future threat to themselves or to other people. Asylum treatment was generally to be the appropriate response to such concerns in this period. Although Castel traces challenges to this approach as dating back to the 1850s, he identifies the 1960s as a period where risk thinking came to change policy objectives. This was seen to be as a result of arguments by 'preventative psychiatrists' in the US campaigning for care in the community. Castel notes that to enhance their credibility, both psychiatrists and social care professionals developed techniques allowing them to identify factors which might lead to future illness at a population level. In doing so, practitioners made a distinction between risk and danger with risk being judged to be, "the effect of a combination of abstract factors which rendered more or less probable the occurrence of undesirable modes of behaviour in the future" (287). His paper went on to predict that psychiatrists would move to a system in which they came to govern risk at a distance through what Castel terms 'the epidemiological clinic'. In other words, monitoring and management would increasingly take place at a population level, reducing the need for face-to-face contact.

Castel's predictions as to the future directions of psychiatric thinking can be seen to be accurate in many respects. A review of the psychiatric literature reveals that by the 1990s the concept of risk had largely come to replace that of dangerousness (Rose, 1998). This change can be seen to have been largely driven by researchers from the MacArthur Research Network on Mental Health and the Law in the US (Monahan, 1981; Steadman and Concozza, 1974). These researchers were concerned about inaccurate predictions of dangerousness and its effect on civil liberties. They noted that the majority of psychiatrists used clinical assessments when making predictions about future danger in which an individual practitioner made predictions based only on his or her own knowledge and experience. They noted that psychiatrists tended to over-predict how dangerous offenders were likely to be in the future with Monahan's study finding that only one of three predictions was accurate. When summarising his findings, Monahan noted that,

> A great deal of research over the past 25 years indicates that the validity of clinical risk assessments of violence is at best, only modestly better than chance. This means that many people hospitalized as dangerous are in fact perfectly safe and that some people discharged from hospital—or never hospitalized at all are tragically violent in the community. We thought that this state of affairs was unacceptable and that it was scientifically possible to do better.
>
> (Virginia Journal, 1999, 21)

As a result of this, researchers from the MacArthur Research network and other mental health researchers sought to develop assessment tools which would improve upon the abilities of individual practitioners. As a result of this, a number of 'actuarial risk assessments' were developed. As the term 'actuarial' implies, these assessments borrowed heavily from the insurance industry and aimed to calculate the likelihood of future outcomes through charting whether an individual exhibits certain risk factors or not. In order to do this, known characteristics of the service user such as their age, gender, mental health characteristics and drug use were compared against statistical data in order to generate a probability statement.

Whilst the use of actuarial risk assessment models is still advocated by some, a number of researchers noted shortcomings with this model of assessment based on concerns that such assessments drew largely on static data (such as gender or age), failed to take into account individual factors and had a low predictive validity when applied to individual cases (Hart and Coke, 2013). Such concerns led to the development of risk assessment models using 'structured professional judgement' in which practitioners are informed by actuarial data but also use their discretion to interpret them to the profile of an individual. Whilst these assessments allow practitioners a degree of freedom, significant emphasis is placed on adherence to evidence-based guidelines as a means to channel decision making (Hart and Cooke, 2013). However, the degree to which such tools have been adopted is debatable. The following section will outline some of the arguments for and against adopting risk assessment tools adopted by academics within the mental health field. This will then provide the context for a discussion of policy and the degree to which structured risk assessments have been adopted within practice.

## PROFESSIONAL DISPUTES OVER THE USE OF RISK MANAGEMENT TOOLS

Governmentality theorists have argued that governments act to monitor and manage populations through the use of professional knowledge. However, professional knowledge is often contested and so attention needs to be paid to tensions within professional groups. As I noted earlier, since Castel's (1991) thesis was published, a wide range of risk assessment tools have been developed. These can no longer be seen to be the specialist concern of forensic mental health services that deal with mentally disordered offenders, and there are now over 150 instruments designed to predict violence in psychiatric populations (Singh et al., 2011). However, expert opinion amongst mental health professionals on the extent to which such tools should be used remains divided, with arguments centring on the ethics of their use. The following section will therefore focus on these tensions in order to provide a context to discussions on the development of mental health policy.

Whilst a range of risk assessment tools have been developed since the 1980s, a number of mental health professionals and researchers remain sceptical about their utility. These individuals have raised a number of concerns about the adoption of standardised risk tools in practice. The first is the predictive validity of risk tools (Large et al., 2014; Ryan et al., 2010; Szmukler and Rose, 2013). Put simply, these writers have highlighted that violent acts by people with a mental health problem are extremely rare once factors such as drug misuse have been taken into account. It is argued that these low base rates have an effect on the prescriptive accuracy of risk instruments, meaning that there is a high probability that the predictions generated by such tools will be incorrect. This then may have serious consequences for service users who are detained or given coercive treatment on the basis of such predicted risk. The use of such tools may also have negative consequences on trust between mental health professionals and service users, with service users being less likely to share personal information in cases where they believe that it will contribute to risk assessments. Second, sceptics have argued that risk assessments discriminate against those with a mental health problem. These authors point out that whilst people with mental health problems may be given compulsory treatment on the basis of professional risk predictions, this is not the case for other offenders without a mental disorder, such as perpetrators of domestic violence (Szmukler and Rose, 2013). Consequently, the use of coercive powers is seen to be unjustified.

By contrast, advocates of risk assessment tools tend to emphasise risk assessment as a public duty. Whilst advocates of risk assessments acknowledge that only a small proportion of people with mental health problems may go on to act violently, they tend to emphasise risk assessment as a science which may be developed to increase accurate predictions of future danger. For example, in his foreword to Anthony Maden's book 'Treating Violence', Professor Louis Appleby (National Clinical Director for Health and Criminal Justice) writes,

> in one sense it does not matter that serious violence by mentally ill people is rare—plane crashes are rare but we expect airlines to do everything they can do to improve safety. The response of mental health services should be similar and the result should be better, more comprehensive packages of care for many patients, prevention of catastrophe for a few.
> (Maden, 2007, v)

Maden himself advocates risk assessment as a necessity. He argues that the public (rightly in his view) demand that mental health professionals control the risk of violence that those with a mental disorder might pose to others. Not grappling with these problems is seen to invite the politicians to impose risk management structures on clinicians which may be ill informed. Although risk assessment is seen to be imperfect, it is advocated as the most accurate means of establishing which individuals are likely to impose a risk to others and of indicating where compulsory treatment is needed. In Maden's view, where a mental disorder is associated with a risk of violence to others then:

> the risk-benefit scales tilt firmly in favour of intervention. No reticence or apology is needed. The mistake of treating too early will always be more acceptable than the mistake of treating too late.
> (Maden, 2007, 161)

From this perspective, risk assessments are seen to be a professional tool through which intervention might be prioritised and compulsory treatment might be justified.

## THE DEVELOPMENT OF RISK RELATED PRACTICES WITHIN MENTAL HEALTH LAW AND POLICY

In the chapter so far I have been concerned to chart how risk assessment tools have been developed as a means of improving risk prediction. I have also considered tensions amongst professionals about the use of such tools. Whilst governmentality theorists have been concerned to chart the way in which professional knowledge acts to shape the way that populations are governed, power is never completely devolved to professionals. Rather governments are concerned to adopt the correct balance between governing too much or too little (Foucault, 1991). Governments may therefore act to influence professional action through the adoption of law and policies. In the following sections, I will set out how mental health law and policy around risk has developed in England. In doing so, I will highlight the way in which policy makers have drawn selectively on professional knowledge, largely emphasising the arguments of professionals in support of risk management tools. In order to understand these developments it is necessary to first take a step back and consider the closure of the asylums and the adoption of 'care in the community'. I will argue that whilst policies set up to enable community care initially placed more responsibility for risk management with the individual, subsequent policies have been adopted to reassure the public that professionals are identifying and managing high-risk groups. I begin by setting out how the policy of care in the community located risk with individual service.

## THE INDIVIDUALISATION OF RISK WITHIN MENTAL HEALTH SERVICES

In 1961, the government's Minister for Health Enoch Powell signalled an intention to close down UK asylums in his speech to the National Association for Mental Health, labelling them 'doomed institutions'. The subsequent Hospital Plan of 1962 recommended that inpatient services should be moved to general hospitals and the freed up resources should be channelled towards community care. This policy held that local authorities would be responsible for providing social care services, whilst health authorities would provide medical care. However, as local authorities and health authorities tended to prioritise poverty relief and hospital-based services respectively, this led to a high level of inertia (Bartlett and Sandland, 2014), meaning that the move from asylum to community care remained slow. Efforts to galvanise care in the community were made by the Conservative Government of the 1980s. The introduction of the NHS and Community Care Act 1990 (DH, 1990a) (NHSCCA) acted to resolve previous funding blocks, making social services rather than health authorities responsible for commissioning and planning long-term care. However, the NHSCCA was also significant in heralding a new form of welfare. The National Health Service Act 1946 and the National Assistance Act had offered a 'cradle to the grave' service based on notions of national insurance locating risk at a societal level rather than with the individual (Kemshall, 2002). The NHSCCA by contrast introduced market principles into the provision of care under a neo-liberal choice agenda. The introduction of the Care Programme Approach in 1991 (DH/SSI, 1991) applied the principles of the NHSCCA to those with a mental health problem seen by secondary services. Through this mechanism, service users were viewed as consumers of care and were encouraged to choose from a range of services provided by the statutory, voluntary or private sectors with the assistance of a care coordinator. Whilst these policies were framed in terms of 'empowerment', they also acted to place greater responsibility for health and welfare decisions with the service user. As such, these measures can be viewed as a form of what Rose refers to as 'prudentialism', in which risk is located at an individual level and individuals are encouraged to measure and monitor their own risks, drawing on professional advice where necessary (Rose, 2000).

Whilst prudentialism operates within the context of neo-liberal choice agendas, it does not signal a total withdrawal of control. Rather, risk management strategies may become focused on those who are seen as unable, unwilling to manage their own risks or may lack the skills to do so. Theses risk management strategies may operate coercively (for example, through detention) or may be aimed at enabling individuals to take responsibility for their risk (for example, through education programmes) in ways that are sanctioned by professionals (Rose, 2000). As I will demonstrate in the following section, public discussion of mental health risk has come to focus on the high level of risk that those with a mental disorder are perceived to pose to the general public. This has led to 'safety-first' policy agendas which have increasingly directed professionals to make assessments of risk integral to their practice and to take steps to control such risks where service users are found wanting.

## THE MOVE TOWARDS 'SAFETY-FIRST' APPROACHES WITHIN MENTAL HEALTH LAW, POLICY AND GUIDANCE

Although the policy of care in the community had been subject to extensive press criticism in the 1980s, these criticisms had tended to position those with a mental disorder as vulnerable. Attention was focused on the lack of support provided to people who had been discharged from the asylums with inadequate funding, service rivalry and poor management being seen as to blame (Alaszewski, 1999; Rose, 2011). A significant shift in public perception took place in the 1990s with an emphasis being placed on the danger that those with a mental disorder might pose towards themselves or others. This shift in emphasis can be seen to have been triggered by two mental health cases which received a high level of press attention. The first was the case of Christopher Clunis, a young black man with schizophrenia. Clunis stabbed and killed a musician named Jonathan Zito, who was unknown to him, in a London tube station in December 1992. The second case was that of Ben Silcott, a mental health service user who was badly mauled after climbing into a lion's enclosure at London zoo two weeks after Clunis attacked Jonathan Zito.

The Silcott case prompted an immediate response from the Conservative Government, who announced a seven-point plan proposing new powers such as supervised discharge (Hallam, 2002). The subsequent Clunis inquiry (Ritchie et al., 1994) aimed to examine the circumstances of Clunis's admission and treatment. The inquiry highlighted a long list of deficiencies in the way that mental health services had been organised. However, what was significant was the way in which the inquiry highlighted Clunis as being illustrative of high-risk service users in the community. For example, the panel wrote:

> we have heard time and again throughout the inquiry that Christopher Clunis is not alone, that there are many more like him living in the community who are a risk either to themselves or others.
>
> (para 42.1.2)

Whilst the panel acknowledged that the majority of people with a mental health problem were not violent, they argued that the continuing success of community care policies relied on the introduction of measures designed to identify and treat the 'significant minority' who posed a danger to themselves or others. A subsequent outcome of the inquiry was a review of the guidance around mental health homicides themselves in which it was established that all future mental health homicides should automatically lead to an inquiry (DH, 1994). Whilst these measures were designed to reassure the public, they had the effect of strengthening public associations between mental disorder and violence with coverage being given before, during and after inquiries (Cairney, 2009). In addition, the findings were often then highlighted by victims groups who would use them as a means for lobbying for greater safety measures.

Following the Clunis inquiry, the Conservative Government issued increasing guidance to professionals outlining the ways in which risk should be assessed and managed. Initial guidance (NHS Executive, 1994) emphasised that risk assessments should be carried out before discharge and should take place within the Care Programme Approach (CPA) (DH, 1990b), which had been designed to provide a coordinated response between health authorities and social services departments. Subsequent guidance advised that an assessment of risk should form part of all mental health assessments (DH, 1995). The New Labour Government furthered directives to professionals around risk assessment. In his letter to the chair of the mental health reference group, the Health Secretary Frank Dobson pledged to expand mental health services but also promised to provide more assertive forms of treatment for a 'small but significant minority' (BBC, 1998). New Labour's reconfiguration of mental health services through the National Service Framework (DH, 1999) aimed to make services 'safe, sound and supportive' both through the expansion of services and through a refocusing of service provision, including greater training for staff around risk assessment.

However, the government also felt more coercive measures were necessary to manage risk. Proposed measures for targeting this population included community treatment orders (which would act to allow compulsory psychiatric treatment in the community) and preventative detention for those diagnosed with a severe and enduring personality disorder through the introduction of a mental health bill. The government's attempts to introduce such measures were met with prolonged opposition from the Mental Health Alliance, a broad grouping of mental health professionals, lawyers and user rights groups. The concerns expressed by members of this group were diverse. User groups were concerned with the increased restrictions being proposed for service users with mental health problems. Whilst some forensic mental health practitioners welcomed new powers to detain those with untreatable severe and antisocial personality disorders, there was significant unease amongst community psychiatrists about the possibility of taking on the role of 'jailor' for such groups (Pilgrim, 2007). In the face of this opposition, plans for a new mental health bill were abandoned and a decision was made instead to introduce an amendment act (DH, 2007a). However, whilst the government offered a number of concessions to the various groups opposing their initial legislation (such as greater access to advocacy and appeals), it maintained its key objective of introducing 'safety-first' legislation with greater calls on professionals to assess and monitor risk (Pilgrim and Ramon, 2009).

Whilst the Mental Health Acts of 1959 and 1983 had allowed for compulsory treatment, the Mental Health Act 2007 was the first to introduce the term 'risk' into the legislation itself.[1] However, the new legislation and the related Code of Practice did not provide guidance to practitioners as to how risk should be defined. Rather the code instructed practitioners to weigh the interests of the patient against considerations of risk and to carry out locally agreed risk assessment policies. Whilst some broad illustrations of what might count as risk were provided (for example that practitioners should look to see whether service users were at risk of suicide, self-harm, self-neglect or reckless conduct when considering compulsory admission) (DH, 2007b, para 4.6), these did not delimit decision making in any way. However, whilst risk was not defined, the new legislation did give practitioners new powers to manage it. The Mental Health Act 2007 (DH, 2007a) broadened the definition of mental disorder and removed a number of exclusions that had existed under the Mental Health Act 1983.[2] These new measures allowed those with severe and antisocial personality disorders to be treated in hospital, even where such treatment would not bring about any improvement in their condition. In addition, community treatment orders were introduced with a view to reducing the amount of 'revolving door patients' who would become mentally unwell after leaving hospital, leading to readmission (Hansard, HL, Vol. 687, cols 656, 657). It was anticipated by the government that such service users would benefit from "a structure designed to promote safe community living" (ibid). This structure took the form of mandatory and discretionary conditions within the community treatment order which might be imposed on service users who had been admitted under section 3 of the MHA (a compulsory admission to hospital for treatment).[3] Consequently, the definitions of risk applied by mental health professionals had a new salience in that they acted to restrict the freedoms that service users in the community who had previously had the freedom to accept or refuse treatment. However, whilst professionals were being provided with new powers to control and manage risk, they were also faced with guidance urging them to enable service users to take risks in their own lives and to avoid defensive risk practice. This guidance was provided as part of the government's drive towards creating services based on notions of recovery which will be examined in the following section.

## RISK AND THE RECOVERY AGENDA

The concept of recovery has developed over the last 25 years and is now one of the key concepts within mental health care. In contrast to the narratives around risk, notions of recovery tend to be optimistic in character, emphasising ways in which those with a mental health problem can retain hope and live a meaningful life. However, definitions of recovery remain contested. In order to provide some context for the discussion in this section, I begin by outlining some of the diverse ways in which recovery has been defined. I then use this analysis as a means to discussing how different versions of recovery impact on risk thinking. I then move on to focus on the way that recovery has been adopted within policy within England with a particular focus on the implications for risk management.

Whilst recovery has become a much used term within the current mental health literature, it has no single or stable definition and a distinct tension remains between biomedical and social models of disability within existing debates. As Watson et al. (2014) note, there is a division between writers who identify recovery as an outcome and those who identify recovery as a process. Where recovery is viewed as an outcome it may be viewed as a remission of symptoms, a clinical improvement or by clinically defined outcome measures (such as whether or not a person agrees to accept treatment). Alternatively, recovery may be viewed as a process or as a 'personal journey'. This version of recovery is illustrated in William Anthony's frequently cited definition in which recovery is seen as (1993, 17):

> a deeply personal unique process of changing one's attitudes, values, feelings, goals and roles. It is a way of living a satisfying, hopeful and contributing life, even with those limitations caused by illness, recovery involves the development of a new meaning and purpose in life as one grows beyond the catastrophic effects of mental illness.

However, this concept of recovery as a process has been interpreted in a number of ways. On the one hand, this concept has been used as a means to promote psychosocial rehabilitation. From this perspective, recovery is not just about symptom remission but may also be aligned to wider rehabilitative goals, such as housing, living skills or an ability for individuals to manage their own mental health (see Watson et al., 2014). However, other authors have been concerned to identify the personal subjective nature of recovery. These authors have challenged the notion of recovery being based on 'recovery from illness' and have argued that recovery should be viewed as the process of 'recovering a life' (Perkins and Slade, 2012). Authors focusing on recovery as a process of 'recovering a life' may either come from the survivor or consumer movements. There are some similarities between the two groups in the sense that both groups seek to challenge professional dominance. However, it is important to note that whilst those coming from a consumer perspective may identify services as being helpful in some instances, survivor groups are distinct in the sense that they challenge the legitimacy of psychiatric constructs altogether (Adame, 2014). From this perspective, psychiatric diagnosis or other professional treatments are viewed as oppressive and the goal of recovery is to achieve separation from the professional mental health system.

These different positions towards recovery have different impacts on the way in which risk may be interpreted and responded to. Whilst the direct focus is not on risk taking, implicit within recovery perspectives is the notion of governance. That is, who should be given the power to define what a mental illness is and to control it? The level of responsibility that professionals should take for identifying risk is then interpreted differently, depending on how recovery is viewed. In cases where recovery is seen to be a biomedical outcome, risk is frequently professionally defined. Whilst authors coming from this perspective do not rule out the value of collaboration, a degree of coercion from professionals may be seen as necessary to enable service users to engage. For example, Silverstein and Bellack write (2008, 1119):

> for people who are severely disabled, highly symptomatic with reality testing difficulties, unwilling to engage in treatment despite severe illness, or at risk of harm to self or others, evidence based-practices . . .

> can help a person regain the ability to self-regulate so that meaningful treatment collaboration is possible.

Seen from this perspective, professionals may need to manage risk in cases where service users might lack the insight to do so for themselves. Other writers focusing on recovery as the process of 'recovering a life' advocate partnership with mental health professionals. In these cases, risk taking may be seen as something which needs to be tolerated by professionals in order that individuals may explore what recovery means to them and eventually obtain it. For example, Deegan writes that,

> in order to support the recovery process mental health professionals must not rob us of the' opportunity to fail. Professionals must embrace the concept of dignity of risk and the right to failure if they are to be supportive of us.
>
> (1996, 97)

From this perspective, recovery is about maximising one's life chances. Whilst professional intervention may still be valued, professionals are asked to permit or facilitate risk taking so that the service user may achieve greater gains in the long run. These approaches may be formalised through shared decision-making initiatives, in which service users make their preferences around risk taking explicit (Adams and Drake, 2006), or through illness self-management programmes in which individuals are encouraged to identify how they would like their illness to be managed (Copeland, 2002). By contrast, psychiatric survivors are suspicious of professional risk assessments on the basis that it acts to legitimise professional models of mental disorder. For example Coleman (2004) argues that mental health professionals act to highlight risk because they are wedded to a model which views mental distress as arising from biological deficit. These notions of risk then act to prevent individuals from recovering, because they continue to identify individuals as 'mentally ill'. Consequently, survivor groups highlight the risks posed to individuals by mental health services, such as the side effects of psychiatric drugs, and advocate a reduction of such risks through the establishment of peer-support services which are separate from professional services (Stastny and Lehmann, 2007).

## THE ADOPTION OF RECOVERY WITHIN MENTAL HEALTH POLICY IN ENGLAND

In the previous section, I outlined the way in which recovery is contested and highlighted different strands within the recovery literature. I also noted that different recovery narratives may see effective risk management as being achieved through professional intervention which might override service user's wishes through partnership agreements or through separation from mental health services. In order to understand how far notions of recovery have altered the way in which risk is assessed and managed within mental health services, I will now examine how recovery has been defined within policy in England. Having done this, I will examine the extent to which theories of recovery affect professional risk judgements.

The concept of recovery first came to light within mental health policy in England through New Labour's National Service Framework (NSF) (DH, 1999). This document set out New Labour's intention to provide a more comprehensive system of care than had existed under the previous administration. Although the document only mentioned the term 'recovery' three times (all in relation to notions of cure), service user involvement was cited as a key principle, and the policy aimed to set out what individuals might expect from mental health providers. The term recovery came to be more firmly aligned with notions of partnership in the Department of Health's (2004) Shared Capabilities Framework. This document extended the notion of user-control and choice. Within this framework, recovery was introduced as a form of partnership working which would enable service users and carers, "to tackle mental health problems with hope and optimism and to work towards a valued lifestyle within and beyond the limits of any mental health problem" (3). The document also acknowledged that recovery should be defined by the individual and not just in terms of cure. Subsequent guidance on recovery issued by the Coalition Government (HM Government, 2011) drew on Anthony's definition of recovery emphasising recovery as a process rather than a remission of symptoms. The document re-emphasised the need for greater service user choice through personal budgets and also outlined the government's intent to view mental health as a public health problem and to increase rates of individual recovery.

Government policy and guidance makes frequent reference to recovery as a process of empowerment (DH, 2004; HM Government, 2011). This sense of empowerment is defined in terms of the ability of individuals to define what their own recovery means to them and to choose the appropriate services to meet this need or to be involved at a community level in commissioning services. However, the degree to which individuals are given the power to define their recovery is limited by professionals who have the power to impose compulsory treatments in some circumstances. These powers may not be immediately obvious, as guidance around risk assessment has increasingly advocated for assessments to be carried out in conjunction with service users and to be based on notions of recovery (DH, 2007c).

However, the guidance draws on a biomedical model of mental disorder. Furthermore, it seeks to standardise the way in which risk is assessed through advocating that all assessments be based on 'structured professional judgement' in which practitioners are informed by actuarial data but also use their discretion to interpret them to the profile of an individual. The adoption of such tools clearly acts to limit the parameters within which recovery can be defined, as these assessments are largely based on medical or psychological constructs and use assessment tools which prioritise evidence in certain ways. Despite the language of service user empowerment, mental health professionals are clearly instructed to monitor whether the risk choices that individuals are taking are acceptable. For example, the Shared Capabilities Framework advocated that professionals should aim to "[empower] the person to decide the level of risk they are prepared to take with their health and safety" (17), but should also control long-term risk behaviours through "medical and psycho-social interventions . . . e.g. through use of medication, anger management, supportive counselling etc." (18).

Similarly, the Best Practice in Managing Risk (DH, 2007c) guidance advises professionals that there will always be circumstances in which professionals have to prioritise concerns about a service users risk over the person's own wishes. Consideration of detention under the Mental Health Act 1983 is highlighted as one option which may need to be considered in such cases. As such, recovery can be seen to have been reduced to a form of prudential decision making (Rose, 2000) in which service users are encouraged to utilise the market in order to individualise and optimise their own care. Whilst this does not prevent a service user from taking risks in their own lives, these freedoms are highly dependent on professional risk judgements.

## THE BALANCING OF RISK AND RECOVERY OBJECTIVES WITHIN MENTAL HEALTH SERVICES

That chapter so far has examined the way that professional knowledge around risk has developed and the way in which policy makers have tried to encourage practitioners to adopt certain risk practices. A criticism of governmentality theory is that it views individuals as easily manipulable and gives insufficient account to human agency (Taylor-Gooby and Zinn, 2006). Whilst individuals may be encouraged or compelled to engage with risk assessment practices, such assessments may not always be applied in their pure form (Horlick-Jones, 2003) and attention therefore needs to be paid to how they are interpreted or applied by practitioners. In the following section, I draw on research evidence in order to evaluate the degree to which risk assessment tools have changed professional practice and consider how far these practices align with recovery objectives. Research in this area remains limited, so the picture presented here is somewhat piecemeal. My objective however is to examine whether recovery objectives can mitigate against a focus on risk within services.

Following the government's guidance to mental health practitioners on risk (DH, 2007c), efforts have been made to encourage mental health trusts to benchmark their practice against the core principles contained in the document (Logan et al., 2011). Whilst case studies indicate that some trusts made considerable efforts to standardise risk assessment practices (Hunt, 2011;

Fountain and McKee, 2011; Strathdee et al., 2011), audits have revealed significant variations in practice amongst professionals (Bowers, 2011; Hunt, 2011). Research by Hawley et al. (2010) in one English county noted a division between professional groups in their attitude to risk assessment pro formas. The study found that whilst inpatient nurses had the most positive views towards risk assessment pro formas, psychiatrists tended to be least enthusiastic with community nurses adopting a more ambivalent stance.

The authors suggest that these differences may be explained by the utility of risk assessment tools for different professional groups, with medics being concerned with issues such as diagnosis and treatment and inpatient nurses being more concerned with issues of safety on the ward. Research by Godin (2004) also reveals ambivalent views amongst community psychiatric nurses. He notes that some nurses embraced the concept of risk assessment, believing that it acted to standardise practice and to justify their decisions, whilst others were more antagonistic towards it. Godin argues that both groups of nurses exhibited resistance to what they saw as the encroaching trend towards actuarialism. This resistance took the form of nurses laying claim to 'intuition' or tacit knowledge as a necessary part of risk assessment.

Whilst standardised risk assessment practice may be resisted by some professionals, research indicates that the increased policy focus on risk does act to frame professional practice. Whilst professionals may not always embrace risk technologies, they are highly aware that law and policy has put increasing demands on them to identify risks. Research in community settings indicates that both psychiatrists (Passmore and Leung, 2002) and mental health social workers (Warner, 2006) worry about the effects of mental health inquiries on their own professional reputations and that these concerns lead to increased defensive decision taking. Workers are aware that inquiries seek to attribute blame to individual workers and imagine how their practice would stand up should a service user that they are caring for go on to harm others (Brown and Calnan, 2013). Whilst workers may be critical of the way in which risks act to shape practice, they often continue to focus on agency risk policies, increased record keeping or multidisciplinary decision making as a means of protecting themselves should an adverse event occur (Robertson and Collinson, 2011; Warner, 2006).

Professionals may also act to protect their professional reputation through identifying who is responsible for managing risk behaviours. For example, social workers in Warner and Gabe's (2004) research were keen to differentiate between cases in which service users suffered from a personality disorder (who were then viewed to be responsible for their own risk behaviours) and service users suffering from a mental illness (who were judged to be incapable of managing their own risks). In addition, professionals may seek to shift the responsibility of managing a service user's risks to another service, such as a Crisis Resolution and Home Treatment Team (Rhodes and Giles, 2014).

Whilst the increase in defensive practice is a common theme within the research literature, it is not the case that professionals act defensively on all occasions. In several research studies, groups of mental health professionals have been critical of the move towards conservative decision making based around risk (Buckland, 2014; Godin, 2004; Rhodes and Giles, 2014; Robertson and Collinson, 2011; Nolan and Quinn, 2012). In making conscious decisions to enable service users to take risks, professionals could be seen to be drawing on some of the recovery principles as set out in policy. That is, that, "risk management should be conducted in a spirit of collaboration and based on a relationship between the service user and their carers that is as trusting as possible" (DH, 2007c, 5).

Research indicates that mental health workers appreciate that service users need to be enabled to take risks and that this process is dependent on a level of trust between service user and professionals (Brown and Calnan, 2013; Robertson and Collinson, 2011). This process of building trust is complicated by the fact that service users may have been given coercive treatment in the past or may view professionals as authority figures (Brown and Calnan, 2013). Mental health workers in Robertson and Collinson's (2011) research indicated that they drew explicitly on strength-based approaches in order to focus on service users' achievements in this way. However, this process was frequently referred to as 'gambling' by staff, with different workers differing in the thresholds of risk they were willing to enable.

Whilst workers in the research projects indicated that they had used principles of partnership in their work, it was often unclear how explicit communication about risk was between service users and professionals. However, research elsewhere (Langan and Lindow, 2004) has indicated that staff often choose not to share risk assessments with service users on the grounds that they 'lacked insight' or that sharing assessments might cause service users to withdraw from services. More recent research with mentally disordered offenders also indicates that information contained in risk assessments is rarely made explicit to service users (Dixon, 2012).

Whilst professionals may act to promote positive risk taking with service users, they are also aware of their own duties to prevent service users from taking harmful risks. As I have argued in previous sections, current guidance to professionals indicates that use of the Mental Health Act 1983 should be considered in cases where there is an immediate risk to others and that this guidance views "knowledge and understanding of mental health legislation . . . [as] an important component of risk management" (DH, 2007c, 5). However, it is important to examine how considerations of risk are applied when mental health professionals make decisions about whether to detain an individual under the Mental Health Act 1983. In order for an individual to be detained under the Mental Health Act 1983 for assessment or treatment, an application must be made by an Approved Mental Health Professional which must be supported by two medical recommendations.

Peay (2003) asked professionals to respond to case vignettes in order to assess how they made judgements about compulsory admission. She noted that decision makers often used a low threshold of risk when deciding to detain based on whether a risk was conceivable (whether it could happen) as opposed to foreseeable (whether it was likely to happen). Buckland's (2014) research into decision making by Approved Mental Health Professionals found that whilst a variety of positions was presented by Approved Mental Health Professionals, these professionals had to make decisions within an assessment about which forms of evidence they chose to prioritise. For example, evidence-based practices and research evidence were used by one Approved Mental Health Professional to validate detention as a means of promoting recovery on the basis that, "people's illnesses are harder to recover from the longer that they're not treated, so the research says" (8).

Whilst the aforementioned account appears to draw on a biomedical model, others in the research were more sceptical of medically oriented explanations of recovery. However, in these instances, a degree of pessimism about recovery was expressed with these participants indicating that they made applications because they could see no other way forward.

## CONCLUSION

This chapter has drawn on governmentality theory as a means of examining the priority given to notions of risk and recovery in mental health policy in the UK and its implications for governance. In setting out mental health policy on risk, government has been concerned to focus professionals' attention on the management of risk. In doing so, they have promoted the use of standardised risk assessment tools. Whilst the government has promoted a policy focus on risk, it has also promoted recovery perspectives. These recovery perspectives have the stated aim of 'empowering' service users to live a hopeful life. However, whilst they give service users the power to define how they would like services to be delivered through the free market, they do not give them the power to challenge dominant medical discourses. Rather, recovery policy acts as a form of prudentialism. That is service users are encouraged to manage their own welfare with the goal of maximising their independence, but these limited rights are dependent on them not being seen to pose a risk to themselves or others.

Factions of mental health practitioners have sought to improve risk assessment practice through developing risk assessment tools. These practices remain contentious, with arguments continuing about their efficacy. Policy makers in England have acted to shape professional practice through providing directives in law, policy and guidance for professionals to adopt such tools. These policies have been promoted on the grounds that practitioners have failed to control a significant minority of service users who pose a risk to others. However, whilst risk is now undoubtedly a central facet of mental health policy, practitioners continue to resist the attempts of governments to standardise their practices.

Nonetheless, concerns by professionals about risk has come to frame professional practice so that practitioners are highly aware of the reputational risk to them should an adverse outcome occur. This then has an effect on the degree to which they are willing to enable service users to define their own recovery. Whilst practitioners might act to enable service users to take positive risks, they are also bound to manage and control their risk taking. In deciding which risks are acceptable, professionals are bound to refer back to legislation which favours a medical model of treatment. This only allows the view of 'recovery as a process' to exist where service users themselves are in agreement with a medical model of mental distress.

## ACKNOWLEDGEMENTS

I would like to thank Professor Nick Gould at the University of Bath for his comments on this chapter.

## NOTES

1. The word 'risk' appears in relation to compulsory treatment in the community and decision making about discharge by the Mental Health Review Tribunal (which makes judgements on legal appeals from detention) (DH, 2007a, sections 17, 20, 41, 43 and 72).
2. The Mental Health Act 2007 (DH, 2007a) adopted a broad definition of mental disorder. This is defined in section 1 of the Mental Health Act 1983 as amended by the Mental Health Act 2007 and is defined as, "any disorder or disability of the mind".
3. Although the government stated that its intent was to target 'revolving door' patients, this was not added as legal criteria, meaning that a Community Treatment Order might be considered after one admission under section 3 of the Mental Health Act 1983 where the necessary criteria are met (outlined in under section 17a of the Mental Health Act 1983).

## REFERENCES

Adame, A. L. (2014). "There needs to be a place in society for madness". The psychiatric survivor movement and new directions in mental health care, *Journal of Humanistic Psychology*, 54 (4) 456–475.

Adams, J. R. and Drake, R. E. (2006). Shared decision-making and evidence-based practice, *Community Mental Health Journal*, 42 (1) 87–105.

Alaszewski, A. (1999). The rise of risk assessment and risk management in the United Kingdom, *International Journal of Public Administration*, 22 (3–4) 575–606.

Anthony, W. A. (1993). Recovery from mental illness: The guiding vision of the mental health service system in the 1990s, *Psychosocial Rehabilitation Journal*, 16 (4) 11–23.

Bartlett, P. and Sandland, R. (2014). *Mental Health Law. Policy and Practice.* Oxford: Oxford University Press.

BBC News (1998). *Health. Dobson Outlines Mental Health Plans* [Online]. http://news.bbc.co.uk/1/hi/health/141651.stm (accessed September 14, 2014].

Bowers, A. (2011). Clinical risk assessment and management of service users. *Clinical Governance: An International Journal*, 16 (3) 190–202.

Brown, P. and Calnan, M. (2013). Trust as a means of bridging the management of risk and the meeting of need: a case study in mental health service provision. *Social Policy & Administration*, 47 (3) 242–261.

Buckland, R. (2014). The decision by approved mental health professionals to use compulsory powers under the Mental Health Act 1983: A Foucauldian discourse analysis. *British Journal of Social Work*, Advance Access 1–14.

Cairney, P. (2009). The 'British policy style' and mental health: Beyond the headlines. *Journal of Social Policy*, 38 (4) 671–688.

Castel, R. (1991). From dangerousness to risk. In: Burchell, G., Gordon, C. and Miller, P. (eds), *The Foucault Effect: Studies in Governmentality.* London: Harvester Wheatsheaf, 281–298.

Coleman, R. (2004). *Recovery: An Alien Concept?* Wormit Fife: P & P Books.

Copeland, M.E. (2002). *Wellness Recovery Action Plan.* West Dummerton, VT: Peach Press.

Deegan, P. (1996). Recovery as a journey of the heart, *Psychiatric Rehabilitation Journal*, 26 (4) 369–376.

Department of Health. (2007a). *The Mental Health Act 2007.* London: Department of Health.

Department of Health. (2007b). *Code of Practice. Mental Health Act 1983.* London: The Stationery Office.

Department of Health. (2007c). *Best Practice in Managing Risk. Principles and Evidence for Best Practice in the Assessment and Management of Risk to Self and Others in Mental Health Services.* London: Department of Health.

Department of Health. (2004). *The Ten Shared Capabilities Framework. A Framework for the Whole of the Mental Health Workforce.* London: Department of Health.

Department of Health. (1999). *A National Framework for Mental Health.* London: Department of Health.

Department of Health. (1995). *Building Bridges. A Guide to Arrangements for Inter-agency Working for the Care and Protection of Severely Mentally Ill People.* London: The Stationery Office.

Department of Health. (1994). *Guidance on the discharge of mentally disordered people and their continuing care in the community. LASSL (94)4*, London: Department of Health.

Department of Health. (1990a). *National Health Service and Community Care Act 1990.* London: Department of Health.

Department of Health. (1990b). *"Care Programme Approach" Circular HC(90)23/LASSL(90)11.* London: Department of Health.

Department of Health/Social Services Inspectorate. (1991). *Care Management and Assessment: Practitioner's Guide.* London: HMSO and Department of Health.

Dixon, J. (2012). Mentally disordered offenders' views of 'their' risk assessment and management plans. *Health, Risk & Society*, 14 (7) 667–680.

Flynn, R. (2002). Clinical governance and governmentality. *Health, Risk & Society*, 4 (2) 155–173.

Foucault, M. (1991). Governmentality. In: Burchell, G., Gordon, C. and Miller, P. (eds), *The Foucault Effect: Studies in Governmentality.* London: Harvester Wheatsheaf, 87–104.

Fountain, L. and McKee, P. (2011). Case Study 3: Learning from Experience—Using Clinical Risk Data to Influence and Shape Clinical Services. In: Whittington, R. and Logan, C. (eds), *Self-Harm and Violence. Towards Best Practice in Managing Risk in Mental Health Services*. Chichester: Wiley-Blackwell, 259–266.

Godin, P. (2004). 'You don't tick boxes on a form': A study of how community mental health nurses assess and manage risk. *Health, Risk & Society*, 6 (4) 347–360.

Hart, S.D. and Cooke, D.J. (2013). Another look at the (Im-) precision of individual risk estimates made using actuarial risk assessment instruments. *Behavioural Sciences & the Law*, 31 (1) 81–102.

Hallam, A. (2002). Media influences on mental health policy: Long-term effects of the Clunis and Silcock cases. *International Review of Psychiatry*, 14 (1) 28–33.

Hansard, HL. Vol. 687, cols 656, 657.

Harrison, S. (2009). Co-optation, commodification and the medical model: Governing UK medicine since 1991. *Public Administration*, 87 (2) 184–197.

Hawley, C.J., Gale, T.M., Sivakumaran, T. and Littlechild, B. (2010). Risk assessment in mental health: Staff attitudes and an estimate of time cost. *Journal of mental health*, 19 (1) 88–98.

HM Government and Department of Health. (2011). *No Health Without Mental Health: A Cross-Governmental Outcome Strategy for People of All Ages*. London: Department of Health.

Horlick-Jones, T. (2003). Managing risk and contingency: Interaction and accounting behaviour. *Health, Risk & Society*, 5 (2) 221–228.

Hunt, K. (2011). Case Study 2: Narrowing the Gap between Policy and Practice. In: Whittington, R. and Logan, C. (eds), *Self-Harm and Violence. Towards Best Practice in Managing Risk in Mental Health Services*. Chichester: Wiley-Blackwell, 251–258.

Kemshall, H. (2002). *Risk, Social Policy and Welfare*. Maidenhead: Open University Press.

Langan, J. and Lindow, V. (2004). *Living with Risk. Mental Health Service User Involvement in Risk Assessment and Management*. Bristol: The Policy Press.

Large, M.M., Ryan, C.J., Callaghan, S., Paton, M.B. and Singh, S.P. (2014). Can violence risk assessment really assist in clinical decision-making?. *Australian and New Zealand journal of psychiatry*, 48 (3) 286–288.

Logan, C., Nedopil, N. and Wolf, T. (2011). Guidelines and Standards for Managing Risk in Mental Health Services. In: Whittington, R. and Logan, C. (eds), *Self-Harm and Violence. Towards Best Practice in Managing Risk in Mental Health Services*. Chichester: Wiley-Blackwell, 145–162.

Maden, A. (2007). *Treating Violence: A Guide to Risk Management in Mental Health Services*. New York: Oxford University Press.

Markowitz, F.E. (2011). Mental illness, crime, and violence: Risk, context, and social control. *Aggression and Violent Behaviour*, 16 (1) 36–44.

Monahan, J. (1981). *The Clinical Prediction of Violent Behaviour*. Washington, DC: Government Printing Office.

NHS Executive. (1994). *Guidance on the Discharge of Mentally Disordered People and Their Continuing Care in the Community*. HSG(94)27. Health Publication Unit: Heywood.

Nolan, D., and Quinn, N. (2012). The context of risk management in mental health social work. *Practice*, 24 (3) 175–188.

Passmore, K., and Leung, W.C. (2002). Defensive practice among psychiatrists: A questionnaire survey. *Postgraduate Medical Journal*, 78 (925) 671–673.

Peay, J. (2003). *Decisions and Dilemmas: Working with Mental Health Law*. Oxford: Hart Publishing.

Perkins, R. and Slade, M. (2012). Recovery in England: Transforming statutory services? *International Review of Psychiatry*, 24 (1) 29–39.

Pilgrim, D. (2007). New 'mental health' legislation for England and Wales: Some aspects of consensus and conflict. *Journal of Social Policy*, 36 (01) 79–95.
Pilgrim, D. and Ramon, S. (2009). English mental health policy under new labour. *Policy & Politics*, 37 (2) 273–288.
Rhodes, P. and Giles, S.J. (2014). "Risky Business": A critical analysis of the role of crisis resolution and home treatment teams. *Journal of Mental Health*, 23 (3) 130–134.
Ritchie, J., Dick, D. and Lingham, R. (1994). *The Report into the Inquiry of the Care and Treatment of Christopher Clunis*. London: The Stationery Office.
Robertson, J.P. and Collinson, C. (2011). Positive risk taking: Whose risk is it? An exploration in community outreach teams in adult mental health and learning disability services. *Health, Risk & Society*, 13 (2), 147–164.
Rose, N. (2011). Historical changes in mental health practice. In: Thornicroft, G., Szmukler, G., Mueser, K. and Drake, R.E. (eds), *The Oxford Textbook of Community Mental Health*. Oxford: Oxford University Press, 9–18.
Rose, N. (2000). Government and control. *British journal of criminology*, 40 (2) 321–339.
Rose, N. (1998). Governing risky individuals: The role of psychiatry in new regimes of control. *Psychiatry, Psychology and Law*, 5 (2) 177–195.
Rose, N., O'Malley, P., and Valverde, M. (2006). Governmentality. *Annual Review of Law and Social Sciences*, 2, 83–104.
Ryan, C., Nielssen, O., Paton, M., and Large, M. (2010). Clinical decisions in psychiatry should not be based on risk assessment. *Australasian Psychiatry*, 18 (5) 398–403.
Silverstein, S.M., and Bellack, A.S. (2008). A scientific agenda for the concept of recovery as it applies to schizophrenia. *Clinical psychology review*, 28 (7) 1108–1124.
Singh, J.P., Serper, M., Reinharth, J. and Fazel, S. (2011). Structured assessment of violence risk in schizophrenia and other psychiatric disorders: A systematic review of the validity, reliability, and item content of 10 available instruments. *Schizophrenia bulletin*, 37 (5), 899–912.
Stastny, P. and Lehmann, P. (2007). *Alternatives Beyond Psychiatry*. Shrewsbury: Peter Lehmann Publishing.
Steadman, H.J. and Concazza, J. (1974). *Careers of the Criminally Insane: Excessive Control of Deviance*. Lexington, DC: Heath.
Strathdee, G., Garnham, P., Moore, J. and Hansjee, D. (2011). Case Study 1: A Four-Step Model of Implementation. In: Whittington, R. and Logan, C. (eds), *Self-Harm and Violence. Towards Best Practice in Managing Risk in Mental Health Services*. Chichester: Wiley-Blackwell, 239–250.
Szmukler, G., and Rose, N. (2013). Risk assessment in mental health care: Values and costs. *Behavioural Sciences & the Law*, 31 (1), 125–140.
Taylor-Gooby, P. and Zinn, J.O. (2006). Current directions in risk research: New developments in psychology and sociology. *Risk Analysis*, 26 (2) 397–411.
Virginia Journal. (1999). *MacArthur Network: Building an Empirical Foundation for the Next Generation of Mental Health Laws* [Online]. https://www.law.virginia.edu/pdf/vajournal/monahan.pdf [accessed November 14, 2014].
Warner, J. (2006). Inquiry reports as active texts and their function in relation to professional practice in mental health. *Health, Risk & Society*, 8 (3) 223–237.
Warner, J., and Gabe, J. (2004). Risk and liminality in mental health social work. *Health, Risk & Society*, 6(4), 387–399.
Watson, D.P., McCranie, A. and Wright, E.R. (2014). Everything Old Is New Again: Recovery and Serious Mental Illness. In: Kohnson, R.J., Ray Turner, R. and Link, B.G. (eds), *Sociology of Mental Health. Select Topics from 40 years: 1970s–2010s*. Cham: Springer International Publishing, 125–139.

# 7 Moving From Gut Feeling to Evidence

## The Case of Social Work

*Gemma Mitchell*

### INTRODUCTION

The rise of evidence-based practice (EBP) in child and family social work in England has been underpinned by a technocratic response to risk and uncertainty (Webb, 2001; Broadhurst et al., 2010) which continues despite a robust critique of EBP in both medicine and social work. This chapter highlights the complex, more informal practices social workers use to respond to the resulting disparity between the messy, uncertain reality of family life and what is deemed 'acceptable' evidence that can help promote change for children and their families. These findings are based on qualitative interviews with thirty-four qualified and unqualified social workers. It will be argued that 'deep expertise' is required in order to share risk knowledges within the same 'epistemic culture' (Knorr-Cetina, 1999). Deep expertise includes 1) acknowledging the importance of what social workers call 'gut feeling' to practice, which is a specific form of tacit knowledge; and 2) an ability to move from what social workers call 'gut feeling' to evidence which is accepted by the profession and also other groups such as the police, health and education. I argue that social workers are able to facilitate this move by sharing their 'gut feeling' with others using what I call 'adequate explication'. Finally, I will argue that a further sign of deep expertise in child and family social work is the ability to reconcile the use of 'gut feeling' with the dominant EBP approach that underpins the official rules and guidance they must follow.

### RISK AND UNCERTAINTY, SOCIAL WORK, TACIT KNOWLEDGE, EVIDENCE-BASED PRACTICE, EXPERTISE

How do social workers make judgements about children and their families in the 'risk society' when the inherent uncertainty involved is only acknowledged in a perfunctory manner by dominant forms of EBP? That is the question at the heart of this chapter. In order to make these judgements, social workers must share information, and in particular, risk knowledges, with others. Those others include experts in other fields, such as medical professionals, police, teachers and solicitors. A vast amount of literature exists within social work (and beyond) on the complexities involved when experts share information with each other, or multi-agency working, as it is commonly known (for example, Reder et al., 2003; Reder and Duncan, 2003; Lyon et al., 2003; Laurence, 2004; Horwath and Morrison, 2007; White et al, 2015, amongst many others). Nevertheless, there tends to be an assumption within this literature that those within the same field can share information in a fairly straightforward manner.

However, once we start to explore how information is shared in practice, we start to see that the picture is more complex than it first appears. For example, what if we interrogate the way risk knowledges are negotiated within what Knorr-Cetina (1999) would call one 'epistemic culture' or community—social work? In order to do so, we need to acknowledge the context those experts are working in—what Beck (1992) calls the risk society. In this chapter, I will explore one element of the often invisible, more informal practices social workers use as a response to uncertainty in the 'risk society'. In particular, I use a social constructionist approach to reveal the ways in which social workers, as experts, rely on gut feeling, intuition and tacit knowledge when making judgements about the messy and uncertain reality of family life. Further, I explore the way in which they might share this type of knowledge to those within the same epistemic community to promote change for children and their families. The findings are based on qualitative interviews with 34 qualified and unqualified social workers. Drawing on the insights of the sociology of scientific knowledge (SSK) tradition and the research findings, I will argue that a sign of what I call 'deep expertise' in child and family social work is the ability to move from what social workers call gut feeling to acceptable, tangible evidence which is accepted by the profession and also other groups such as the police, health and education.

## SOCIAL WORK, THE RISK SOCIETY AND EVIDENCE-BASED PRACTICE

In the risk society, through a process Beck (1992) calls 'reflexive scientisation', our faith in experts, and science itself, is undermined, thus expert judgements are constantly called into question. Moreover, since the early 1990s, there has been a shift (officially at least) from a needs-based to a risk-based assessment approach in child and family social work (Kemshall, 2002). Webb (2006) argues that in practice, need and risk have been conflated, leading to the 'risk' of 'harm' to children being a central focus of this epistemic community's work.[1] This includes deciding whether a child is at risk or not, what level of risk that is (if there is any) and what to do as a result of those judgements.[2] As part of this shift, social work is heavily audited using standardised, technocratic techniques as a response to an increased sense of uncertainty and decreased faith in this group of experts (Parton, 1996; Webb, 2006; Broadhurst et al., 2010). These developments have been heavily influenced by the rise of EBP, which can be documented not only in medicine but also in child and family social work (Webb, 2001; Adams et al., 2009; Gray et al., 2009).

Here, the term EBP refers not to the use of research in social work per se, but to a particular, dominant form of EBP, which is rooted in the assertion that social workers are better equipped to make informed judgements by basing them on past research and current rules and guidance. Dominant EBP also utilises an 'evidence hierarchy' (Gray et al., 2009: 11), with systematic reviews and randomised controlled trials (RCTs) seen as the 'gold standard' and qualitative research viewed as least reliable forms of evidence. This hierarchy of evidence leads to the promotion of 'risk reduction technologies' which are based on a techno-rational approach to decision making (Webb, 2001; Broadhurst et al., 2010). In this context, it is tempting to assert, as Lord Laming has acknowledged, that all social workers need to do is 'just do it' (Laming, 2009). That is, follow the rules, incorporate what the research says, do what countless serious case reviews have told them to, and expert judgement and decision making will improve.

However, much criticism has been made of EBP in medicine (for example Bazarian et al., 1999; Timmermans and Angell, 2012) and social work (Taylor and White, 2001; Webb, 2001; Broadhurst et al., 2010, Gray et al., 2009, amongst many others). Moreover, risk and uncertainty scholars more generally have argued that the response to uncertainty is more complex than this assertion to 'just do it' allows (Zinn, 2008; Brown, 2013). Further, the SSK literature and many within the social work community, such as O'Sullivan (2005); Adams et al. (2009) and Helm (2010; 2011), have argued that this focus on specific forms of evidence and basing current judgements and decisions on past exemplars[3] ignores the role of professional judgement—when in practice, we need both. Although Gambill, a proponent of EBP, recognises that it should not attempt to remove clinical expertise altogether, she argues that EBP 'is essentially a way to handle uncertainty in an honest and informed manner, sharing ignorance and knowledge' (Gambill, 2006: 340). However, under conditions of uncertainty, 'missing information, time constraints, vague goals and changing conditions' (Klein, 1998: 14) abound, and more than one version of reality can be 'true' at any one time (Taylor and White, 2001). Therefore, the EBP-based approach Gambill advocates does not exist in practice (see, for example, Klein, 1998; Cimino, 1999; Horlick-Jones, 2005; Gillingham and Humphreys, 2010; and Timmermans and Angell, 2012).

Despite a wealth of research, and one of the key findings of the Munro review (2010, 2011a, 2011b)[4] being an emphasis on professional judgement rather than yet more rules and red tape, the social work profession is still guided by a dominant EBP perspective. Moreover, this approach is underpinned by fear, 'moral panic' (Warner, 2011) and 'a cycle of crisis and reform' based on specific, collective emotional politics (Warner, 2011: 1). This remains the case even if policy and guidance make token claims of understanding the inherent uncertainty involved in the profession. Overall, the matter of contention is not the use of research in social work per se, but the narrow definition of evidence which currently shapes dominant EBP discourses in England (Gray et al, 2009; White, 2013). This definition tends to ignore more 'humane' approaches which emphasise so called 'soft skills' and a development of professional knowledge and expertise, particularly with regards to relationship-building (Taylor and White, 2001; Featherstone et al., 2014). Moreover, there is a lack of genuine acknowledgement in dominant EBP discourses of the inherent uncertainty involved when making judgements about the risk of harm to children. This in turn leads to more informal strategies social workers use to respond to this uncertainty being rendered invisible.

This is important because we know from SSK literature that more formal rules and guidance, in particular when used to respond to uncertainty, are only useful to a certain extent. This is because rules and guidance are based on a finite number of past exemplars (Bloor, 1997). Thus, when making a decision on a new case, experts must 'make the next step' (Bloor, 1997) and go beyond these more formal documents by deploying professional judgement. Therefore, we can learn from past mistakes and apply those lessons from individual cases to new rules and guidance, but this will never overcome the inherent uncertainty in this area of expertise. Moreover, a sign of what I call 'deep' expertise is the ability to move away from consciously following rules and guidance and instead move this process to the unconscious (Collins, 2010; Dreyfus and Dreyfus, 1986). As Marie, one of my interviewees, states:

> I think they [rules and guidance] can provide a useful framework and that can be quite freeing as long as you don't think that the rules and guidance are the only things that you need to follow. But I think as long as you see it as being something . . . to base your practice around, I think that's good. As long as you're not then feeling as if you're completely limited by that, and I suppose if you're given guidance about how to do a visit and all you do is go out and answer those questions without, it's a bit like, it's easy to go out and gather information, that's simple, anybody could do that. I could send anybody off the street with a list of questions to go and answer. You've got to be able to take it one stage further and then know how to assess that situation and analyse it and think about what dilemmas might appear—the strengths and vulnerabilities of those people might be on the basis of it. And I would say the same about frameworks and policies and procedures—you can follow them all, but they will never be able to actually help you with those really, really tricky situations, because there isn't a policy and procedure for those one off situations that occur.

(Marie, qualified social worker with supervisory responsibilities, over fifteen years' experience)

This chapter adds to existing research on more informal, less visible practices that help social workers deal with risk and uncertainty when working with children and their families. This includes Taylor and White (2000; 2001); Ferguson (2009); Broadhurst et al. (2010); Helm (2010; 2011) and O'Sullivan (2011), amongst others. One part of these more informal responses is what participants call 'gut feeling', something that is portrayed negatively in certain areas of social work policy and media representation, or what Helm (2010: 121) calls the 'what's bad' literature. I support Klein (1998), Fook et al. (2000); Horlick-Jones (2005); O'Sullivan (2005), Gigerenzer (2007); Ferguson (2009) and Helm (2010) amongst others in arguing that what social workers call 'gut feeling' can be an effective part of judgement and decision making. Taylor and White's influential work has identified how professionals put forward 'truth claims' (Taylor and White, 2000: 6), which include moral judgements about service users' lives (Taylor and White, 2001). Further, it has been argued by O'Sullivan (2005) that explicating our reasoning in social work, including the use of gut feeling, is important.

I build on this research by carrying out a detailed exploration of what social workers mean when they refer to gut feeling. Leaving aside any normative judgements about social work practice, I argue that what participants refer to as 'gut feeling' is what Collins (2010) calls 'collective tacit knowledge'. Moreover, this form of knowledge is an important part of a social worker's toolkit when responding to risk and uncertainty. Further, I use a sociological analysis to explore what has, until now, been a largely invisible process—how this type of knowledge is shared within the same epistemic community. I call this process 'adequate explication'. Crucially, adequate explication enables collective tacit knowledge to be a more visible part of social work judgement, thus enabling social workers to move from what they call gut feeling to evidence in order to promote change for children and their families.

First, clarity will be provided on three terms—gut feeling, intuition and tacit knowledge. Building on existing research emphasising the importance of gut feeling in relation to judgement and decision making, I will use Collins's (2010) typology of tacit knowledge to argue that we need to go back to the *social* when exploring gut feeling as used by experts in practice. I will then move away from Collins's focus on the full explication of tacit knowledge and argue that, in this context, 'adequate' explication is sufficient. I will explore how, through adequate explication, social workers can make what they call gut feeling a more visible part of their judgement, and thus move from this type of tacit knowledge to acceptable evidence that can promote change for children and their families. Moreover, even where, in some cases, gut feeling is not even partially explicable, it is still a useful part of social work practice. Finally, I will argue that a sign of deep expertise in child and family social work is the ability to acknowledge the role of gut feeling as a form of collective tacit knowledge within this epistemic community and reconcile this with the dominant EBP approach that underpins the official rules and guidance they must follow. Prior to the aforementioned, there will be a brief outline of the methodology.

## METHODOLOGY

The findings presented in this chapter are based on thirty-four interviews with practising qualified and non-qualified social workers. No social work students have been included because the focus is on experts in one epistemic community, rather than a comparison between novices and experts, which has been explored previously in relation to social work (for example, Fook et al., 2000; O'Connor and Leonard, 2014). A combination of purposive and snowball sampling was used to recruit participants. The main objective was to recruit as many different levels of experience and seniority as possible, therefore specific individuals were contacted initially to access these different groups. Following this, snowball sampling helped the researcher increase the number of participants. Data were analysed using an abductive approach, an iterative process where going back and forth between reading and data analysis is essential in order to promote creativity and originality (Timmermans and Tavory, 2012). The research complies with University of Leicester ethics regulations.

## GUT FEELING

Throughout the research, it was interesting to hear social workers talk about gut feeling and the centrality of this concept to many participants' judgement. The importance of gut feeling to the participants came to light as data was being collected; therefore, gut feeling was discussed with thirty social workers. Two participants said gut feeling was not part of their practice, and the remaining twenty-eight stated it was important to them, although they differed in relation to whether they accepted it as part of 'professional' judgement and decision making. Moreover, I was surprised to find that this difference affected whether they were able to move from gut feeling to acceptable evidence, which is the way that social workers are able to promote change for children and their families—but how? In order to attempt to answer this question, I will begin by providing clarity on terms used, followed by examples from social workers themselves. It is only then that I will explore how they make the move from what they call gut feeling to acceptable evidence.

First, I should be clear about three terms I am using in this chapter—gut feeling, intuition, and tacit knowledge. It is easy to get stuck on the problem of defining concepts such as these. For example, tacit knowledge is often conflated with practice wisdom, when in fact practice wisdom refers to more general processes than tacit knowledge alone (O'Sullivan, 2005). This confusion over different terms is a legitimate problem, but because the focus here is on how social workers share their knowledge with others, the discussion of this topic will be necessarily brief. I will begin by defining gut feeling, on account of it being the term participants used the most and identified with.

When trying to define gut feeling, one comes across difficulties and disagreements from the start. For example, the *Collins English Dictionary* defines gut feeling as 'an instinctive feeling, as opposed to an opinion based on facts' (Gut Feeling, 2014). It is deceptively simple and a definition that many proponents of EBP might agree with. However, this interpretation is based on what Webb (2001) describes as an unhelpful dichotomy between facts and values. It is also part of what Helm (2010: 121) calls the 'what's bad' literature within social work, which, in terms of gut feeling, portrays this kind of thinking as inherently bad, biased and problematic (Helm, 2010). More specifically, although participants refer to gut feeling and intuition interchangeably (and gut feeling is the term used much more often), gut feeling refers to the embodiment of intuition—it is a sensory experience resulting from a specific type of thinking (Helm, 2010; Gigerenzer, 2007). What is intuition? Gigerenzer neatly describes it as unconscious intelligence:

> 1. that appears quickly in consciousness,
> 2. whose underlying reasons we are not fully aware of, and
> 3. is strong enough to act upon.
>
> (Gigerenzer, 2007: 16)

From now on, gut feeling will be used to refer to both intuition and gut feeling, because it is the term participants used the most. To be clear, when using the term gut feeling, I am referring to unconscious intelligence as Gigerenzer describes it. Gigerenzer challenges the dominant view that gut feeling cannot be understood—he argues that it can and explores this by using a psychological approach, arguing that gut feeling is a combination of heuristics and 'evolved capacities of the brain' (Gigerenzer, 2007: 18). This psychological turn is popular in the social work community, although work on heuristics is often used (in direct opposition to Gigerenzer) to demonstrate the bias inherent in gut feeling (Helm, 2010). However, it is not 'irrational' or inherently biased. Like all other forms of reasoning, it has its flaws, but it also has the potential to be a useful, robust part of judgement and decision making (Helm, 2010).

With regard to this chapter, the important point about gut feeling is that it is inherently difficult to share. In other words, as Reber (1995) has argued, it is a form of tacit knowledge (Zinn, 2008). This is where Collins's work on this subject is so useful, because it helps us go back to the *social*, in order to understand gut feeling from a sociological standpoint. Tacit knowledge is often thought of as a rather static form of knowledge which is impossible to share. This makes apprehension about the use of gut feeling in social work understandable. However, Collins's (2010) typology helps us to understand that tacit knowledge is knowledge that is *either* difficult or impossible to explicate. Therefore, the only thing all tacit knowledge has in common is that it hasn't been made explicit—whether it can or not is a separate matter entirely and is the basis for Collins's typology.[5]

Collins has written extensively on the subject of tacit knowledge (for example, Collins, 1974, 1985, 2001, 2010), although he acknowledges that his earlier work was often based on too vague a definition of the concept (2010). In his influential book, *Tacit and Explicit Knowledge* (2010), Collins draws on but extensively reworks Polanyi's (1966) original creation of the term. Here, the most important part of Collins's argument is the assertion that some forms of tacit knowledge can be made explicit. Therefore, the three types of tacit knowledge which make up his typology are based on how easy or difficult they are to explicate. Collins refers to the three types as relational (weak), somatic (medium) and collective (strong).[6] Briefly, relational knowledge is tacit due to the nature of social relations in any given situation and can be explicated if these change, and somatic tacit knowledge is tacit because the makeup of the human body and brain and is difficult but not impossible to explicate (Collins, 2010). Collective tacit knowledge is the type that is most relevant here, which I discuss below.

## GUT FEELING AND COLLECTIVE TACIT KNOWLEDGE

We all have collective tacit knowledge which we learn through socialisation as 'social parasites' (Collins, 2010: 138). As social workers are part of one 'epistemic culture' (Knorr-Cetina, 1999), they share much of this collective knowledge, thus they have what Collins calls 'social fluency' in this particular group (Collins, 1998). Moreover, social workers in England are in the process of mastering (due to its fluid, ever changing nature, it can never be fully mastered) the collective tacit knowledge of this community. This form of tacit knowledge is located in the collective, rather than the individual (Collins, 2010). Thus psychological explanations of gut feeling will only take us so far. We need to acknowledge the vital role the social context plays in determining why we might get a gut feeling in response to a situation in the first place. Within this epistemic community, individuals will acquire certain types of collective tacit knowledge which allow them to perform the role of social worker. Importantly, this knowledge is contingent, therefore we cannot say 'do this when x happens', because every situation is different and requires a unique response. Let's apply this to child and family social work. Let me give three examples which illustrate that gut feeling in this context is a form of collective tacit knowledge. Claire describes how, in one case, she just knew something was 'wrong':

> There was nothing guttural about it, you could just see it, you know, and everybody would know it.
>
> (Claire, qualified social worker with some supervisory responsibilities, less than five years' experience)

Claire is referring to collective tacit knowledge that she believes 'everyone' would know. Clearly she is referring to knowledge she has learned through socialisation in England and, most importantly, as part of her experience as a social worker. More experienced participants were able to be more specific when talking about gut feeling:

> I think it's how they [service users] relate to you. Eye contact. How relaxed they are in your company. How often they keep distracting you from a certain question. Or they repeatedly answer in the same way and will not move off of a topic and stay with what they think are safe topics. They will disclose something quite minor so you don't look at the major thing.
>
> (Jenny, unqualified social worker with more than fifteen years' experience)

Jenny is able to explain why she might get a gut feeling, which is a form of collective tacit knowledge—she would not know that 'staying with safe topics' is meaningful without her emersion into the social work sphere through practice. Further, many participants who shared their thoughts on gut feeling referred to it as a sense of something being 'incongruent':

> Sometimes it's straightforward because people, what people are saying and the way they're saying it—sort of like the non-verbal way they're saying it—actually there's no incongruence with that. But then occasionally I'll visit families where I feel as if what they're saying and the way they're saying it is not congruent and that's when I probably, my little early warning indicators kind of like start beeping away . . . because I start noticing things that don't seem quite right and that's when I'll probably ask more questions, but maybe still come away not feeling one hundred per cent confident with the information I've been given. And think about whether that's going to be something that's going to be problematic later or not.
>
> (Sandra, qualified social worker with some supervisory responsibilities, over fifteen years' experience)

Sandra only knows something is 'incongruous' through her practice experience and knowledge. This supports Collins's (2010) point about the *social* nature of tacit knowledge. Thus, in this context, gut feeling is not 'natural' or located in the individual—it is learned through language and practice in specific epistemic communities (Collins, 2011). Moreover, the rules are infinite and constantly changing, so the mechanisms of why a social worker might get a specific gut feeling in any given context are not explicable. Thus we can acquire collective tacit knowledge through our emersion in the social work sphere, but Collins argues that we cannot *fully* explicate it due to its fluid, contingent nature.

I have argued that gut feeling in this context is a form of collective tacit knowledge, which requires a sociological analysis. However, to complicate matters further, a piece of tacit knowledge can be one, two or even three of the types Collins describes. That a piece of tacit knowledge can be more than one type of tacit knowledge at the same time makes deciding when it is possible to fully explicate a piece of tacit knowledge—for the purposes of this discussion, a gut feeling—extremely complex. For example, a social worker has what they call a gut feeling about a case. If we focus on full explication, we would have to decide, first, what we mean by explication, as Collins provides four meanings of the term 'explicable' (Collins, 2010: 81). Next, we would have to decide what type (or types) of tacit knowledge that gut feeling was. I have argued that gut feeling is always a form of collective tacit knowledge in this context. But if it is also relational, for example, then there are different categories of relational tacit knowledge, and we would have to decide which one it is, then respond appropriately. If it is solely collective tacit knowledge, then, according to Collins, it cannot be fully explicated.[7] So what then? As we can see, focusing on full explication raises as many questions as it answers.

To summarise, Collins has highlighted the social nature of tacit knowledge, which helps us better understand that what social workers call gut feeling is located in the collective, rather than the individual, and thus a sociological analysis is crucial. Collins also helps us understand that some forms of tacit knowledge can be explicated. Thus, when thinking about how social workers move from collective tacit knowledge to evidence (which they do), it might seem useful to focus on explication of that knowledge. Clearly, however, this is incredibly complex and not very practical for experts when making judgements in practice. Full explication, therefore, is not a reasonable goal for social workers. I will argue that, instead, social workers aim for what I call 'adequate' explication, which focuses on the move from collective tacit knowledge to evidence.

## ADEQUATE EXPLICATION OR 'SHARING GUT FEELING WITH OTHERS'

Adequate explication is a social worker's pragmatic response to the impossible task of full explication. In this sense, this group of experts, when sharing risk knowledges with one another, have something in common with biobank scientists. Those scientists, according to Demir and Murtagh (2013) respond to the problem of sharing and working with data from different biobanks through harmonisation (combining data in a way that facilitates comparison). This process places an emphasis on 'epistemic adequacy' rather than full precision (Demir and Murtagh, 2013). Here, although the focus is on the challenges that arise when sharing risk knowledges within the same epistemic community; equal value is placed on the advantages of epistemic adequacy.

Let's look at some examples of adequate explication and how this helps social workers move from collective tacit knowledge to evidence. Yasmin refers to an example of what she calls a gut feeling that can be shared with others and is thus viewed as acceptable evidence:

> I think sometimes just talking to professionals can reinforce your opinion or if you've made a decision and you're thinking is this the right one you can talk to someone else and actually they've got the same concerns as you but it's putting it into words. Because sometimes I think it's quite difficult when you're working with people. You know there's something not right but you can't put it into words. And that's one of the families I'm working with at the moment. There's something that's not right about the daughter. There's something about her behaviour that's off. And I knew that as soon as I went on the first visit. And it was quite good because I went with a colleague and we both said there's something not right about that girl . . . It was her facial expressions, how she was talking, the way in which she was talking, her lack of eye contact. There was something off about her. I don't know what it is but there's something off about her. So that's why I've done a referral and I was able to, with the school, get loads of examples about what it is.
>
> (Yasmin, unqualified social worker, over fifteen years' experience)

Yasmin explains how difficult it is to put this collective tacit knowledge into words and can only go so far as 'there was something off about her'. However, she is able to give physical, concrete examples of body language in order to share that form of knowledge with others. But this does not mean it is evidence that will be accepted by others as 'proof' that something is wrong. She had to go one step further, get 'loads' of examples with others, and it was only then that she could share this information as 'evidence'. Therefore, adequate explication was sufficient, because it meant she was able to move from collective tacit knowledge to evidence that could promote change for the child.

Erin provides an example of having a gut feeling and being able to partially share that with others, but she also demonstrates that just because she has shared it does not mean it is automatically seen as acceptable evidence—this requires further work:

> There was a situation before where sometimes you've got no evidence to prove what you're thinking and what you're feeling but you just know something's not quite right. I suppose then again it might be because of your theory and your knowledge and what you learn in training and things like that. I had a situation where we had no disclosures but just the relationship between this [child] and [adult]—my gut feeling was there's something not right here [concrete, explicit examples] and

> although the child never made any disclosures and I had no evidence, there was no previous offending, nothing to suggest that [adult] was a sexual offender my gut instinct is [adult is] grooming this child, if something hasn't happened something's going to happen and that was just a feeling that I had but I didn't have anything to back it—well I had stuff to back it up like [concrete, explicit examples] but I had no disclosure, no history to really take that [to court].
>
> (Erin, qualified social worker, less than ten years' experience)

Erin could 'adequately' explicate her gut feeling, but this example of collective tacit knowledge was not considered to be 'acceptable' evidence. Erin dealt with this by putting her concerns in writing to the family. When concerns are put in writing in this way, it is generally called a 'written agreement'. Written agreements are somewhat controversial and are not legally binding but aim to provide a physical, explicit piece of 'evidence' about the risk of harm to a child. For example, if a family signs the agreement but does not adhere to the conditions outlined, this can be used as a piece of evidence to support a social worker's judgement. By using this strategy, Erin was able to move from collective tacit knowledge to a formal document which could be used as part of (alongside other forms of reasoning) her evidence that the child was at risk of 'significant harm'.

It is important to state that it is not always possible to even partially or adequately explicate collective tacit knowledge. Here is an example of where it was not possible to share a piece of collective tacit knowledge, but the worker was still able to draw on it (alongside other forms of knowledge) in order to promote change for the child. Zoe, a social work manager, refers to an example of a child who was running away from home. The allocated social worker was concerned about the child's emotional well-being, and both the manager and the social worker wanted the child to be placed in local authority care:

> It was a struggle . . . but we knew something was, we were waiting for it, so when we had a disclosure there was no surprise to us but it helped higher management understand why then the child needed to be in court proceedings . . . It took a long time from the beginning until the end and we aren't at the end we're still in it but to get to where we felt we were more confident in act—we couldn't prove what we knew was true. And we still can't prove it . . . so we are still working with what we think is best for that child.
>
> (Zoe, social work manager, over ten years' experience)

Zoe was not able to explicate her gut feeling—and still isn't. It took the passing of time and her professional persistence for the decision she wanted—the child placed into local authority care—to be made. Therefore, what social workers refer to as gut feeling (which we now know is a form of collective tacit knowledge) is just as flawed as any other form of reasoning (Helm, 2010). Again, I am leaving aside any normative judgements about whether this decision was 'right' or 'wrong'—the outcome could have been different. But this is the nature of responding to uncertainty. Social workers have to make a judgement, and collective tacit knowledge is one of the resources they draw on in order to do so.

I have argued that gut feeling is a form of collective tacit knowledge. Moreover, in some cases, this knowledge can be 'adequately' explicated, and we are able to see how social workers are able to share what many think of as 'unshareable' knowledge with others as part of their response to risk and uncertainty. In other cases, this knowledge cannot be explicated—meaning it is simply, as Helm (2010) has argued, just as fallible as other forms of judgement. Nevertheless, even when it is not explicable, collective tacit knowledge is still useful—as we can see in the earlier example, it was still part of Zoe's professional judgement. Therefore, I argue that in the first instance, it is preferable to attempt to explicate collective tacit knowledge but that we should be realistic about the extent to which this is possible. In other words, social workers should aim for 'adequate' rather than full explication. Where this is not possible, it should still be acknowledged as an influence on that worker's judgement. If this happens, in both cases, collective tacit knowledge is rendered more visible, and why certain judgements and decisions are made over others is clearer to the wider epistemic community.

Acknowledging the role collective tacit knowledge plays in social worker judgement can be difficult when the dominant EBP perspective promotes what Broadhurst et al. (2010: 1047) call a 'standardising, technocratic' approach, which is based on a rather narrow definition of what is considered 'acceptable' evidence (Gray et al., 2009; White, 2013). So how do expert social workers reconcile the EBP based rules and guidance they must follow with the collective tacit knowledge used by many on a day-to-day basis? And what implications does this have for social work judgement?

## RECONCILING TWO WORLDS: EBP AND COLLECTIVE TACIT KNOWLEDGE

I have argued that the technocratic approach to judgement and decision making advocated by the traditional EBP approach (Webb, 2001; Broadhurst et al., 2010) renders collective tacit knowledge invisible, when it is, in fact, a central part of the social work response to risk and uncertainty. I argue that the participants' ability to reconcile these two worlds—that is, the EBP-based rules and guidance they must follow and the collective tacit knowledge they also rely on—is a form of deep expertise. This is important because it makes collective tacit knowledge, when used, a more visible part of social work judgement, thus making it easier for others to understand why a particular judgement has been made. Whether participants could do this depended not on the seniority of their position but on their level of experience and professional confidence—or, as O'Connor and Leonard (2014) call it, 'professional voice'. In the next example, Nita illustrates that collective tacit knowledge and an EBP approach to evidence are able to coexist in practice and begins with her thoughts on gut feeling:

> It is really hard to quantify, but you do [use gut feeling]. Experience plays into that, just sometimes how people react to you, and you can't kind of legislate for that gut feeling when you knock on the door when you just know there's something wrong. I mean there was an example only [recently about a child with physical injuries]. And some social workers might have gone out to see the [physical injury], listened to the explanation [given by parent/carers], and then walked away thinking that's fine. This social worker said I just had a really uneasy feeling about how [parent/carer] reacted . . . said they just had a horrible feeling. So we persuaded them to let us have a medical and this [child] had [more extensive injuries]. And [the worker] doesn't really know what made them think there was more to it than that because the actual black and white evidence was this [physical injury] and [the parent/carer's explanation].
>
> Researcher:
>
> So if someone ever comes to you and they say to you oh I've just got a feeling about something, how do you respond to that and deal with that?
>
> Participant:
>
> Sometimes it's exploring with people why they had that feeling, because when you explored it with this social worker—why they had that feeling—it was more than just a feeling in the end because there was something about how [parent/carer] had behaved . . . So when you explore it with people sometimes they can explain what, there are things that they can think about that actually caused that, that gut feeling. And sometimes you just do have to explore it a little bit further but sometimes you have to find the evidence to either back up your gut feeling or not. As the case may be really. But I don't think you can ever dismiss it out of hand but it has to have some evidence to go alongside it before you can progress. But sometimes working on your gut feeling can be what you need to do. But not to do it in that kind of way where everything you do confirms that because sometimes you can go along on that conformational bias can't you and just look for your evidence to confirm your feeling. So it's about using those discussions, using supervision to just explore that and reflect on that and encourage workers to do that.
>
> (Nita, qualified social work manager, over fifteen years' experience)

In Nita's practice, then, collective tacit knowledge and an EBP-based approach to evidence can coexist, thus neither one is minimised or rendered invisible. By providing a space for collective tacit knowledge amongst other forms of reasoning, Nita is able to include this type of knowledge in her judgement in a reflexive manner. In the following example, Patricia is also able to maintain a balance and emphasises the move from gut feeling to acceptable evidence:

> Yeah, I mean, it [gut feeling] does happen quite a lot. It's happened with me, as a social worker and as a supervisor. I think if you've got a gut feeling you have to follow it up, but you also have to evidence, you know, social work's evidence based, you have to evidence your information—it is how to evidence gut feelings. But I think if you have a gut feeling that something isn't right in that family then you have to follow it through and you have to exhaust, you know, all the chances and opportunities. You maybe need to follow up with other agencies, you maybe need to go back and do another visit, you maybe need to do whatever you can to eliminate that or if you can't eliminate it, then you're going to have to look at other options available to you. But I think it's quite a balance really, gut instinct and evidence, because your gut instinct might not be able to provide the evidence, it might just be something isn't right here but I don't know what. But I do feel that you do need to—gut instinct's I think's quite relevant, so I would go back and I would check things out that you weren't happy about. If mum's saying the child's in the bedroom all the time and you never, you know, you haven't seen that child on two visits then you keep going back until you see that child, you don't just—, you have to, as research says, [there's] lots of disguised compliance and you need to be very mindful of that, so it's quite important.
>
> (Patricia, social work manager, over fifteen years' experience)

It is important to highlight Patricia's point that what she calls gut feeling is not inherently 'right' or 'wrong'—it is simply another form of reasoning she uses to form the basis of her professional judgement. Moreover, for Patricia and other participants, collective tacit knowledge can be described as a form of evidence that something needs to be explored further. The difficulty with using the term 'evidence' is that, when participants refer to this, they are using the narrow definition provided by the dominant form of EBP (as referred to above). Therefore, collective tacit knowledge and 'evidence' are in this context seen as separate categories, but they are categories that those with deep expertise recognise do not have to be oppositional. In other words, they have a more flexible, fluid definition of what constitutes 'acceptable' evidence, which has developed from their experience of responding to the inherent uncertainty involved when making judgements about children who are deemed to be 'at risk' of 'harm'.

I have argued that a measure of 'deep' expertise is participants' ability to reconcile their use of collective tacit knowledge with the broader EBP-based rules and guidance they must follow. This is important because a lack of clarity in this area leads to specific knowledge being rendered less visible and understanding social work judgement extremely difficult. To summarise, when social workers are clear about the use of gut feeling, which is a form of tacit knowledge, in practice, and are confident about its place in their professional judgement, this knowledge becomes more visible. Moreover, it is only when collective tacit knowledge is rendered more visible that it can be placed under scrutiny and, where necessary, challenged by others. In this way, it is possible for what social workers call gut feeling to be part of 'acceptable' evidence that can promote change for children and their families.

## CONCLUSION

By providing an in-depth exploration of what participants mean when they talk about gut feeling, I have argued that what they are referring to when they use this term is what Collins (2010) calls collective tacit knowledge. Collins's (2010) typology of tacit knowledge helps us go back to the social and to understand that gut feeling is located in the collective rather than the individual, and thus a sociological analysis of its place in this epistemic community is vital. However, the dominant EBP approach and its narrow definition of what constitutes 'acceptable' evidence renders these more informal practices in child and family social work less visible. What Gray et al. (2009: 11) refer to as the 'evidence hierarchy' thus has a detrimental effect on our understanding of the way in which social workers respond to risk and uncertainty in their day-to-day practice.

This chapter adds to existing literature on less visible, more informal responses to risk and uncertainty in child and family social work by identifying the move social workers must make from collective tacit knowledge to 'acceptable' evidence, and how they do so. Therefore, in order to increase our understanding of the judgements social workers must make—why one might view one child as at risk of 'significant harm' and not another, for example—we must make a concerted effort to try and broaden our understanding of what constitutes 'acceptable' evidence. Moreover, by refusing to prioritise one form of reasoning or type of evidence over another, we acknowledge that all forms of judgement—including gut feeling—are flawed (Helm, 2010) and thus should be subject to scrutiny.

Alongside an attempt to broaden our definition of what constitutes 'acceptable' evidence in child and family social work, we need to acknowledge the existing strategies social workers are using when a hierarchy of evidence remains in place. In other words, we can learn from social workers with deep expertise about how they make the move from collective tacit knowledge to 'acceptable' evidence. This allows us to use these insights to demonstrate how more informal practices, such as the use of collective tacit knowledge, can be rendered more visible, thus increasing our understanding of expert responses to risk and uncertainty in practice.

I have argued that social workers with deep expertise recognise that collective tacit knowledge is part of their 'toolkit' when responding to risk and uncertainty. I have argued that it is not 'irrational' or inherently biased. Like all other forms of reasoning, it has its flaws, but it also has the potential to be a useful, robust part of judgement and decision making (Helm, 2010).

I have drawn on Collins's (2010) emphasis on the social nature of tacit knowledge. However, I have moved away from Collins's focus on full explication and argued that we should be realistic about the extent to which this is possible in social work practice. In other words, we should aim for 'adequate' rather than full explication. Where this is not possible, it should still be acknowledged as an influence on that worker's judgement. If this happens, in both cases, collective tacit knowledge is rendered more visible and why certain judgements and decisions are made over others is clearer to the wider epistemic community. As well as not aiming to fully explicate this form of reasoning, social workers with deep expertise recognise the fallibility of collective tacit knowledge and are reflexive in their practice. Further, another sign of deep expertise is the ability to reconcile the use of collective tacit knowledge with the existing dominant EBP-based approach, particularly in relation to evidence.

I agree with Helm (2010) that gut feeling, as a form of collective tacit knowledge, is central to practice where we face uncertainty and are time-poor. But even when we do this, we still need a way of making our judgements and decisions 'acceptable' to the wider epistemic community (and beyond). Social workers cannot just say 'I had a feeling' in order for others to understand and accept (or not) our judgements. This simply keeps the strategies they use to share risk knowledges invisible. Therefore, future research possibilities include further exploration of the way in which social workers help their colleagues understand what their gut feeling means. Participants have argued that we need to identify responses to risk and uncertainty prior to statutory social work involvement (for example, when children are not considered to be 'at risk' but there are concerns for their well-being). Moreover, we have seen that knowledge sharing within a particular epistemic community is not straightforward. Thus next steps could include using these insights to explore the response to risk and uncertainty by different epistemic communities (such health, education, the legal profession and so on), which could contribute to the literature on multi-agency working. However, I would argue that before we can make this step, we need to further explore the more informal strategies social workers use when making 'risky' judgements and decisions about children and their families.

## NOTES

1. I refer to the current meaning of harm in child and family social work in England. Briefly, harm is split into four categories—sexual, physical and

emotional abuse and neglect. Of course, this definition changes dependent on time and space. For a more in-depth discussion of the contingent nature of how we define harm to children, see Hacking (1991).

2. Within child and family social work, a common term is 'likely or actual significant harm' which derives from section 31 of the Children's Act (1989).
3. Child and family social work policy develops in response to reviews into prominent child deaths or past exemplars (Reder et al., 2003; Corby, 2006). The Munro review (2010, 2011a, 2011b) was the first of its kind not to be a response to a specific child death (Parton 2012), although it is arguably heavily influenced by the wider response to the death of Peter Connelly in 2009.
4. The Munro review was commissioned by the coalition government within two weeks of the 2010 election. Eileen Munro is a professor at the London School of Economics and a qualified social worker who has written extensively on social work practice. The review is divided into three parts. Part 1, entitled 'A Systems Analysis', set out the main problems Munro identified in child protection practice in England (Munro, 2010). The second part, 'The Child's Journey', argued that social work had become too focused on following formal procedures rather than asking if children were being helped (Munro, 2011a). The final part, 'A Child-Centred System', recommended placing more emphasis on professional judgement, acknowledging uncertainty in child protection practice, reducing overly complicated guidance and procedures, and prioritising early interventions with children and their families (Munro, 2011b). The review looked at other agencies, including health, education, probation and the police, but placed social work at the centre of the response to child maltreatment (Parton, 2012).
5. See Sternberg (1999) for a useful summary of tacit knowledge in organizations, including examples of how tacit knowledge may be explicated, why organizations resist acknowledging the role of tacit knowledge and how tacit knowledge and explicit knowledge interact.
6. For a thorough critique of Collins's typology and Collins's response, see Soler et al. (2013).
7. Soler and Zwart (2013) argue that, according to Collins's typology, collective tacit knowledge can be partially explicated. Collins (2013) disagrees, and this disagreement is based on what is meant by 'explicable'. It is an interesting debate, but what is important here is that 'explicable' means an ability to share knowledge to the extent that this knowledge can become acceptable evidence. Thus whether social workers are sharing what Collins (2010) calls the underlying mechanisms of collective tacit knowledge or simply 'providing "hints or "coaching rules"' (Collins, 2013: 173) to enable the acquisition of this knowledge is not important in this context.

## REFERENCES


Adams, K.B, Matto, H.C. & LeCroy, C.W. (2009) Limitations of evidence-based practice for social work education: unpacking the complexity, *Journal of Social Work Education*, 45 (2): 165–186.

Bazarian, J., Davis, C., Spillane, L., Blumstein, H. & Schneider, S. (1999) Teaching emergency medicine residents evidence-based critical appraisal skills: a controlled trial, *Annals of Emergency Medicine*. 34 (2):148–154.

Beck, U. (1992) *Risk Society: Towards a New Modernity,* London: Sage.

Bloor, D. (1997) *Wittgenstein, Rules and Institutions,* London: Routledge.

Broadhurst, K., Hall, C., Wastell, D., White, S. & Pithouse, A. (2010) Risk, instrumentalism and the humane project in social work: identifying the informal logics of risk management in children's statutory services, *British Journal of Social Work*, 40: 1046–1064.

Brown, P. (2013) Risk and social theory—a new venture and some new avenues, *Health, Risk & Society* 15 (8): 624–633.

Cimino, J.J. (1999) Development of expertise in medical practice, in Sternberg, R.J. & Horvath, J.A. (eds.) *Tacit Knowledge in Professional Practice: Researcher and Practitioner Perspectives*, Mahwah: Laurence Erlbaum Associates, 101–120.

Collins, H. (1974) The TEA set: tacit knowledge and scientific networks, *Science Studies,* 4: 165–186.

Collins, H. (1985) *Changing Order: Replication and Induction in Scientific Practice,* London: Sage.

Collins, H. (1998) Socialness and the undersocialised conception of society, *Science, Technology and Human Values*, 23 (4): 494–516.

Collins, H. (2001) Tacit knowledge, trust and the Q of sapphire, *Social Studies of Science,* 31 (1): 71–85.

Collins, H. (2010) *Tacit and Explicit Knowledge*, London: University of Chicago Press.

Collins, H. (2011) Language and Practice, *Social Studies of Science,* 41 (2): 271–300.

Collins, H. (2013) Refining the tacit, *Philosophia Scientiæ,* 17 (3) 155–178.

Corby, B. (2006) *Child Abuse: Towards a Knowledge Base,* 3rd edition, Maidenhead: Open University.

Demir, I. and Murtagh, M.J. (2013) Data sharing across biobanks: epistemic values, data mutability and data incommensurability, *New Genetics and Society,* 32 (4): 350–365.

Dreyfus, H.L. & Dreyfus, S.E. (1986) *Mind over Machine: The Power of Human Intuition and Expertise in the Era of the Computer*, New York: Free Press.

Featherstone, B., Morris, K., & White, S. (2014) *Reimaging Child Protection: Towards Humane Social Work with Children and Families,* University of Bristol: Policy.

Ferguson, H. (2009) Walks, home visits and atmospheres: risk and the everyday practices and mobilities of social work and child protection, *British Journal of Social Work*, 40 (4): 1100–1117.

Fook, J., Ryan, M. & Hawkins, L. (2000) *Professional Expertise: Practice, Theory and education for Working in Uncertainty*, London: Whiting and Birch.

Gambill, E. (2006) Evidence-based practice and policy: choices ahead, *Research on Social Work Practice,* 16 (3): 338–357.

Gigerenzer, G. (2007) *Gut Feeling: The Intelligence of the Unconscious,* London: Penguin.

Gillingham, P. & Humphreys, C. (2010) Child protection practitioners and decision-making tools: observations and reflections from the frontline, *British Journal of Social Work*, 40 (8): 2598–2616.

Gray, M., Plath, D. & Webb, S. (2009) *Evidence-Based Social Work: A Critical Stance*, Abingdon: Routledge.

Gut Feeling. (2014) in *Collins English Dictionary,* retrieved from: http://www.collinsdictionary.com/dictionary/english/gut-feeling

Helm, D. (2010) *Making Sense of Child and Family Assessment How to Interpret Children's Needs*, London: Jessica Kingsley.

Helm, D. (2011) Judgements or assumptions? The role of analysis in assessing children and young people's needs, *British Journal of Social Work*, 41 (5): 894–911.

Horlick-Jones, T. (2005) Informal logics of risk: contingency and modes of practical reasoning, *Journal of Risk Research*, 8 (3): 253–272.

Horwath, J. & Morrison, T. (2007) Developing multi-agency partnerships to serve vulnerable children and their families, *Child Abuse and Neglect*, 31 (1): 55–69.

Kemshall, H.J. (2002) *Risk, Social Policy and Welfare*, Buckingham: Open University Press.

Klein, G. (1998) *Sources of Power*, Cambridge, Massachusetts: MIT.

Knorr-Cetina, K. (1999) *Epistemic Cultures: How the Sciences Make Knowledge*, Cambridge: Harvard University Press.

Laming, H. (2009) *The Protection of Children in England: A Progress Report*, London: The Stationery Office.

Laurence, A. (2004) *Principles of Child Protection: Management and Practice*, Maidenhead: Open University.

Lyon, C.M., De Cruz, P., Cobley, C., Petrie, S., & Reid, C. (2003) *Child Abuse*, 3rd edition, Bristol: Jordan.

McNeece, C.A. and Thyer, B.A. (2004) Evidence-based practice and social work, *Journal of Evidence-Based Social Work*, 1 (1): 7–25.

Munro, E. (2010) *The Munro Review of Child Protection, Part One: A System's Analysis*, London: Department for Education.

Munro, E. (2011a) *The Munro Review of Child Protection: Interim Report: The Child's Journey*, London: Department for Education.

Munro, E. (2011b) *The Munro Review of Child Protection: Final Report: A Child-Centred System*, London: Department for Education.

O'Connor, L. & Leonard, K. (2014) Decision making in children and families social work: the practitioner's voice, *British Journal of Social Work*, 44 (7): 1805–1822.

O'Sullivan, T. (2005) Some theoretical propositions on the nature of practice wisdom, *Journal of Social Work*, 5 (2): 221–242.

O'Sullivan, T. (2011) *Decision Making in Social Work*, 2nd edition, Basingstoke: Palgrave Macmillan.

Parton, N. (1996) *Social Work, Social Change and Social Theory*, London: Routledge.

Parton, N. (2012) The Munro review of child protection: an appraisal, *Children and Society*, 26 (2): 150–162.

Polanyi, M. (1966) *The Tacit Dimension*, London: Routledge and Kegan Paul.

Reber, A. (1995) *Implicit Learning and Tacit Knowledge: An Essay on the Cognitive Unconscious*, New York: Oxford University Press.

Reder, P. & Duncan, S. (2003) Understanding communication in child protection networks', *Child Abuse Review*, 12 (2): 82–100.

Reder, P., Duncan, S., & Gray, M. (2003) *Beyond Blame: Child Abuse Tragedies Revisited*, London: Routledge.

Soler, L. and Zwart, S.D. (2013) Collins's taxonomy of tacit knowledge: critical analyses and possible extensions, *Philosophia Scientiæ*, 17 (3): 107–134.

Soler, L., Zwart, S.D. & Catinaud, R. (eds.) (2013) Tacit and explicit knowledge: Harry Collins's framework, *Philosophia Scientiæ*, 17 (3): 5–178.

Sternberg, R.J. (1999) What do we know about tacit knowledge? Making the tacit become explicit, in Sternberg, R.J. & Horvath, J.A. (eds.) *Tacit Knowledge in Professional Practice: Researcher and Practitioner Perspectives*, Mahwah: Lawrence Erlbaum Associates, 231–236.

Taylor, C. & White, S. (2000) *Practising Reflexivity in Health and Welfare: Making Knowledge*, Buckingham: Open University Press.

Taylor, C. & White, S. (2001) Knowledge, truth and reflexivity: the problem of judgement in social work', *British Journal of Social Work*, 1 (1): 37–59.

Timmermans, S. & Angell, A. (2012) Evidence-based medicine, clinical uncertainty, and learning to doctor, in Broom, A. & Adams, J. (eds.) *Evidence-Based Healthcare in Context: Critical Social Science Perspectives*, Farnham: Ashgate, 23–42.

Timmermans, S. & Tavory, I. (2012) Theory construction in qualitative research: from grounded theory to abductive analysis, *Sociological Theory*, 30 (3): 167–186.

Warner, J. (2011) Social work, class politics and risk in the moral panic over Baby P, *Health Risk and Society,* 15 (3): 217–233.

Webb, S.A. (2001) Some considerations of the validity of evidence based practice in social work, *British Journal of Social Work,* 31 (1): 57–79.

Webb, S.A. (2006) *Social Work in a Risk Society: Social and Political Perspectives*, Basingstoke: Palgrave Macmillan.

White, S. (2013, September) *Social Work Judgement and the Politics of Evidence: A Cautionary Tale*, Paper Presented at Professional Judgement Conference, London.

White, S., Wastell, D., Smith, S., Hall, C., Whitaker, E., Debelle, G., Mannion, R. and Waring, J. (2015) Improving practice in safeguarding at the interface between hospital services and children s social care: A mixed-methods case study, *Health Services and Delivery Research*, 3 (4). Retrieved from: http://dx.doi.org/10.3310/hsdr03040

Zinn, J. (2008) Heading into the unknown: everyday strategies for managing risk and uncertainty, *Health, Risk and Society*, 10 (5): 439–450.

# 8 Regulating for Safer Doctors in the Risk Society

*John Martyn Chamberlain*

## INTRODUCTION

> Modern individuals are not merely "free to choose", but obliged to be free, to understand and enact their lives in terms of choice.
>
> Rose (1999: 87)

The analysis of medicine and risk is indelibly linked to a core disciplinary concern within sociology with the nature of 'good governance' and 'good citizenship' (Rose 1999). This chapter discusses recent developments in medical governance in relation to two key 'schools of thought' concerned with the analysis of risk in today's society—respectively, the 'risk society' and the 'governmentality' perspectives (Lupton 1999). In doing so, my aim is not to offer a definitive critical analysis of these viewpoints concerning medical risk. To do so would take up considerably more space than is available. Rather, I seek to achieve two interrelated goals by highlighting points of agreement between the risk society and governmentality perspectives. First, I aim to reinforce the importance of paying close attention to the type of subject-citizen promoted by 'liberal mentalities of rule' as they seek to minimize risks threatening the wealth, health, happiness and security of the population (Rose and Millar 1992). Second, I aim to establish areas for further empirical investigation in relation to medical governance. For in spite of repeated calls for investigation into doctors' training and regulatory arrangements (i.e. Elston 1991, 2004), little empirical research has been published on this topic (Chamberlain 2008).

Sociologists who concerned themselves with the analysis of expertise at the beginning of the twentieth century by and large possessed an uncritical acceptance of professional practitioners' altruistic claims to place the needs of their clients above their own material self-interests (McDonald 1995). In doing so, they reflected the social mores of the time, which dictated that the good patient play a subservient role during doctor-patient encounters, in much the same way that the good citizen knew their place within the established oligarchic governing order (Moran 2004). But times have changed. Over the last four decades, sociologists have become more critical of professional practitioners altruistic claims (Friedson 2001). An ever-growing series of high-profile malpractice cases—such as the general practitioner Harold Shipman who murdered over 215 of his patients—have reinforced to sociologists the need to advocate the adoption of more open, transparent and publicly accountable governing regimes (Davies 2004). Furthermore, the public now expects to play a significant role in treatment decision making and planning, just as they expect to have their voices heard and opinions listened to by their democratically elected political leaders (Lupton 1999). They refuse to accept the legitimacy of the traditional elitist and paternalistic view of professional and state forms of governance, which dominated Western societies until relatively recently (Moran 2004). As the following discussion of the rise of the risk society will highlight, underlying recent reforms in medical governance is a more fundamental shift in the conditions under which good governance and good citizenship can be practiced as a result of the economic and political re-emergence of liberalism (Rose and Miller 1992).

## THE POLITICAL RE-EMERGENCE OF LIBERALISM

> I think we've been through a period where too many people have been given to understand that if they have a problem, it's the government's job to cope with it. "I have a problem. I'll get a grant". "I'm homeless, the government must house me". They're casting their problem on society. And, you know, there is no such thing as society. There are individual men and women, and there are families. And no government can do anything except through people, and people must look to themselves first. It is our duty to look after ourselves, and then to look after our neighbour.
>
> Thatcher (1987: 10)

The 1970s saw the renewal of liberalism as an economic and political ideology, with its emphasis on enterprise and individualism, advocacy of 'rolling back the state' and belief in the ability of the discipline of the market to promote consumer choice, improve service quality and minimise risk (Elston 1991). The neo-liberalism of Margaret Thatcher's conservative government of 1979 possessed an overriding concern for the '3 Es'—economy, efficiency and effectiveness—and had its ideological roots in classical liberalism (Rhodes 1994). This emerged in the seventeenth and eighteenth centuries, through the works of a variety of writers, such as Thomas Hobbes, John Stuart Mills, Adam Smith, Thomas Locke, Jeremy Bentham and Herbert Spencer. The concept of 'possessive individualism' lies at the heart of classical liberalism (Macpherson 1962). Macpherson (1962) argues that for these thinkers, the individual and her capabilities 'pre-figure' the circumstance into which she is born. In short, her talents and who she is owes nothing to society, rather she owns herself, and she is morally and legally responsible for herself and herself alone. She is naturally self-reliant and free from dependence on others. She need only enter into relationships with others because they help her pursue her self-interests. According to this viewpoint, society is seen as a series of market-based relations made between self-interested subjects who are actively pursuing their own interests. Only by recognising and supporting this position politically and economically will the greatest happiness for the greatest number be achieved. Classical liberalism is a critique of state reason which seeks to set limits on state power (Peters 2001).

A very real problem here is that frequently individual members of society do not start their lives equally. This fact led social reformers in the nineteenth and twentieth centuries to advocate changes in working conditions, poor relief and public health. A huge literature was produced by social activists of the time, such as Henry Mayhem, linking inequality and poverty to disease and death (White 2001). Furthermore, contra the ethos of liberalism, John Maynard Keynes argued for a strong interventionist role for the state in regulating the market, protecting working and living conditions, as well as promoting public health. Adopting Keynesian economics to control the tendency of capitalism to operate in 'boom and bust' cycles formed an important part of the foundation of the post-Second World War welfare state in the United Kingdom (Green 1987). However, large fluctuations in oil prices and economic recessions occurred in most Western economies in the 1970s. This led to the labour government of 1976 devaluing the pound and seeking the support of the International Monetary Fund (IMF) (Graham and Clark 1986). The IMF provided credit and loan arrangements that in turn led to a political recognition of the need to introduce competitive practices into the workings of the welfare state. This eventually led to the privatisation of previously publicly owned industries, such as electricity, rail and water (Cutler and Waine 1994). Concurrently, the ideas of a number of prominent 'liberalist' social commentators such as Friedrich Hayek (1973) and Milton Friedman (1962)—who both advocated a liberal market-based system instead of state-dominated welfare provision—became increasingly influential within the political arena, particularly after the collapse of the Soviet Union. This led to Fukuyama (1992) arguing that the 'end of history' had occurred, and the only contender for legitimate government was now liberal democracy. Integral to which was the economic necessity of free-market capitalism.

## THE RISE OF THE RISK SOCIETY

> Each person's biography is removed from given determinations and placed in his or her own hands.
>
> Beck (1992: 135)

Whether they agreed with Fukuyama or not, these changes reinforced to sociologists that tied up with the political re-emergence of the 'enterprise culture' of liberalism was a renewed focus on the individual, particularly the idea that the individual alone possesses ultimate responsibility for herself, as the apparent gradual withdrawal of the state from welfare provision forces her "to make the transition from dependent, passive welfare consumer to an 'enterprise self' " (Burchell 1996: 85). For the idea that an individual's life is her own enterprise may mean she has to submit herself to an endless process of self-examination, self-care and self-improvement. But it also means that she is now "free from the social forms of industrial society—class, stratification, family [and] gender status" (Beck 1992: 87). Her life is no longer mapped out for her. Who she is, and who she could possibly be, is no longer defined by her locality, her occupation, her gender or even her religious affiliation. This does not mean that inequalities no longer exist, only that they can no longer so easily be attributed to the traditional sociological categories of class, race, age or gender (Beck 1992). So her identity is fluid and negotiable, detached from traditional social structures and cultural mores; she is able to reflexively construct her life biography as she sees fit. She is in a very real sense the creative artist of her life.

For risk theorists such as Beck (1992) and Giddens (1990, 1991), a key defining feature of modern society—or 'late' or 'high modernity' as they call it—is that there has been "a social impetus towards individualisation of unprecedented scale and dynamism . . . [which] . . . forces people—for the sake of their survival—to make themselves the centre of their own life plans and conduct" (Beck and Beck-Gernsheim 2002: 31). In *Risk Society*, Beck (1992) argues that as capitalist-industrial society gives way under the tripartite forces of technology, consumerism and globalisation, there is a 'categorical shift' in the nature of social structures and, more importantly, the relationship between the individual and society. Furthermore, as working conditions change, and the technology and communication revolutions continue at pace, more than ever before individuals are required to make life-changing decisions concerning education, work, self-identify and personal relationships in a world where traditional beliefs about social class, gender and the family are being overturned (Lupton 1999). This state of affairs leads to a concern with risk management entering centre stage within society's institutional governing apparatus, as well as individual subject-citizen's personal decision-making process (Mythen 2004).

Risk theorists argue that throughout human history societies have always sought to 'risk manage' threats, hazards and dangers. But these management activities have been concerned with natural risks, such as infectious diseases and famine. However, in today's technologically adv
individuals are seen to be both the producers and minimiser
dens 1990). That is, within the conditions of high moderni
and large seen to be solely the result of human activity (Myth
events previously held to be natural disasters, such as floo
are now held to be avoidable consequences of human acti
be 'risk managed' (Lupton 1999). Hence society's institut

bodies need to become ever more collectively self-aware of their role in the creation and management of risk (Beck and Beck-Gernsheim 2002). While for individuals uncertainties now litter their pathway through life to such an extent that it appears to be loaded with real and potential risks. So they must seek out and engage with a seemingly ever-growing number of information resources, provided by a myriad of sources, as they navigate through their world. In the risk society "[we] find more and more guidebooks and practical manuals to do with health, diet, appearance, exercise, lovemaking and many other things" (Giddens 1991: 218).

A key defining feature of the risk society is the demystification of science and technology, as well as a growing uncertainty about truth and claims to truth (Mythen 2004). Advances in communication technology—such as the mobile phone, the Internet and the twenty-four-hour news channel—have not just made individuals constantly aware of the risks associated with modern living, they also reinforce the limitations of technical and expert knowledge to cope with and even solve them (Lupton 1999). So much so that

> attitudes of trust, as well as more pragmatic acceptance, scepticism, rejection and withdrawal, uneasily co-exist in the social space linking individual activities and expert systems. Lay attitudes towards science, technology and other esoteric forms of expertise, in the age of high modernity, express the same mixture of attitudes of reverence and reserve, approval and disquiet, enthusiasm and antipathy, which philosophers and social analysts (themselves experts of a sort) express in their writings.
>
> (Giddens 1991: 7)

Within the risk society, a sense of growing (perhaps even mutual) distrust characterises the relationship between the public and experts (Giddens 1999). At the same time, a pervasive and seemingly increasingly necessary reliance on an ever-growing number of experts appears to be a key feature of individuals' personal experience of everyday life (Mythen 2004). Consequently, expert authority can no longer simply stand on the traditional basis of position and status. Not least of all because individuals' growing need to manage risk and problem solve their everyday lives, to make choices about who they are and what they should do, means that personal access to the technical and expert knowledge of the elite is now regarded as an inherent right. No longer the sole preserve of those elite few who have undergone specialist training. As Giddens (1991: 144–146) notes:

> technical knowledge is continually re-appropriated by lay agents . . . Modern life is a complex affair and there are many 'filter back' processes whereby technical knowledge, in one shape or another, is re-appropriated by lay persons and routinely applied in the course of their day-to-day activities . . . Processes of re-appropriation relate to all

aspects of social life—for example, medical treatments, child rearing or sexual pleasure.

Risk society theorists frequently observe that modern individuals increasingly find themselves having to make 'risk-laden' choices "amid a profusion of reflexive resources: therapy and self-help manuals of all kinds, television programmes and magazine articles" (Giddens 1992: 20). In doing so, they echo the views of authors operating from a governmentality perspective (Lupton 1999). For both focus upon how in today's society individual acts of self-surveillance and self-regulation are not only central to the formation of a person's sense of personal identity but also the management of risk at the individual and group levels and therefore can be said to be a key mode by which the population is governed 'at a distance' without recourse to direct or oppressive intervention (Rose and Miller 1992).

## GOVERNMENTALITY AND 'NEO-LIBERAL MENTALITIES OF RULE'

> Modern selves have become attached to the project of freedom, have come to live in terms of [that] identity, and to search for means to enhance that autonomy.
>
> Rose (1990: 250)

A key point of difference between the governmentality and risk society perspectives lies in their conception of the individual-subject. For it is arguable that in spite of noting that an individual's sense of self is now arguably more than ever before a product of her own making, risk society authors nevertheless seem to often stay wielded to the idea of the subject as an autonomous actor possessing a coherent core self (Elliott 2001). Consequently, they often adopt a "positivist ego psychology, which is hostile to any notion that the self is complexly structured and differentiated" (Peterson 1997: 190).

Indeed, on occasion Giddens in particular seems to accept that the concept of the sovereign individual self lies at the heart of society to such a degree that he could be accused of being an uncritical apologist for liberalism's 'possessive individualism' and concurrent advocacy of a self-reliant 'enterprise culture', with its focus upon encouraging "autonomous, productive, individuals" (du Guy 1996a: 186). In contrast, following Foucault, governmentality theorists firmly historicise their conception of the individual by discursively locating it within the history of Western thought through critiquing the post-enlightenment conception of the rationally autonomous subject (Peters 2001). They advocate an alternative viewpoint whereby individual subjectivities are neither fixed nor stable but rather are constituted in and through a spiral of power-knowledge discourses—generated by political objectives, institutional regimes and expert disciplines—whose primary aim is to produce governable individuals (Deleuze 1988).

Aside from this noticeable difference, the risk society and governmentality perspectives share much in common. Both argue that there has been a profound shift in 'the nature of the present' (Rose 1992: 161) and the way "[we] come to recognise ourselves and act upon ourselves as certain kinds of subject" (Rose 1992: 16). Due in no small part to the re-emergence of liberalism and the growing ascendancy of the concept of the enterprise self throughout all spheres of modern social life (Gordon 1996). For example, Burchell (1996) argues that neo-liberalism's dual advocacy of the self-regulating free individual and the free market has led to "the generalisation of an 'enterprise form' to all forms of conduct" (Burchell 1996: 28). Similarly, du Guy (1996a, 1996b) argues that enterprise—with its focus upon energy, drive, initiative, self-reliance and personal responsibility—has assumed a near-hegemonic position in the construction of individual identities and the government of organisational and everyday life. Enterprise, he concludes, has assumed "an ontological priority" (du Guy 1996a: 181). Consequently, as Burchell (1993: 275) notes:

> one might want to say that the generalization of an "enterprise form" to all forms of conduct—to the conduct of organisations hitherto seen as being non-economic, to the conduct of government, and to the conduct of individuals themselves—constitutes the essential characteristic of this style of government: the promotion of an enterprise culture.

The risk society and governmentality perspectives both focus upon the changing relationship between individuals and experts during the last four decades. The re-emergence of liberalism in the 1970s reactivated classical liberalism's concern with the liberty of the individual, advocacy of free markets and call for less direct government. It emphasised the entrepreneurial individual, endowed with freedom and autonomy as well as a self-reliant ability to care for herself and, furthermore, driven by the desire to optimise the worth of her own existence (Rose 1999). Governmentality theorists such as Rose (1993: 285) argue that this has led increasingly to the relocation of the authority of expertise from the political into the economic sphere where it is increasingly "governed by the rationalities of competition, accountability and consumer demand". Rose argues that during the nineteenth and twentieth centuries, the increasingly rational, experimental and scientific basis of modern forms of expertise led to them becoming integral to the exercise of political authority. So much so that experts gained "the capacity to generate 'enclosures', relatively bounded locales or fields of judgement within which their authority [was] concentrated, intensified and rendered difficult to countermand" (Rose 1996: 50). However, as a result of the rise of the enterprise self, the enclosures are now being "penetrated by a range of new techniques for exercising critical scrutiny over authority—budget disciplines, accountancy and audit being the three most salient" (Rose 1996: 54).

Power (1997) and Rose (1999) emphasise the enormous impact of the trend in all spheres of contemporary social life towards audit in all its guises—with its economic concern with transparent accountability and standardisation—particularly for judging the activities of experts. This is because two technologies are central to the promotion of the enterprise self at the organisational and individual levels. A 'technology of agency', which seeks to promote the agency, liberty and choices of the individual as they strive for personal fulfilment, and a 'technology of performance', which seeks to minimise risk by setting norms, standards, benchmarks, performance indicators, quality controls and best practice standards in order to survey, measure and render calculable the performance of individuals and organisational structures (Dean 1999). As Dean (1999: 173) notes:

> from the perspective of advanced liberal regimes of government, we witness the utilisation of two distinct, yet entwined technologies: technologies of agency, which seek to enhance and improve our capabilities for participation, agreement and action, and technologies of performance, in which these capabilities are made calculable and comparable so that they might be optimised. If the former allow the transmission of flows of information from the bottom, and the formation of more or less durable identities, agencies and wills, the later make possible the indirect regulation and surveillance of these entities. These two technologies are part of a strategy in which our moral and political conduct is put into play within systems of governmental purposes.

Bound up with the technologies of agency and performance of the enterprise culture is what can be called a progressive and insipid process of 'contractualization' (Burchell 1993). Here in a concerted effort to manage risk, institutional roles and social relations between individuals are increasingly defined in terms of explicit contract, or at the very least, 'in a contract like way' (du Guy 1996a). For the promotion of the enterprise form involves the creation of processes where subjects and their activities are "reconceptualised along economic lines" (Rose 1999: 141). Gordon (1991: 43) argues that entrepreneurial forms of governance rely on contractualization as they seek "the progressive enlargement of the territory of economic theory by a series of redefinitions of its object". That is, entrepreneurial forms of governance 're-imagine' the social sphere as a form of economic activity by contractually a) reducing individual and institutional relationships, functions and activities to distinct units b) assigning clear standards and lines of accountability for the efficient performance of these units and c) demanding individual actors assume active responsibility for meeting performance goals, primarily by using tools such as audit, performance appraisal and performance-related pay (du Guy 1996a). Here judgement and calculation are increasingly undertaken in economic cost-benefit terms, which gives rise to what Lyotard (1984: 46) terms "the performativity principle". Whereby the performances of individual subjects and organisations serve as measures of productivity or output, or displays of 'quality' and the ability to successfully minimise risk, so "an equation between wealth, efficacy and truth is thus established" (Lyotard 1984: 46).

## REFORMING MEDICAL GOVERNANCE

> [Technologies of Performance] . . . subsume the substantive domains of expertise (of the doctor, the nurse, the social worker, the school principal, the professor) to new formal calculative regimes.
>
> Dean (1999: 169)

Osborne (1993) discusses how since the re-emergence of liberalism there has been a gradual reformulation of health-care policy and practice, so that 'the field of medicine' is, to a greater degree than ever before, simultaneously both governed and self-governing. A key part of this process is the subjection of the activities of medical practitioners to an additional layer of management and new formal 'calculative regimes' (Rose and Miller 1992), such as performance indicators, competency frameworks and indicative budget targets (Rose 1993). This process began with the 1979 conservative administration, which possessed a firm neo-liberal commitment to 'rolling back the state' and introducing free-market philosophies within the public and private spheres (Dean 1999). Thatcherism emphasised the entrepreneurial individual, endowed with freedom and autonomy, and a self-reliant ability to care for herself and driven by the desire to optimise the worth of her own existence (Rose 1993). For example, the conservative home secretary Douglas Hurd stated in 1989 that "the idea of active citizenship is a necessary complement to that of the enterprise culture" (quoted in Barnett 1991: 9). A new form of citizenship was being promoted by the changing conditions caused by the re-emergence of liberalism and having a direct effect upon medical governance. Indeed, reviewing National Health Service (NHS) reform during the mid-1990s, Johnson (1994: 149) noted that "government-initiated change has, in recent reforms, been securely linked with the political commitment to the "sovereign consumer". In the case of reform in the National Health Service, this translates "[to a] stress on prevention, the obligation to care for the self by adopting a healthy lifestyle, the commitment—shared with the new GP—to community care". This state of affairs did not end with the election of 'new labor' in 1997 (Dean 1999). Although generally critical of many of their conservative predecessors' health policies, under the guise of treating "patients as equal partners in the decision-making process" (Department of Health 2000: 2) new labour introduced a comprehensive, management-led system of clinical governance into the NHS, designed to set and monitor standards governing health-care delivery (Department of Health 1998).

Clinical governance is officially defined as "a framework through which the NHS organisations are accountable for continuously improving the quality of their services and safeguarding high standards of care by creating an environment in which excellence in clinical care will flourish" (Department of Health 1998: 33). Clinical standards are set nationally by the National Institute for Clinical Excellence (NICE), which was established in 1999. This body makes recommendations on the cost effectiveness of specific treatments and disseminates clinical standards and guidelines, based upon evidence-based research, for compulsory use by doctors. It also plays a role in developing what are called National Service Frameworks (NSFs), which look at the pathways between primary (i.e. community based) to secondary (i.e. hospital based) care followed by certain patient types (i.e. those suffering from heart disease, diabetes or mental health issues) to identify activity levels and productivity figures and improve service resource allocation. The local implementation of the NSF guidelines and NICE clinical standards are monitored by what was first called the Commission for Health Improvement (also established in 1999), which has more recently been renamed the Commission for Healthcare Audit and Inspection (CHAI). CHAI is empowered to visit hospital and primary care trusts and ensure they are following good clinical governance guidelines. It awards star ratings, similar to those given to hotels, and likewise scores them based on their performance against set criteria, for example, length of time patients spend on a waiting list. CHAI is supported in its activities by the National Patient Safety Agency (NPSA), which was established in 2002 and focuses on promoting good health-care practice.

Given new labour's reforms, it is unsurprising that in his review of NHS reform, Light (1998: 431–432) stated that: "the national framework for performance management is extensive. The White Papers propose establishment of evidence-based patterns and levels of service, clinical guidelines, and clinical performance review, in order to ensure patients of high uniform quality throughout the service". Furthermore, Slater (2001: 874) believes that NHS reforms in general, and clinical governance in particular, have established "a rationalistic bureaucratic discourse of regulation which reveals itself through increasingly extensive rule systems, the scientific measurement of objective standards, and the minimisation of the scope of human error. Behind it lies a faith in the efficacy of surveillance as a directive force in human affairs". This new rationalistic-bureaucratic discourse, with its focus on the surveillance and management of risk through standard setting and transparent performance monitoring, has presented a significant challenge to the authority of medical elites, such as the royal colleges and medical schools, who have traditionally been left alone to oversee the arrangements surrounding medical training and discipline (Stacey 2000). To ensure their continued 'fitness for purpose' medical elites have had to adapt and adopt more open, transparent and inclusive governing regimes, which furthermore rely upon a risk-focused, best-evidenced approach to medical governance (Lloyd-Bostock and Hutter 2008). This has required medicine's training programmes, disciplinary mechanisms and regulatory inspection regimes possess clear standards that can be operationalised into performance outcomes against which the 'fitness to practice' of members of the profession can be regularly checked in a transparent and accountable manner (Irvine 2003, 2006).

## HAROLD SHIPMAN AND THE 2008 HEALTH AND SOCIAL CARE ACT

The 2008 Health and Social Care Act can be said to represent a watershed in the regulation of the medical profession in the UK. Certainly on the surface it seems to have effectively ended 150 years of exclusive medical control over the General Medical Council (GMC) (Chamberlain 2012). But it would be incorrect to say that medical control of the GMC went completely unchallenged for a century and a half. As the twentieth century progressed, a series of high-profile medical malpractice cases reinforced the need to introduce a more stringent system of checks and balances to entrenched medical power and autonomy (Gladstone 2000). For instance, in the 1990s, the Royal Bristol Infirmary case saw several children die due to botched procedures, which the surgeons involved tried to cover up (and were by and large successful in doing so until a medical colleague finally came forward to report what had happened). Bristol led to significant changes to National Health Service (NHS) governance and performance monitoring systems, including the adoption of clinical governance frameworks to guide health-care delivery, alongside the introduction of annual NHS performance appraisal for consultants and general practitioners (Chamberlain 2009). Bristol also reinforced to medical elites, such as the royal colleges, that they needed to adopt more open and transparent governing regimes which included all the stakeholders involved, i.e. patients and other health-care professions (Davies 2004). Consequently, they set about establishing clearer practice standards that could be operationalised into performance outcomes against which the fitness to practice of members of the profession could be regularly checked (Black 2002). As the then chairman of the GMC, Donald Irvine, noted (2001: 1808), "the essence of the new professionalism is clear professional standards".

Yet the fact of the matter is that the internal reforms initiated by medical elites during this period were felt to be inadequate by the victims of medical malpractice. A tipping point was reached with the case of Harold Shipman, a general practitioner from Hyde in Greater Manchester. During a criminal career spanning three decades, Shipman was able to use his position of trust to murder over 215 of his patients (Stacey 2000). The watching public, already horrified as Shipman's story began to unfold, were at a loss to understand why it was not until well after his conviction that the GMC finally struck him off the medical register. It appeared the GMC was acting to protect the rights of Shipman instead of to respect the memory of his victims. This sense of bewilderment rapidly turned to anger when it became clear that Shipman had come before a GMC fitness to practise panel previously for prescription abuse (Gladstone 2000). The GMC had had its chance to stop Shipman from practising medicine, but had decided to let him continue. Whatever the reasons behind the GMC's decision, the families of Shipman's victims, patient rights advocacy groups, the media and even government ministers all began to call for far-reaching reforms to medical regulation (Smith 2005).

Undoubtedly, the Shipman case played a pivotal role in reinforcing the need to address medical control of the GMC (Chamberlain 2014). Smith (2005: 1174), at the end her subsequent governmental review of the Shipman case, was "driven to the conclusion that, for the majority of GMC members, the old culture of protecting the interests of doctors lingers on". She also said that "it seems . . . that one of the fundamental problems facing the GMC is the perception, shared by many doctors, that it is supposed to be 'representing' them. It is not, it is regulating them . . . In fact the medical profession has a very effective representative body in the BMA, it does not need—and should not have—two" (Smith 2005: 1176). In 2007, the Health and Social Care White Paper was announced as a result of Smith's report. This subsequently passed through parliament as the 2008 Health and Social Care Act. The Act introduced several key reforms in medical regulation. Non-medical lay members now have to make up half of the GMC membership. Furthermore, an independent system overseen by the Public Appointments Commission was introduced to elect GMC members, while the grounds on which fitness to practise cases are judged was also changed. Such cases have traditionally been judged on the criminal standard: beyond all reasonable doubt. A situation that frequently led commentators to argue the GMC's disciplinary procedures first and foremost protected doctors (Allsop 2006). But the Act required that such cases now be judged on the civil standard of proof—on the balance of probability. It is argued that this will enable underperforming doctors to be more easily stopped from practising medicine. While to enhance impartiality and the independence of the hearing process, the Act also required cases be heard by an independent adjudicator, not by members of the GMC (Chamberlain 2012).

The Act also introduced what was called a 'GMC affiliate' (later known as a 'Responsible Officer'). This person operates at a local NHS level to coordinate the investigation of patient complaints. They also work with NHS management, the GMC and the royal colleges to implement, at a local level, new arrangements for ensuring every doctor is fit to practise in their chosen specialty. This process is called revalidation (Donaldson 2006). Since the Bristol case, doctors have undergone an annual developmental check of their performance as part of the conditions of their NHS employment contract (Black 2002). But Smith (2005: 1048) felt that this process would not have flagged up Shipman as a risk to patients and did "not offer the public protection from underperforming doctors". Smith argued for the need for a more stringent and rigorous performance appraisal system. As a result, the Act made it compulsory for doctors to pass revalidation to stay on the medical register. The revalidation process involves a mixture of clinical audit, direct observation, simulated tests, knowledge tests, patient feedback and continuing professional development activates (Donaldson 2008). Although originally planned for introduction in 2010, the development and piloting process took somewhat longer than expected, with revalidation finally being introduced naturally on a 'roll-out' basis in late 2012. It is now expected that this process will be completed by the end of 2016 at the latest.

It is certainly the case that the introduction of revalidation has caused fear and anxiety amongst some quarters of the profession. However, no matter how long this process takes, medical elites have had to accept that the risk management of the activities of doctors will no longer be solely undertaken 'in house' by them alone (Stacey 2000). This in no small part is why the GMC and royal colleges are emphasising the developmental, cyclical nature of revalidation. To some extent, this state of affairs is to be expected, as there is a somewhat natural tension between bureaucratic managerial systems of surveillance and control, which seek to standardise working practices to make them measurable and predictable, and professions such as medicine, which emphasise practitioner autonomy in the form of freedom of judgment based around the possession of specialist knowledge and expertise alongside a recognition of the inherently messy nature of the real world of professional practice. But what is fundamentally different is that, more than ever before, there is interprofessional cooperation and managerial and lay involvement in the regulation of medical expertise (Chamberlain 2014).

## LIBERAL MENTALITIES OF RULE AND 'POSITIVE' AND 'NEGATIVE' LIBERTY

> [Under liberal mentalities of rule] a person's relation to all his or her activities, and indeed his or her self, is . . . given the ethos and structure of the enterprise form.
>
> Rose (1999: 138)

Policy developments such as revalidation reinforce the need to undertake a dedicated research programme into medical governance. It is widely acknowledged that such a programme is needed as their currently is a lack of published research on the topic (Gray and Harrison 2004). Yet sociologists need to keep in mind that current changes in medical governance take place against the background of a broader societal shift in the grounds under which the legitimate governance of the population can be practised (Rose 1999). Governmentality theorists remind us that changes in how expertise operates are directed towards the object of good governance—the population in general and the individual subject-citizen in particular—as much as they are experts themselves (Rose 1999). For changes in how good citizenship is practised are bound up with shifts in the conditions under which good governance operates. In terms of Berlin's (1969) famous dichotomy of 'positive' and 'negative' liberty, although liberal mentalities of rule may appear at first to promote 'negative liberty' (i.e. the personal freedom of the individual-subject to decide who they are and discover what they want to be), in reality they promote 'positive liberty' (i.e. that is a view of who and what a citizen-subject is and should be).

It certainly can be argued that a key facet of advanced liberal society is its central concern with disciplining the population without recourse to direct or oppressive intervention. Yet liberal mentalities of rule seek to promote good citizenship by discursively constructing and promoting subjective positions for subject-citizens to occupy in relation to the form of the enterprise self. Typically, this is associated with a 'bundle of characteristics', such as energy, resilience, initiative, ambition, calculation, self-sufficiency and personal responsibility (Rose 1996). For the world of enterprise valorises the autonomous, productive, self-regulating individual, who is following his or her own path to self-realisation, and so it requires that of all society's citizens "come to identify themselves and conceive of their interests in terms of these . . . words and images" (du Guy 1996a: 53).

## CONCLUSION

As was touched upon earlier, the concept of the self as enterprise requires that the possession of an essential core self is taken as the central feature of personal identity (Rose 1990, 1993, 1996, 1999). How else could individuals be expected to become responsible for themselves and the care of their bodies and not be a burden on the state? The very notion of the enterprise self requires a political commitment to the idea that all individuals are capable of self-fulfilment. This is the core mechanism by which the self-regulatory capabilities of the individual can be enhanced and entwined with the key objectives of governance—the security, health, wealth and happiness of the general population (Barry, Osborne and Rose 1996). Consequently, failure to achieve the goal of self-fulfilment is not associated with the possession of a false idea of what it means to be human, or that individuals do not possess an essential core self which is the 'real' and 'true' them for all eternity. Rather, it is the fault of poor choices, a lack of education or the 'dependency culture' created by the welfare state (Dean 1999). It is the result of 'learned helplessness', which in itself can be resolved with "programmes of empowerment to enable [the individual] to assume their rightful place as self-actualizing and demanding subjects of an "advanced" liberal democracy" (Rose 1996: 60). The sociological analysis of medicine and risk needs to focus upon this point as it considers the type of citizen and forms of subjectivity promoted and sustained by the governing regimes of the risk society (Peterson and Bunton 1997). For it is arguable that under the guise of advocating personal freedom and minimal forms of government as the 'natural way of things', liberal mentalities of rule run the risk of promoting a highly limiting view of what it is to be a human being, let alone a good citizen, within today's increasingly complex social world.

## REFERENCES


Barnett, M. (1991) *The Politics of Truth* Cambridge: Polity.

Barry, A, Osborne, T and Rose, N. (1996) *Foucault and Political Reason* University College London Press.

Beck, U. (1992) *Risk Society: Towards a New Modernity* London: Sage.

Beck, U and Beck-Gernsheim, E. (2002) *Individualization: Institutionalized Individualism and its Social and Political Consequences* Sage Publications.

Berlin, I. (1969) Two Concepts of Liberty, in I. Berlin (2002 editor) *Four Essays on Liberty* Oxford University Press.

Burchell, G. (1993) Liberal Government and Techniques of the Self *Economy and Society* 22 (3): 267–282.

Burchell, G. (1996) Liberal Government and Techniques of the Self, in Barry, A, Osborne, T and Rose, N. (editors) *Foucault and Political Reason* University College London Press 155–177.

Burchell, G, Gordon, C and Miller, P. (1991, editors) *The Foucault Effect: Studies in Governmentality* Harvester Wheatsheaf.

Chamberlain, J.M. (2008) *Governing Medicine—A Study of Doctors Educational Practices* Unpublished PhD Thesis, The University of Liverpool.

Chamberlain, J.M. (2009) *Doctoring Medical Governance: Medical Self-Regulation in Transition* New York: Nova Science Publishers.

Chamberlain, J.M. (2012) *The Sociology of Medical Regulation: An Introduction* Springer: New York and Amsterdam.

Chamberlain, J.M. (2014) Reforming Medical Regulation in the United Kingdom: From Restratification to Governmentality and Beyond *Medical Sociology* 8 (1) 32–43.

Cutler, A and Waine B. (1994) *Managing the Welfare State* Oxford: Berg.

Davies, C. (2004) Regulating the Health Care Workforce: Next Steps for Research *Journal of Health Services Research and Policy* 9 (Supplement 1): 55–61.

Dean, M. (1999) *Governmentality: Power and Rule in Modern Society* Sage Publications.

Deleuze, G. (1988) *Foucault* University of Minnesota Press.

Department of Health. (1998) *A First Class Service: Quality in the New NHS* DOH London.

Department of Health. (2000) *The NHS Plan* DOH London.

Donaldson, L. (2006) *Good Doctors, Safer Patients* London: Department of Health.

Donaldson, L. (2008) *Revalidation the Next Steps* London: Department of Health.

du Guy, P. (1996a) Organising Identity: Entrepreneurial Governance and Public Management, in Hall, S and du Guy, P. (editors) *Questions of Cultural Identity* Sage Publications 121–133

du Guy, P. (1996b) *Consumption and Identity at Work* Sage Publications.
Elliott, A. (2001) *Concepts of the Self* Cambridge Polity Press.
Elston, M.A. (1991) The Politics of Professional Power: Medicine in a Changing Medical Service, in Gabe, J, Calman, M and Bury, M (editors) *The Sociology of the Health Service* Routledge 67–88.
Elston, M.A. (2004) Medical Autonomy and Medical Dominance, in Gabe, J, Bury, M and Elston, M.A. (editors) *Key Concepts in Medical Sociology* Sage Publications 33–44.
Friedman, M. (1962) *Capitalism and Freedom* University of Chicago Press.
Friedson, E. (2001) *Professionalism: The Third Logic* Cambridge Polity Press.
Fukuyama, F. (1992) *The End of History and the Last Man* Penguin.
Giddens, A. (1990) *The Consequences of Modernity* Cambridge Polity.
Giddens, A. (1991) *Modernity and Self-Identity: Self and Society in Late Modernity* Cambridge Polity.
Giddens, A. (1999) Risk and responsibility *Modern Law Review* 62(1): 1–10.
Gordon, C. (1991) Governmental Rationality: An Introduction in Burchell, G, Gordon, C and Miller, P. (editors) *The Foucault Effect: Studies in Governmentality* Harvester Wheatsheaf 3–15.
Gordon, C. (1996) Foucault in Britain in Barry, A, Osborne, T and Rose, N (1996) *Foucault and Political Reason* University College London Press 23–34.
Graham, D and Clark, P. (1986) *The New Enlightenment The Rebirth of Liberalism* Macmillan.
Gray, A and Harrison, S. (2004, editors) *Governing Medicine: Theory and Practice* Open University Press.
Green, D. (1987) A Missed Opportunity?, in Green, D, Neuberger, J, Young, M and Burstal, M. (editors) *The NHS Reforms: Whatever Happened to Consumer Choice?* London Institute of Economic Affairs 45–55.
Harrison, S. (2004, editors) *Governing Medicine: Theory and Practice* Open University Press.
Hayek, F. (1973) *Law, Legislation and Liberty* Routledge and Kegan Paul.
Irvine, D. (2003) *The Doctors Tale: Professionalism and the Public Trust* Radcliffe Medical Press.
Irvine, D. (2006) Success Depends Upon Winning Hearts and Minds *BMJ* 333: 965–966.
Johnson, T.J. (1994) Expertise and the State, in Gane, M and Johnson, T.J. (editors) *Foucault's New Domains* Routledge 139–152.
Light, D.W. (1998) Managed Care in a New Key: Britain's Strategies for the 1990s *International Journal of Health* Sciences 28 (3): 427–444.
Lloyd-Bostock, S and Hutter, B. (2008) Reforming Regulation of the Medical Profession: The Risks of Risk Based Approaches *Health, Risk and Society* 10 (1): 69–83.
Lupton, D. (1999) *Risk* Routledge.
Lyotard, J F. (1984) *The Postmodern Condition A Report on Knowledge* University of Manchester Press.
Macpherson A. (1962) *The Political Theory of Possessive Individualism* Oxford Clarendon Press.
McDonald, K.M. (1995) *The Sociology of the Professions* Sage.
Moran, M. (2004) Governing Doctors in the British Regulatory State, in Gray, A and Gray, A and Harrison, S. (editors) *Governing Medicine: Theory and Practice* Open University Press 27–36.
Mythen, G. (2004) *Ulrich Beck: A Critical Introduction to the Risk Society* London: Pluto.
Osborne, T. (1993) On Liberalism, Neo-Liberalism and the Liberal Profession of Medicine *Economy and Society* (22) 3: 345–356.
Peters, M. (2001) *Poststructuralist, Marxism and Neo-Liberalism: Between Theory and Practice* Rowman and Littlefield.

Peterson, A. (1997) Risk, Governance and the New Public Health, in Peterson, A and Bunton, R. (editors) *Foucault Health and Medicine* Routledge 87–99.
Peterson, A. and Bunton, R. (1997, editors) *Foucault Health and Medicine* Routledge.
Power, M. (1997) *The Audit Society* Oxford University Press.
Rhodes, R. (1994) The Hollowing Out of the State: The Changing Nature of Public Services in Britain *Political Quarterly* 65: 138–151.
Rose, N. (1990) *Governing the Soul: The Shaping of the Private Self* Routledge.
Rose, N. (1992) Governing the Enterprise Self, in Heelas, P and Morris, P. (editors) *The Values of the Enterprise Culture* Routledge 123–144.
Rose, N. (1993) Government, Authority and Expertise in Advanced Liberalism *Economy and Society* 22 (3): 283–299.
Rose, N. (1996) Governing Advanced Liberal Democracies in Barry, A, Osborne, T and Rose, N. (1996) *Foucault and Political Reason* University College London Press 189–211.
Rose, N. (1999) *Powers of Freedom: Reframing Political Thought* Cambridge University Press.
Rose, N. and Miller, P. (1992) Political Power Beyond the State: Problematics of Government *British Journal of Sociology* 43 (2): 173–205.
Slater, B. (2001) Who Rules? The New Politics of Medical Regulation *Social Science and Medicine* (52): 871–883.
Smith, J. (2005) *Shipman: Final Report* London: Department of Health.
Stacey, M. (1992) *Regulating British Medicine* John Wiley and Sons.
Stacey, M. (2000) The General Medical Council and Professional Self-Regulation, in Gladstone, D. (editor) *Regulating Doctors* Institute for the Study of Civil Society 23–45.
Thatcher, M. (1987) Interview *Women's Own,* October 1987: 8–10.
The Secretary of State for Health. (2007) *Trust, Assurance and Safety—The Regulation of Health Professions in the 21st Century* London: Stationary Office.
White, K. (2001) *The Early Sociology of Health* London Routledge.

# 9 Health Experts Challenge the Safety of Pesticides in Argentina and Brazil

*Renata Motta and Florencia Arancibia*

## INTRODUCTION

Motivated by high international commodity prices, many countries in the Global South are expanding their agrarian borders and converting their soils to agrarian commodities production with intensive use of machinery and new technologies, including genetically modified (GM) seeds tolerant to agrochemicals. Indeed, the technological package composed of GM seeds and agrochemicals, particularly pesticides,[1] are a constitutive component of large-scale contemporary agrarian production and deemed indispensable to the challenge of feeding the world. Together with the expansion of GM crops, the world market for pesticides is on the rise. This chapter explores this development in the case of Argentina and Brazil.

From the point of view of state regulation, the legal basis for introducing agrarian biotechnologies into the market is situated in the context of innovation policy. This assumes the beneficial aspects of innovation and no state interventions other than in the areas of health and the environment. However, assessing potential detrimental health and environmental effects of new technologies is not an easy task. Potential negative effects are usually latent (Beck 2008), and regulatory agencies require complex risk analysis to determine their magnitude and nature.

The type of knowledge produced by this risk analysis is quite different from basic science. Jasanoff called it "regulatory science" (1990) and has shown how flaws in its production process can determine conclusions that are based on incomplete data or co-opted by powerful stakeholders. Frequently, approved technologies produce unpredicted and critically detrimental effects on public health and the environment once in use. Moore (Moore et al. 2011) describes three recent, intertwined global trends in the regulatory field: a. regulation is increasingly taking place within international governance bodies; b. the influence of multinational corporations—and their backing by industrial science—has increased; and c. the regulation of technology is framed in a discourse of scientism that utilizes the authority of the scientific field (Moore et al. 2011: 11).

These transnational science-based regulatory frameworks usually downplay the risks derived from the adoption of new technologies. One consequence is an asymmetrical distribution of health and environmental risks. This is what Beck (2008) calls a "global inequality of risk": a radical asymmetry between those who take the risks and profit from them and those who are assigned to them, suffer the "unforeseen side effects" of the decisions of others, and perhaps even pay with their lives. Often it is the case that the danger is exported geographically to countries or regions whose elites see a selfish opportunity and whose populations have no means to resist the adoption of a hazardous technology. Indeed, the rural poor in export countries suffer the biggest burden of the negative consequences of an expansive, profitable, and chemical-intensive agriculture commodity production.

How can the detrimental effects of the dominant agrarian model ignored by current regulatory frameworks be acknowledged? What are the potential contributions from medicine and science in these attempts? Pesticides provide a good entry point to discuss the role of science and medicine in the construction of a regulatory order that legitimizes the dominant model of agrarian development as well as in challenging it and constructing alternatives. This chapter addresses these questions and contributes to this discussion by analyzing the struggles of Argentinean and Brazilian health professionals and scientists to challenge the dominant discourse that agrochemicals are safe and explores their demands for a scientific and political recognition of the negative consequences on health and the environment.

The argument is structured in five parts. We start by situating the problem of how regulatory science contributes to legitimizing agrarian practices with intensive use of pesticides that have a high and nonassessed negative health and environmental impact, conceptualized in the literature as "undone science" (Frickel et al. 2010, Hess 2009, 2010). In face of health and environmental impacts, health professionals play an important role in challenging regulatory science and producing knowledge that supports claims from local populations concerning their struggles against agrochemicals (Part I). We then present the cases of Argentina and Brazil, describing the data on the use of pesticides and their regulation (Part II). The following two sections describe the role of health professionals in support of grassroots movements fighting agrochemicals in Argentina (Part III) and Brazil (Part IV). The conclusion draws the lessons on the role of science and health professionals in the disputes over agrarian models and therefore agrarian futures, a relevant issue in the global agenda of food security (Part V).

## REGULATORY SCIENCE AND UNDONE SCIENCE ON HEALTH IMPACTS OF NEW TECHNOLOGIES

In a global knowledge economy, political decision makers seek scientific advice to analyze the risks and benefits of new technological developments

(Moore et al. 2011). Regulation of technology "is often framed, particularly at the international level, in a discourse of scientism that utilizes the authority of the scientific field but also depoliticizes the regulation of new technologies" (Moore et al. 2011: 11). In this context, regulatory science (Jasanoff 1990)—a new type of knowledge—gains a new relevance. Jasanoff (1990) calls the type of knowledge produced to serve as bases for regulatory decisions "regulatory science," to distinguish it from basic science. Science used in the policy process differs from research science both in context and content.

In terms of its content, regulatory science includes three different types of scientific activity: 1. knowledge production, 2. knowledge synthesis, 3. prediction (Jasanoff 1990: 77). In terms of its contexts, regulatory science is not conducted in academic settings, which determines the heavy involvement of government and industry in the process of producing and certifying knowledge. Institutional pressures may influence researchers' attitudes to issues of proof and evidence. At the same time, the validation process based on peer review is more complicated and less reliable in the case of regulatory science. The potential for bias is more pronounced, as scientists serving on peer-review panels may either be formally affiliated with particular interest groups or otherwise have a stake in the outcome of the regulatory process. And, as Jasanoff has pointed out, "regulatory agencies could stack the deck in favor of one or another viewpoint by selecting peer reviewers with known opinions on these issues" (Jasanoff 1990: 81). Also, often the production of this knowledge is driven by political pressure. While scientists working in academic settings usually have unlimited time for testing hypothesis, scientists working to meet policy needs are under constant pressure to deliver results quickly. In policy, a decision to wait for more data might imply a decision not to act. Since experts are often forced to provide advice quickly, it is common that new technologies are released on the market even without enough empirical data and when the levels of risks are uncertain (Hess 2010, Moore et al. 2011).

Since regulatory frameworks are based on scientific assessments, communities exposed to technological hazards willing to challenge current regulations have to first prove the mistakes of regulatory science. But in order to do this, they need alternative knowledge, which most of the time is not available. Given that research agendas are influenced by the industry, "undone science" can become a critical issue (Frickel et al. 2010, Hess 2009, 2010). The concept of "undone science" denotes absence of scientific research that social movements or civil society organizations discover when attempting to make epistemic claims in the political field—such as the safety of a new technology or an industrial process (Hess 2007, Woodhouse et al. 2002). In other words, it is the absence of knowledge that could help a social movement or civil society organization to resist policies that are not beneficial and thus promote change. In this context, it is critical to study efforts made to get "undone science" done (Hess 2010).

Since the 1960s, pesticides have been widely used and have been constantly under the scrutiny of regulatory science. For most of the products, the toxicological classifications by the World Health Organization (WHO) apply scientific studies provided by the same companies that sell the pesticides. The methodology used by these studies (DL50) only takes into account lethal damage, determined by giving rats a single dose or multiple doses over a relatively short period of time. The acute oral DL50 is the amount of substance that, if ingested one time, causes death in 50 percent of test animals. This dose is expressed as mg/kg of the test animal's weight (Commission of the Universidad Nacional del Litoral 2010). DL50 only measures mortality at short time exposure, not morbidity after long periods of exposure. Hence a whole set of toxicological health damages (subacute lethal, long-term lethal, acute sublethal, chronic sublethal) are not measured. Interestingly, WHO explicitly states that their toxicological classifications of phytosanitary products should only be used as a guide and that they are not responsible for any negative effect of the practical application of such a classification.

As a consequence, regulatory science might oversee the critical effects of pesticides on rural communities. In fact, a few experiments conducted by independent scientists from various countries have revealed links between pesticide exposure and cancer, as well as a range of reproductive health ailments, including miscarriages, birth defects, infertility, delayed pregnancies (Antoniou and Fagan 2012, Arbuckle, Lin, and Mery 2001, Axelrad, Howard, and McLean 2003, Benachour and Séralini 2009, Dallegrave et al. 2003, Hardell, Eriksson, and Nordstrom 2002, Marc, Mulner-Lorillon, and Bellé 2004, Marc et al. 2005, Marc, Bellé, et al. 2004, McDuffie et al. 2001, Paganelli et al. 2010, Richard et al. 2005, De Roos et al. 2005, Seralini et al. 2012) (Dallegrave et al. 2003). In the last years, scientists, health experts, and social movements have called attention to "undone science" and the health impact of pesticides in Argentina (Arancibia 2013a, 2013b) and Brazil (Carrizo and Berger 2012; Porto and Milanez 2009).

## PESTICIDES IN ARGENTINA AND BRAZIL: CONSUMPTION AND REGULATION

Argentina and Brazil are classified as having a high commodity dependence, with commodity exports (in millions of US dollars) accounting for, respectively, 67 percent and 63 percent of merchandise exports, from which agrarian products destined for feed and food correspond to 76 percent (Argentina) and 52 percent (Brazil) (UNCTAD 2012). Both countries experienced a substantial increase in pesticides consumption over the last two decades. Such an increase is related to the introduction of the technological package formed by genetically modified (GM) seeds tolerant to pesticides.

Following the USA, Brazil, and Argentina are, respectively, the second and the third largest producers of genetically modified crops (Table 9.1).

The first transgenic trait to be widely adopted, and one that still occupies the first ranking in cultivation, is herbicide tolerance. Its most famous application is the Roundup Ready Soy (RR soy), developed by Monsanto. It has been genetically modified to be resistant to the application of the herbicide glyphosate. Roundup is the brand of the herbicide product that has elaborated with glyphosate as the main active ingredient registered and patented by Monsanto. Thus the company has developed a technological package: the seed is to be used in conjunction with the pesticide.

This genetic modification to give seeds herbicide tolerance allows for a shift in agricultural practices in the application of pesticides. Given the tolerance of the GM seeds and the whole soy plant, it becomes possible to apply pesticides in many phases of the cultivation cycle, whereas before this would have endangered the entire crop, while all other plants (considered to be pests) would die. In this sense, this trait does not promise the reduction in pesticide use but rather makes the work more time efficient.[2] In short, genetic modification enables a more radical conversion to industrial agriculture, which is highly dependent on machinery and industrial inputs such, as fertilizers, pesticides, and patent protected seeds.

Argentina and Brazil are, like many other developing countries, heavily dependent on the agricultural sector. In 1996, Argentina pioneered the adoption of GM soy, and other varieties of GM seeds—corn, cotton—soon followed. The adoption was surprisingly fast and widespread, and it marked a turning point (Vara 2005). Since then, the agricultural sector has embarked

*Table 9.1 Global Areas of Biotech Crops in 2013 by Country (Million Hectares)*

| Position | Country | Area (millions Hectares) | Biotech Crops |
|---|---|---|---|
| 1 | United States | 70.1 | Maize, soybean, cotton, canola, squash, papaya, alfalfa, sugar beet |
| 2 | Brazil | 40.3 | Soybean, maize, cotton |
| 3 | Argentina | 24.4 | Soybean, maize, cotton |
| 4 | India | 11.0 | Cotton |
| 5 | Canada | 10.8 | Canola, maize, soybean, sugar beet |
| 6 | China | 4.2 | Cotton, papaya, poplar, tomato, sweet pepper |
| 7 | Paraguay | 3.6 | Soybean, maize, cotton |
| 8 | South Africa | 2.9 | Maize, soybean, cotton |
| 9 | Pakistan | 2.8 | Cotton |
| 10 | Uruguay | 1.5 | Soybean, Maize |

*Source*: Adapted from James 2014

on a pathway of change in which intensive, high input commodity crop production has become dominant, a trajectory that many other developing countries are encouraged by seed and pesticide companies to follow. In Brazil, the same GM soy was approved in 2005. The almost ten-year lag between Argentinean and Brazilian conversion of the majority of its soy fields to GM soy, in 1999 and 2009 respectively, is explained by a long dispute over Brazilian policy for agrobiotechnology (Motta 2014).

Argentina and Brazil have led the increase in area planted with (GM) soy in South America in the last 20 years. In 2010, Brazil was responsible for 50 percent of the area cultivated with the crop and Argentina for 40 percent. Accordingly, the two countries lead also in terms of volume produced: Brazilian volume oscillated in the last 20 years between 50 to 62 percent of the total regional volume and Argentinean production from 30 to 45 percent (Catacora-Vargas et al. 2012).

In Argentina and Brazil, the increase of GMOs production was accompanied by an increase in volume of pesticides. In the last decade, Brazil surpassed the USA as the world's leading consumer of pesticides. In 2010, it represented 19 percent of world market, whereas the USA represented 17 percent (Carneiro et al. 2012). The increase in volume of pesticide has been higher than the increase in area planted in both countries. Table 9.2 below shows the increase in pesticide use. Argentina experienced a much higher

*Table 9.2 Pesticide Consumption in Argentina and Brazil in Millions of Liters*

| | Argentina | Increase | Brazil | Increase |
|---|---|---|---|---|
| 1997 | 123,84 | ... | ... | ... |
| 1998 | 132,35 | 7% | ... | ... |
| 1999 | 127,47 | –4% | ... | ... |
| 2000 | 147,72 | 16% | ... | ... |
| 2001 | 142,31 | –4% | ... | ... |
| 2002 | 151,28 | 6% | 599,5 | ... |
| 2003 | 198,46 | 31% | 643,5 | 7% |
| 2004 | 228,05 | 15% | 693 | 8% |
| 2005 | 234,21 | 3% | 706,2 | 2% |
| 2006 | 252,43 | 8% | 687,5 | –3% |
| 2007 | 254,06 | 1% | 686,4 | 0% |
| 2008 | 225,22 | –11% | 673,9 | –2% |
| 2009 | 260,54 | 16% | 725 | 8% |
| 2010 | 313,42 | 20% | 827,8 | 14% |
| 2011 | 335,89 | 7% | 852,8 | 3% |
| 2012 | 317,17 | –6% | ... | |
| Total increase | (1997–2012) | 156% | (2002–2011) | 42% |

*Source*: Carneiro et al. 2012; Group 2014

relative increase: from 2002 to 2011, increase in pesticide use amounted to 156 percent, whereas in Brazil it was 42 percent, also significant.

## REGULATING PESTICIDES: AGRARIAN PRODUCTION VERSUS HEALTH AND ENVIRONMENTAL PRODUCTION

Three types of knowledge are considered when regulating pesticides: agronomical performance, human toxicology, and environmental toxicology (Pelaez, Silva, and Araújo 2013). The relative weight of each type of knowledge varies from country to country, according to the socio, political, and economic context. Due to the importance of agrarian production for the economy in Argentina and Brazil, there are strong political and economic stakes in favor of agronomical criteria. A good indicator for assessing the weight of each is the type of governmental body that has decision-making powers in pesticides regulation. In terms of human and environmental toxicology, both countries register pesticides based on the toxicological product classifications made by the World Health Organization. However, the international standard is just a starting point for state regulation, which should take into account the concrete contexts of pesticide use. As stated in the previous sections, the WHO does not hold responsibility for the damage or effects of the practical use of pesticides.

In Argentina, though the approval, registration, and commercialization of pesticides are under the jurisdiction of the federal government, their use is the jurisdiction of provincial and municipal governments. This means that only the federal government can ban the commercialization of a pesticide, while only the provinces and municipalities can define the "wrong use" or "wrong place to use it" (for example, through the definition of environmental protection areas). National regulations, mainly based on the agronomic criterion, have been and are very permissive, and no substantial changes have been registered in the past years. In fact, the only governmental body in charge is the National Service of Sanitation and Food Quality (SENASA), subordinate to the ministry of agriculture. Neither the National Ministry of Health nor the secretary of environment has a voice on this issue. More progress was made at the local level, where environmental and public health criteria have been increasingly incorporated in the last years. New provincial laws and municipal (county) ordinances establishing "pesticide-free zones" around populated areas (restricting ground and aerial sprayings) were enacted to fill the gaps of the national regulatory framework (Vara, Piaz, and Arancibia 2012). However, the toxicological classification established by SENASA-WHO still provides the basis of these local norms (which establishes stricter limits for the use of more toxic products).

In Brazil, pesticide regulation has shifted from a very permissive to a more restrictive framework as a result of environmental, public health, and agronomical performance criteria, in which all three governmental bodies are involved: the ministries of agriculture, health, and environment (Pelaez, Terra, and Silva 2010).

The national pesticide bill (Bill 7802/89) established stricter rules for registering pesticides, such as limiting new register to substances that are equally or less toxic to those on the market; foreseeing the possibility of canceling registration by request of civil society; traceability from agrochemicals from production to final use by means of a register of all involved; obligation of agronomic prescription for selling agrochemicals; rules for packaging, labeling, and new sanctions and liability rules (Pelaez et al. 2010). These new rules have affected the interests of influential associations of agrarian producers and national chemical industries. These actors not only contrapose a stricter enforcement of the current regulations but also provide constant pressure to exclude the attributions of the environment and health bodies in making toxicology assessments in favor of the sole competence of the ministry of agriculture in making a decision, one that is based on agronomic efficiency (Coutinho 2013).

However, new rules in Brazil and Argentina were not accompanied by an increase in human and material resources to improve the state capacity to enforce and sanction them (Pelaez et al. 2010), Vara, Piaz, and Arancibia 2012). The gap between the law and its application is a constant challenge, considering the vast cultivated area in both countries and the rapid extension of their agrarian borders, which cannot be separated from a larger volume of pesticide use. In addition, the concentration of decision-making powers in regulating agrochemicals in the executive power has paved the way for lobbyists from chemical industries and agrarian producers to take action, particularly through the ministry of agriculture, their main spokesperson in the executive power.

In sum, in light of contrasting positions between those who favor the increase in large-scale production of agrarian commodities and of those concerned with or affected by the negative health and environmental consequences, pesticide regulation in general, and regulatory science in particular, have become a target of political struggles in Argentina and Brazil. On the one hand, actors from agribusiness quantify the rise in pesticide consumption as a sign of market growth, technological incorporation, and economic productivity. On the other hand, various scientists and health professionals have hypothesized that such substantial and steady increase in pesticide use as the underlying cause for many health and environmental problems among rural communities in these countries—some of which had been already acknowledged by international experiments. These experts initiated a series of independent clinical, experimental, and epidemiological research proving the poisonous effects of pesticides in an effort to get undone science done (Hess 2010). Some experts worked collectively and in close collaboration with grassroots movements and participated in local campaigns against the unrestricted use of pesticides. The following two sections will describe how concerned scientists and health professionals challenged the safety of pesticides in Argentina and Brazil respectively.

ARGENTINA

The first complaints about illnesses associated with pesticides in Argentina were raised at the beginning of the 2000s and involved a group of mothers, a biologist, and a clinical physician from a suburban neighborhood bordering soybean farms in the city of Córdoba (Arancibia 2013a). A group of mothers, who came to be known as Mothers of Ituzaingó, identified an unusual increase in the cases of cancer and reproductive problems among their children and neighbors. They shared their concern with Dr. Raúl Montenegro, a biologist from the National University of Córdoba, and offered an hypothesis on the association between these illnesses and pesticide exposure (Montenegro 2002, 2003). At the same time, they requested changes in local regulations to restrict their use in close proximity to their houses. Ignored by local authorities, and together with Dr. Mario Carpio, they pursued an epidemiological survey, which showed more cases of cancer in the neighborhood than what provincial health authorities had acknowledged (Municipalidad de Córdoba—Secretaría de Salud—Equipo de trabajo UPAS 28 2013). Though the official recognition of poisoning effects of pesticides in the neighborhood took years, these early claims became the first steps that sparked a national campaign against the unrestricted use of pesticides.

In 2004, the Mothers of Ituzaingó together with Grupo de Reflexión Rural (GRR),[3] Union of Popular Assemblies (UAC),[4] and the NGO CEPRONAT launched the national campaign "Stop the Sprayings." One of the outcomes of the campaign was the publication of a book titled *Fumigated Peoples* in 2009. The book contained data provided by physicians and scientists who had studied the problem of pesticides as well as testimonies from victims. In this context, concerned scientists and rural physicians produced new independent clinical, experimental, and epidemiological research (undone science) proving the poisonous effects of pesticides in various GM crops–producing provinces of Argentina. In the next sections, we consider the "undone science" generated in this context and, in particular, a turning point experiment and the foundation of the Network of Physicians of Fumigated Villages-REDUAS.

## Getting Undone Science Done

Indeed, over the years, physicians and scientists from different GM crop–producing provinces across Argentina had been denouncing the poisoning effects of pesticides and produced different types of scientific evidence. Pediatrician and neonatologist Dr. Rodolfo Páramo showed that in the hospital where he was employed, a rural village in the province of Santa Fe (Malabrigo), the annual rate of birth defects was critically higher than the national average. He demonstrated how, in 2006, 12 cases of birth defects were found per 200 newborns (0.06), whereas the national rate was one per 85,000 newborns (0.001) (REDUAS—Médicos de Pueblos Fumigados 2010).

Geneticist Dr. María Fernanda Simoniello from the National University of Litoral in the province of Santa Fe, analyzed genotoxic and oxidative damage in a group of horticultural workers. She evaluated the DNA damage, modifications in oxidative balance, and exposure biomarkers in groups of individuals occupationally exposed to mixtures of agrochemicals. The study involved 105 farmworkers (indirectly exposed) and pesticide applicators (directly exposed) from the horticultural belt of Santa Fe and 112 donors from the same area who had no exposure to pesticides in their workplace as the control group. Subjects directly and indirectly exposed to pesticides showed enzymatic alterations, modifications in oxidative balance, and genotoxic damage when compared to the control group (Simoniello et al. 2008; Simoniello et al. 2010).

Furthermore, biochemist Dr. Raúl Lucero, geographer Dr. Mirta L. Ramírez, intensive care physician, Dr. María del Carmen Seveso, and pediatrician Dr. Analía Otaño from the province of Chaco pointed to a critical increase in the provincial annual rates of birth defects and cancer, which they associated to the steady spread of areas cultivated with GM crops in the period between 1994–2009. While in 1997/1998 they found 19.1 cases of birth defects per 10,000 newborns, in 2008/2009 they found 85.3 per 10,000. While in 1991 children cancer rate was 8.03 per 100,000 children, it was 15.7 per 100,000 in 2007 (Ramírez et al. 2012; REDUAS—Médicos de Pueblos Fumigados 2010).

Pediatrician Dr. Hugo De Maio, Chief of Surgery Division from the Pediatric Provincial Hospital Madariaga in the province of Misiones, stated that while the provincial historic average rate was 0.1 birth defects per 1000 newborns (0.001), at his hospital he found 7.2 per 1000 (70 percent higher) in 2008 (REDUAS—Médicos de Pueblos Fumigados 2010). This hospital was the only one equipped to treat birth defects in the province, so it received all the cases. De Maio also applied a neurocognitive test to children younger than one year and found that children coming from agricultural areas where they had been exposed to pesticides performed worse than children from the capital city.

Geneticist Dr. Gladys Trombotto, from the Maternity and Neonatal Unit of the National University of Córdoba (UNC), assessed 110,000 births over a ten-year period, and found a two and threefold increase in congenital and musculoskeletal defects respectively between 1971 and 2003 (Trombotto, 2009). At the same time, compared to the international average, percentages of birth defects were critically higher. For the period 2004–2008 the European Registry of Birth Defects showed 23.3 percent of cases in 69,635 pregnancies (EUROCAT 2012), the Latin American (ECLAM 2010) showed 26.6 percent in 88,000 pregnancies, and the maternity ward at UNC showed 37.1 percent (ECLAM 2010) with increasing tendency.

Geneticists Dr. Delia Aiassa and Dr. Fernando Mañas monitored genotoxicity in a group of 80 people exposed in relation to a control group. The analysis of their health status showed that 50 percent of the participants in the exposed group reported persistent symptomatology associated with respiratory (sneezing, coughing, bronchospasm, etc.), dermatological and/or mucocutaneous (skin and eye itching, tearing, pigmentation, etc.), digestive (vomiting), and neurological problems (headache and dizziness). The indicators of genetic damage observed in the exposed group were all significantly increased in comparison to the reference group in the three tests used. The results indicated that genetic damage could be attributed to exposure to various chemical substances (Aiassa et al. 2012; Mañas, Peralta, Gorla, Bosh, and Aiassa 2009).

Ecotoxicologist Dr. Rafael Lajmanovich has demonstrated that the run-off of agricultural pesticides has serious consequences on amphibian's survival and health. Indeed, agricultural activities not only deprive some species of healthy environments but also produce biochemical negative responses, hematological disturbances, testicular damage, and morphological abnormalities (Attademo, Peltzer, Lajmanovich, Cabagna, and Fiorenza 2007; Casco et al. 2006; Izaguirre, Lajmanovich, Peltzer, Soler, and Casco 2000; R C Lajmanovich, Sánchez-Hernández, Stringhini, and Peltzer 2004; Rafael C Lajmanovich, Attademo, Peltzer, Junges, and Cabagna, 2011; Lorenzatti et al. 2004; Peltzer et al. 2008; Peltzer, Lajmanovich, and Beltzer 2003). Investigating how pesticides affect the survival and different biology traits of anuran amphibians is especially important considering the importance of amphibians in the food webs of diverse ecosystem communities, as well as biological indicators of environmental health.

A new subnational comparative epidemiological study on health effects of pesticide exposure across three GM soy–producing provinces (Córdoba, Santa Fe, and Chaco) is currently underway and coordinated by Dr. Damian Verseñazzi from the National University of Rosario, Dr. Cristina Arnulphi from the National University of Córdoba, and Dr. María del Carmen Seveso from the Hospital of Chaco in collaboration of a group of students from the National University of Buenos Aires. In 2009, the results of a new experiment proving detrimental effects of glyphosate on the development of embryos were published on the front page of a famous national newspaper, which marked a critical turning point in the overall struggle over pesticides in Argentina.

## An Experiment on Embryos Reaches the Media

In April 2009, the front page of the national newspaper *Página 12* published new experimental findings by Dr. Andrés Carrasco, embryologist from the National Commission of Science and Technology (CONICET) and head of the Molecular Embryology Lab at the National University of Buenos Aires. His findings showed that glyphosate causes malformations in embryos (Aranda 2009a). Dr. Carrasco's results confirmed what rural communities had been saying for years. In an interview, Dr. Carrasco said that further studies should be conducted immediately to analyze other damages caused by glyphosate, and its use should be banned or at least strongly limited (Aranda 2009b). In the interview, he argued that science is urged by powerful economic interests, and not by the quest for truth and the welfare of the people.

Even if Dr. Carrasco's findings were not the first experimental results on detrimental effects of glyphosate on public health, previous experiments published in scientific journals in English or French were inaccessible for the Argentine lay public. The fact that the study was published in Spanish in a massive national newspaper made a difference, and his findings quickly garnered public attention. The government was forced to address the debate on pesticides and explain the lack of protective regulations. The Defense Ministry (where Dr. Carrasco was head of the Research Department), prohibited the use of glyphosate on lands and urban areas belonging to the ministry. Although the area was relatively small, it was an important political gesture. Not surprisingly, the initiative came up against strong opposition: high-ranking public officers and powerful agribusiness men launched a strong delegitimizing campaign against Dr. Carrasco. In the following years, he faced censorship, withdrawal of funds, reprimands, threats, and even physical repression.

In the days after, *La Nación*, the oldest national newspaper known for defending the interests of rural elites, published five articles challenging the validity of Carrasco's research (Motta and Alasino 2013). In addition, the minister of science and technology questioned the scientific validity of the results on television, due to the fact that they were first published in a massive newspaper instead of a scientific journal. He also defended the use of glyphosate-based herbicides and highlighted that the Ministry of Agriculture approved its use a long time ago based on worldwide experiences (Barañao in Huergo 2009).

Soon after the minister's TV appearance, more than 600 intellectuals and scientists, as well as NGOs and indigenous movements from various countries produced a manifest in support of Carrasco and demanded a real detachment of science from lucrative interests and international corporations: when the results of a study on the effects of a widespread agrochemical used in Argentina are being challenged, we support a university-scientific system autonomous from large corporate economic interests (Alerta 2009).

At the same time, the Committee on Ethics in Science and Technology recommended the creation of a scientific interdisciplinary council within CONICET in order to review and evaluate available international and national scientific evidence on the effects of glyphosate. A report was published in July 2009. Epidemiological studies show some pesticides (including glyphosate) were associated with miscarriages and loss of fertility. There is no scientific data in Argentina.

> (. . .) It has been mentioned the increase in birth defects and abnormal development associated to the use of glyphosate in fumigators' and rural worker children. (. . .) Different environmental factors can intervene in

> the process of endocrine disruption. It is difficult to establish a causal relationship between exposition to chemical substances and illness or alterations of human health (. . .). There is not enough data on the effects of glyphosate on human health in Argentina. It would be important to promote the development of pertinent studies.
>
> (Comision Nacional de Investigacion sobre Agroquímicos 2009: 94–95)

Agribusiness firms produced most of the scientific studies quoted. Neither Carrasco's study nor studies by other physicians and scientists were taken into account. In August 2010, Dr. Carrasco's results were published in an international journal of toxicology (Paganelli et al. 2010). Yet none of those who challenged the validity of Dr. Carrasco's results, based on the fact that the results had been published in the mass media, withdrew their criticism. In fact, the same month the worst episode of censorship took place in a rural village in the Province of Chaco. Before the beginning of a talk that Dr. Carrasco was to deliver to the neighbors, a "gang" of 100 men showed up and threatened him (Amnesty International 2010).

## Physicians of Fumigated Villages—REDUAS

In August 2010, scientists and physicians who had been researching pesticide-related illnesses, among them Dr. Carrasco, Dr. Páramo, Dr. Otaño, Dr. De Maio, Dr. Trombotto, Dr. Lucero, Dr. Seveso, and Dr. Simoniello, held a meeting at the School of Medical Sciences at the National University of Córdoba to present the empirical results of their research. The idea was born in a national campaign meeting within the campaign "Stop the Sprayings" and became possible by convincing the university to host and fund the event. The meeting was a success. It became the first conference on the detrimental health effects of pesticides hosted at a renowned national university; and it gathered many more attendants than expected, not only experts but also lay public.

A summary of all the presentations of the conference was published as a printed report, available as well online on REDUAS's webpage. The report was introduced by a declaration signed by the participants. It noted that for ten years rural populations of soy-production areas have been claiming to political authorities, the judiciary system, and public opinion that their health is threatened by agrochemical spraying. And in order to create a space for analysis and academic reflection on the state of fumigated villages, listen and help the members of health teams at rural hospitals that have been denouncing and facing this problem, the School of Medicine at the National University of Córdoba called this first national meeting of physicians and experts (Ávila Vázquez and Nota 2010).

On the last day of the meeting at the National University of Córdoba, some of the physicians decided to establish the University Network of

Environment and Health-Physicians of Fumigated Villages (REDUAS), coordinated by Dr. Medardo Ávila Vázquez. The goals of Physicians of Fumigated Villages were defined as:

> To link, coordinate and enhance scientific research, health care, epidemiological analysis and the promotion and defense of the right to collective health, performed by different teams working in ten different provinces of Argentina and who are mobilized because of the problem of the damaging effects on health brought upon by the fumigation and spraying, systematically more than 300 million of liters of insecticides over 12 million people that coexist with sewn fields of agro-industrial crops. In order to advance in this sense, it is proposed to contribute to the public debate out of the necessity to construct productive practices which allow for the happy survival of the entire human race on earth's surface and for the public, private and collective responsibility of the defense of these ecological conditions. (. . .) Considering the right to health as one of the social values that we should try to favor when we analyze or make political-economic decisions, we find it necessary to broaden the diffusion of scientific knowledge available and many times ignored; provide this generation with new data as well as experimental and epidemiological research; and give power to the voice of those health teams, researchers, and habitants in general whose rights are effected by environmental attacks generated by productive practices which are ecologically aggressive.
>
> (REDUAS n.d. 17)

After the first national meeting, two other meetings of REDUAS were held at the National University of Rosario in the Province of Santa Fe. With more than 20 professionals involved, REDUAS set out to organize workshops, deliver talks, and communicate national and international scientific news on health effects of pesticides on their webpage and social media.

## BRAZIL

In 2011, on April 7, World Health Day, an alliance of civil society organizations and social movements launched the nationwide Permanent Campaign Against Pesticides and For Life. It aimed at fighting pesticide use associated with agribusiness and promotes an alternative model of agrarian development, based on agroecology and peasant farming. The campaign is a joint result of wide alliances among different sectors in civil society: 1) social movements and networks; 2) schools, universities, and research institutes; 3) trade unions and professional organizations; 4) NGOs, associations, cooperatives, and civil society entities; 5) student movements; and 6) politicians. In the scientific and medical community, the prominent National

Cancer Institute, the Fundação Oswaldo Cruz and the Associação Brasileira de Saúde Coletiva (Brazilian Association of Collective Health, ABRASCO) joined the campaign, along with many universities and research centers.

Evidence that agrochemicals negatively influence health was a starting point of the campaign and therefore the participation of scientists and physicians is fundamental to its actions and success. Indeed, the campaign resulted from two parallel yet converging processes: grassroots mobilization among the rural poor, and health professionals producing and communicating empirical findings. Regarding the former, social movements from the state of Ceará, a region of fruit production for export, were fighting locally the effects of agrochemicals in the health of workers, communities, mothers, as well as the environmental contamination. They brought the issue to the national assembly of Via Campesina, the international peasant movement. Via Campesina Brazil then organized the National Seminar on Agrochemicals, in September 2010, in which the movement decided to launch a national campaign.

At the same time, scientists and health professionals also started their own mobilization against pesticides. ABRASCO provided the main organizational base in which networks of health professionals started a critical engagement with the issue and worked on defining strategies on how to employ their main resource, namely, expertise. Indeed, the campaign relies on two types of scientific evidence to back their claims: first, the damage caused by agrochemicals among producers and consumers and second, the possibility of feeding the population with agroecology. Scientists and health professionals affiliated with ABRASCO, from various disciplines and based in different regions in Brazil, played a key role in collecting existing scientific studies and conducting new studies on both issues. Their engagement culminated with the launching of a dossier in 2012, in three volumes. The next part of this article will focus on how they addressed the "undone science" related to the health impact of pesticides. First, it will present the history of ABRASCO and of its involvement in the issue and then show their contribution to build "undone science" and challenge regulatory science.

## Antecedents

Founded in 1979, ABRASCO is an association of research institutes, universities, training bodies, and public services, as well as individual professionals working on social medicine and public health. The goal is to strengthen dialogue between research, education, and training but also to provide a better articulation of the technical-scientific community with health services, civil society, and public bodies. ABRASCO has been active in the processes of political redemocratization in Brazil, taking part in the first national health conference and influencing the creation of a public health system in the federal constitution that was approved in the new democratic period. Since then, ABRASCO plays an active role in participatory democracy in Brazil, where it is committed to proposing public policies that foster public health. A wide-ranging program of congresses, seminars, and workshops inform their role. The national congresses organized by ABRASCO bring together around 7,500 health experts and professionals.

In terms of knowledge production, it edits renowned scientific journals with high impact factors. ABRASCO states that part of its mission is to strengthen knowledge production and improve the elaboration of public policies in health, education, science, and technology to address the health problems of the Brazilian population. The association has a democratic organizational structure and a decentralized structure of working groups and thematic networks.

The Thematic Group on Health and Environment (GTSA) set the pesticide issue on the agenda of ABRASCO and created a series of events to promote the debate. In 2010, the general assembly of the first Brazilian Symposium in Health and Environment (a second edition followed in 2014) approved a motion calling for a greater involvement of the members with the pesticides including: research, technologies, capacity building, support bodies and institutions committed to the health promotion of Brazilian society, social movements to protect health and environment and to promote zones free of pesticides, and the promotion of agroecological transition for a healthy and sustainable production and consumption. ABRASCO gives its support to the National Permanent Campaign against Pesticides and for Life (Carneiro et al. 2012).

In April 2011, a similar motion was approved at the Fifth Brazilian Congress of Social and Human Sciences on Health, also organized by ABRASCO. In November of the same year, during the Seventh Brazilian Congress of Epidemiology, the GTSA organized a workshop to propose that ABRASCO members, commissions, and working groups join efforts to produce a dossier on the health impact of pesticides. The working groups on nutrition, workers' health, and health promotion joined the call and participated in elaborating the dossier. In their presentation of the dossier, they wrote that their aim was to alert, by means of scientific evidence, national public authorities and society in general for the elaboration of public policies that can protect and promote human health and that of ecosystems affected by agrochemicals. ABRASCO adopted different forms of action: recompilation of information, conduction of their own research, as well as lobbying. Here we concentrate on their actions to address "undone science" on the health impact of agrochemicals.

## The Dossiers on "Undone Science"

The dossier titled, *A Warning about the Health Impacts of Agrochemicals*, was published in three separate volumes, each with a specific focus and each launched in a different event in the year of 2012 in order to call attention to each topic at once. The first, *Agrochemicals, Food and Nutritional*

*Safety, and Health*, was released in April at the World Nutrition Congress, in Rio de Janeiro. The second, *Agrochemicals, Health, and Sustainability* was launched during the People's Summit for Social and Environmental Justice, a civil society forum parallel to the Rio+20 United Nations Conference on Sustainable Development, in June. The third, *Agrochemicals, Knowledge, and Citizenship*, was launched in November at the Tenth ABRASCO Public Health Congress. The authors explained that they opted for a quick answer instead of a thorough compilation, since the motivation in collecting information was to mobilize society (Carneiro et al. 2012). In the following, we explore how these experts have: (a) defined what is undone science on health impacts of agrochemicals in Brazil, (b) conducted studies to get "undone science" done, and (c) made policy recommendations to reform regulatory science.

## DEFINING "UNDONE SCIENCE" ON THE HEALTH IMPACT OF AGROCHEMICALS IN BRAZIL

In Dossier I, the section "Challenges to Science" provides a summary of the critiques of regulatory science, which includes: pesticide regulation is based on fragile and insufficient scientific evidence of the absence of damage; it is reductionist and supports the use of agrochemicals, at the same time as it hinders a more comprehensive knowledge of causes of human intoxication. The authors emphasize two areas of "undone science": assessments of multi-exposure and chronic effects. First, experimental methods can only assess one toxic substance and one route of exposure, whereas in the real world people are exposed to multiple substances via multiple routes (oral, dermal, inhalation). Second, these methods only assess acute exposure. Thus data is only collected for serious intoxication, such as death and emergencies, whereas little is known about the "subclinical" symptoms of chronic intoxication, to which most people are exposed. In addition, health professionals and institutions lack capacity to identify such effects. They conclude that these are the limitations of decontextualized research—that is, research not based on contexts that happen in the real world but instead designed in the context of approving the wide-scale use of chemicals—that is, in the context of regulatory science (Carneiro et al. 2012).

In Dossier 2, the section "Gaps in Knowledge" reiterates multi-exposure as an area of "undone science" in toxicology, calling attention to the possible synergies between products that might generate toxicity, even when respecting the established legal limits of each product. In addition, this section of the dossier emphasizes the context of vulnerability in which populations that are exposed to agrochemicals live, including socioeconomic conditions affecting public health.

In toxicology, risk assessment is conducted as a scientific method on the potential adverse effects derived from human exposure to dangerous agents or situations. Usually only exposure to one substance is taken into consideration, in a decontextualized way. In the real processes of production/work as well as consumption, there is contact with more than one chemical substance, with the concomitant aggravation by other potential dangers or lifestyles (Augusto et al. 2012).

"Undone science" is detailed in Dossier 3 in two further subsections. The section "Challenges in Toxicology" lists four areas to advance regulatory science. The first is to have adequate laboratorial technologies to monitor residues in water, air, soil, and food. The second is to establish appropriate indicators of occupational exposure that can assess long-term exposure to small dosages, which is the reality of most rural workers. The third is to assess effects of simultaneous exposure to various pesticides and chemical substances. The fourth is the need for independent studies on the health and environmental effects of the cultivation and consumption of GMOs (Rigotto et al. 2012).

The section "Diagnostics on Impacts of Agrochemicals" identifies three nodes of "undone science." Regarding epidemiological studies on acute intoxications, there is no knowledge on their frequency and characteristics in Brazil and, due to methodological differences, available studies cannot be compared. Therefore, they call for the need of a multi-sited study, on different agricultural contexts and geographical regions, supported by public research grants. Second, there are few studies on chronic diseases and none brings together different contexts and products. Such a study should be carried out, one that builds on the findings of the study on acute intoxications. Finally, there is a lack of qualitative studies on the impacts of agrochemicals. These should be conducted by social scientists, with priority to cases of environmental injustice (Rigotto et al. 2012).

## STUDIES TO MAKE UNDONE SCIENCE DONE

As explained by the organizers of the dossiers, there was an urgent need to compile existing information to support their claims that there was enough scientific evidence to take preventive measures in order to avoid further health damage by agrochemicals. Though they acknowledged that further thorough research should be conducted to address the knowledge gaps. With this aim, they first compiled national scientific studies conducted, among others, by the authors of the dossier and/or ABRASCO members. They then elaborated on a cartography of existing research in Brazil on the topic. Dossier 1 presents the studies in the section "Scientific Evidence of Health Risks," organized in six subsections.

The first relates to data on residues of agrochemicals in food. In 2011, a national monitoring program from the Brazilian Agency for Health Surveillance found that 63 percent of the food samples showed residues from agrochemicals and 28 percent were above the allowed limits or using nonapproved products. The second consists of a recompilation of international scientific evidence of health damage from agrochemicals. One table summarizes the acute and chronic health damages for each agrochemical; one table lists the effects of agrochemicals that motivated their ban or restriction in other countries, while they are still in use in Brazil.

The third type of evidence comprises data on contamination of water for human consumption and of rain. Against the background of a lack of official data and weak monitoring, covering only 10 percent of approved products in a context of expansion of number and types of substances allowed in legal parameters for water quality, ABRASCO researchers collected data from two states with higher pesticide use, Ceará and Mato Grosso (Neto 2010). Building on this, a fourth study focuses on workers' health and environmental contamination in fruits and shrimps culture in Ceará. With public grants and financial support from the health ministry, a research coordinated by Rigotto (Rigotto 2010) found poly-exposure to many agrochemicals in all samples collected. A further study confirmed contamination of the subsoil water.

The two latter types of evidence are results from research conducted in Mato Grosso by the Federal University (UFMT) and analyzed the contamination of water and of breast milk. In 2006, there was a "chemical rain" in São Lucas do Rio Verde, a location of intensive agrarian production, when aerial spraying destroyed 180 sites of medicinal plants and greens and caused acute intoxication of children and elderly (Pignati, Machado, and Cabral 2007). Between 2007 and 2011, researchers controlled water samples, detecting high exposure (occupational, environmental, and through food ingestion) to agrochemicals (136 liters/year per capita in 2010). Further findings established that aerial spraying disrespected legal distances to villages and water reservoirs; there was contamination in schools by various agrochemicals in drinking water, rain, and air; and there were lakes with residues of agrochemicals and fauna with higher levels of malformation. Finally, evidence of contamination of breast milk was also found in São Lucas do Rio Verde and in cow's milk in four states in Brazil (Moreira, Peres, Pignati, and Dores 2010).

Dossier 3 presents a "Cartography of Scientists Working on Agrochemicals and Health in Brazil (2007–2012)." It offers the results from research in a national database and consists of quantitative and qualitative data on the topics, methodologies, and areas of available research. The main goal was to search for possible partnerships to make "undone science," in particular to conduct nationwide epidemiological studies and monitoring studies of residues in water, soil, and food. The cartography shows that from all scientists working on agrochemicals in Brazil, only a few have made experimental (2 percent), epidemiological, or (3 percent) toxicological studies (10 percent), nor did many scientists conduct research on the products under toxicological reassessment by the health regulatory agency. Among these, the most studied was glyphosate (10 percent of research), of which

74 percent focused on agronomic performance, while only 2 percent on toxicity. Based on this information, the authors of the dossier argue that existing research concentrates on the expansion of use to new crops and pests. They conclude that, although there are almost 5,000 scientists in Brazil working on agrochemicals, there lacks institutional incentives to research the health and environmental impacts (Rigotto et al. 2012).

## POLICY RECOMMENDATIONS TO REFORM REGULATORY SCIENCE

The Dossier 1 ends with ten recommendations to address agrochemicals as a public health problem. Points 3 and 10 are related to the "undone science" that is constructed by current regulatory science:

> 3. Encourage and support the production of knowledge and technical/scientific capacity on the issue of pesticides in its various dimensions, facing the theoretical and methodological challenges (. . .)
> 10. Consider for the registration and re-evaluation of pesticides evidence on: epidemiological; chronic effects, including low concentrations and multi-exposure; clinical signs and symptoms in populations exposed, pathological and predictive indicators.
>
> (Carneiro et al. 2012: 18–24)

The organizers of Dossier 2 argue that there is lack of available and systematized data and knowledge on health and environmental effects of agrochemicals. However, there is enough evidence to demonstrate the link between exposure and increase in cancer, allergies, and endocrine deregulation. Recalling examples of state omission and delays to act (such as asbestos, benzeno, DDT), they argue that the existing evidence on the detrimental health effects of pesticides are sufficient warnings to demand governmental protective responses. For regulatory science in particular, Dossier 2 states the need of revising concepts used in toxicology and its assumptions on linear relationship of dose/effect. According to the authors, certain types of substances, such as carcinogenic and immunotoxic, cannot be said to have "acceptable and safe exposure limits," for instance (Augusto et al. 2012). For pesticide regulation in general, the dossier calls for stronger surveillance and monitoring of health effects.

> Considering the fragmentation of data; diversification of diffuse sources; little information on degradation, transformations, derivatives and human exposure; that environmental monitoring focuses primarily on fluid media (air, water) and frequently forgets soil, sediment, and

> human consumption products, it is necessary to establish (. . .) monitoring indicators/surveillance.
>
> (Augusto et al. 2012)

The recommendations are: to identify gaps in toxicity test data, in data on surveillance/exposure, and in information on environmental externalities and to identify the magnitude of impacts and identify priority impacts in sentinel groups and children (Augusto et al. 2012). With such data, scientists will be able to advance in making "undone science" done.

## CONCLUSION

Although agricultural biotechnology has brought important economic benefits to Argentina and Brazil, over the years, rural populations have increasingly pointed to the related health problems, what they perceive as a direct result of the increased use of pesticides. The claims of rural communities have been almost entirely ignored by local and national governments, as well as the science and technology industry. In fact, the domestic science and technology systems have played a key role in facilitating that pathway of agricultural intensification, and agronomic formal knowledge creation is now almost exclusively orientated towards the support of further development in this realm. Ignored by governmental authorities, some communities initiated grassroots movements in order to advocate for more protective regulations to restrict the use of pesticides and to promote alternative agricultural practices (agroecology, organic farming) (Arancibia 2013a, 2013b, Carrizo and Berger 2012, Porto and Milanez 2009).

A growing number of physicians, scientists, and health experts have joined social movements' claims against the unrestricted use of pesticides in Argentina since 2002. These experts produced various types of studies showing the poisoning effects of pesticides and challenged the official toxicological classifications of pesticides determined by SENASA. The publication of the results of an experiment on birth defects associated with glyphosate (main ingredient of Roundup) in 2009 brought the problem of pesticides to the national political agenda. In 2010, some experts founded the Network of Environment and Health-Physicians of Fumigated Villages (REDUAS). In the eyes of public opinion, REDUAS became an important expert benchmark on the issue of pesticides and rural public health.

In Brazil, the launching of the Permanent Campaign Against Pesticides and For Life in 2011 was a fundamental step in the social mobilization on the health effects of pesticides, providing the organizational basis to network existing local struggles and to stimulate new local and regional initiatives. In 2014, during the International Day Against Pesticide Use, on December 3, there were simultaneous mobilizations in 27 Brazilian cities. The campaign sealed an alliance between social movements and the scientific community, which brought significant resources to support the movements' claims. The ABRASCO Dossier provided scientific evidence of the negative health and environmental impacts of pesticides and identified critical issues for undone science to be done. Since its publication in 2012, the authors and the spokespersons from the campaign are invited for interviews on the issue and have published articles in blogs and newspapers (Carneiro 2015, Folgado 2013, Paula 2015, Tubino 2013). Among the achievements of the campaign, they consider the National Policy for Agroecology and Organic Production, established in 2012; the health ministry's plan of health surveillance of populations exposed to agrochemicals; and local bill projects to forbid products.

There is a political dispute between two types of science when it comes to the health and environmental effects of pesticides. On the one hand, there is regulatory science, which is dominant because it is used by the state and also legitimized by international organizations such as the WHO. It relies on studies made by interested industries and consists of laboratory studies that only assess acute intoxication. On the other hand, the examples presented in this chapter on "undone science" present a different type of science. Independent researchers working at public universities and research institutes conduct this science. Their research is concerned with the contexts in which pesticides are actually applied. It consists of complementary data (epidemiological, experimental, clinical), assessing chronic diseases and long-term impacts of small dosages, multi-exposure to various chemical substances, and monitoring residues in the air, soil, water, and food.

The two cases outlined in this article show how personal and collective efforts as well as institutional resources are required to produce "undone science." According to Hess, 'undone science can get done, but it tends to get done in subordinate positions of a research field, where funding is limited and reproduction of a network (getting students into positions that can produce students) is difficult' (Hess 2010: 6). At the same time, it seems that even if producing "undone science" is a critical first step for challenging official regulatory science, scientific evidence is not enough on its own. The production of "undone science" is an important resource for social movement actions, but making it "official" requires further struggle. In both countries, powerful stakeholders have challenged the validity of research and experts still have to defend their findings. As Martin (1999) and (Delborne, 2008) have stated, affronting powerful economic interests usually implies a high cost for scientists producing "undone science." The fierce delegitimizing campaign against Dr. Carrasco in Argentina is the clearest example. Having important consequences over economic profits, the regulation of biotechnology is a field of strong social contention. A tough and long-term political struggle seems to be required in order to overcome the power of official regulatory science.

## NOTES

1. Agrochemicals is a generic term for the various chemical products used in agriculture. In most cases, agrichemical refers to the broad range of pesticides. It may also include synthetic fertilizers, hormones, and other chemical growth agents and concentrated stores of raw animal manure. Pesticides are substances meant for attracting, seducing, and then destroying or mitigating any pest. The term "pesticide" includes all of the following: herbicide, insecticide, insect growth regulator, nematicide, termiticide, molluscicide, piscicide, avicide, rodenticide, predacide, bactericide, insect repellent, animal repellent, antimicrobial, fungicide, disinfectant (antimicrobial), and sanitizer.
2. Some authors include the method of no till farming (siembra directa) as part of the technological package launched with GM seeds. No tillage means that machines sow the seeds without previously revolving land, which saves labor and protects soil against erosion.
3. GRR was founded in the mid-nineties by intellectuals and experts from different disciplines (social sciences, agronomic engineering, and economics). The group opposed the hegemonic agricultural model based on the export of transgenic commodities, which, according to them, was causing severe health and social problems.
4. UAC is a self-defined nonpartisan and autonomous national network of horizontal groups of neighbors involved in social-environmental struggles across Argentina.

## REFERENCES

Aiassa, D., Mañas, F., Bosch, B., Gentile, N., Bernardi, N., & Gorla, N. (2012). Biomarkers of genetic damage in human populations exposed to pesticides. *Acta Biológica Colombiana*, *17*(3), 485–510. Retrieved from http://www.scielo.org.co/scielo.php?script=sci_arttext&pid=S0120-548X2012000300003&lng=en&nrm=iso&tlng=es

Alerta, V. de. (2009). *Declaración*. Retrieved from http://voces-de-alerta.blogspot.com.ar/

Amnesty International. (2010). *Amnesty International Web Page*. Retrieved January 2, 2015, from http://www.amnesty.org/en/library/asset/AMR13/005/2010/en/303e9ee6-9138-405f-97fc-ed58965b76d0/amr130052010en.html

Antoniou, M., & Fagan, J. (2012). GMO Myths and Truths genetically modified crops (June). London: Earth Open Source.

Arancibia, F. (2013a). Challenging the bioeconomy : The dynamics of collective action in Argentina. *Technology in Society*, *35*, 72–92.

Arancibia, F. (2013b). Controversias científico-regulatorias y transgénicos en la Argentina. In T. Molina & M. Vara (Eds.), *Riesgo, Política y Alternativas Regulación y la Discusión Pública* (pp. 309–357). Buenos Aires, Argentina: Prometeo.

Aranda, D. (2009a, April 13). El tóxico de los campos. *Pagina 12*. Retrieved from http://www.pagina12.com.ar/diario/elpais/1–123111–2009–04–13.html

Aranda, D. (2009b, May). Lo que sucede en Argentina es casi un experimento masivo. *Página 12*. Retrieved from Lo que sucede en Argentina es casi un experimento masivo

Arbuckle, T.E., Lin, Z., & Mery, L.S. (2001). An exploratory analysis of the effect of pesticide exposure on the risk of spontaneous abortion in an Ontario farm population. *Environmental Health Perspectives*, *109*(8), 851–857. Retrieved from http://www.pubmedcentral.nih.gov/articlerender.fcgi?artid=1240415&tool=pmcentrez&rendertype=abstract

Attademo, A. M., Peltzer, P. M., Lajmanovich, R.C., Cabagna, M., & Fiorenza, G. (2007). Plasma B-esterase and glutathione S-transferase activity in the toad Chaunus schneideri (Amphibia, Anura) inhabiting rice agroecosystems of Argentina. *Ecotoxicology (London, England)*, *16*(8), 533–539. doi:10.1007/s10646–007–0154–0

Augusto, L.G.S., Carneiro, F., Pignati, W., Rigotto, R.M., Friedrich, K., Faria, N.M., . . . Guiducci Filho, E. (2012). *Agrotóxicos, saúde, ambiente e sustentabilidade. Dossiê ABRASCO: Um Alerta sobre os Impactos dos Agrotóxicos na Saúde*. Rio de Janeiro: ABRASCO. Retrieved from http://www.abrasco.org.br/UserFiles/File/ABRASCODIVULGA/2012/DossieAGT.pdf

Ávila Vázquez, M., & Nota, C. (2010). *1° ENCUENTRO NACIONAL DE MEDICXS DE PUEBLOS* (pp. 1–40). Córdoba.

Axelrad, J.C., Howard, C. V., & McLean, W.G. (2003). The effects of acute pesticide exposure on neuroblastoma cells chronically exposed to diazinon. *Toxicology*, *185*(1–2), 67–78. Retrieved from http://www.ncbi.nlm.nih.gov/pubmed/12505446

Beck, U. (2008). World at risk: The new task of critical theory. *Development and Society*, *37*(1), 1–22.

Benachour, N., & Séralini, G.-E. (2009). Glyphosate formulations induce apoptosis and necrosis in human umbilical, embryonic, and placental cells. *Chemical Research in Toxicology*, *22*(1), 97. Retrieved from http://pubs.acs.org/doi/abs/10.1021/tx800218n

Carneiro, F. (2015, January 17). Produção agroecológica tem capacidade de alimentar população com qualidade.

Carneiro, F., Pignati, W., Rigotto, R.M., Augusto, L.G.S., Rizollo, A., Muller, N., . . . Mello, M.S. de. (2012). *Agrotóxicos, segurança alimentar e nutricional e e saúde. Dossiê ABRASCO: Um Alerta sobre os Impactos dos Agrotóxicos na Saúde*. Rio de Janeiro: ABRASCO. Retrieved from http://www.abrasco.org.br/UserFiles/File/ABRASCODIVULGA/2012/DossieAGT.pdf

Carrizo, C.S., & Berger, M. (2012). The international peasant movement and the struggle for environmental justice in Brazil: An interview with Cleber Folgado from Movimiento de Pequeños Agricultores (MPA), Vía Campesina, Brazil. *Environmental Justice*, *5*(2), 111–114.

Casco, V.H., Izaguirre, M.F., Marín, L., Vergara, M.N., Lajmanovich, R.C., Peltzer, P., & Soler, A.P. (2006). Apoptotic cell death in the central nervous system of Bufo arenarum tadpoles induced by cypermethrin. *Cell Biology and Toxicology*, *22*(3), 199–211. doi:10.1007/s10565–006–0174–1

Catacora-Vargas, G., Galeano, P., Zanon Agapito—Tenfen, S., Aranda, D., Palau, T., & Nodari, R. (2012). *Report: Soybean Production in the Southern Cone of the Americas: Update on Land and Pesticide Use*. Cochabamba: Virmegraf. Retrieved from http://www.genok.com/news_cms/2012/july/report-soybean-production-in-the-southern-cone-of-the-americas-update-on-land-and-pesticide-use/158

Comision Nacional de Investigacion sobre Agroquímicos, C. (2009). *Evaluación de la información científica vinculada al glifosato en su incidencia sobre la salud humana y el ambiente*. Buenos Aires, Argentina.

Coutinho Jr., J. (2013, January 24). Por pressão ruralista, governo pretende criar uma comissão técnica para analisar e registrar novos agrotóxicos | Portal EcoDebate. *EcoDebate*. Retrieved from http://www.ecodebate.com.br/2013/12/10/por-pressao-ruralista-governo-pretende-criar-uma-comissao-tecnica-para-analisar-e-registrar-novos-agrotoxicos/

Dallegrave, E., Mantese, F.D., Coelho, R.S., Pereira, J.D., Dalsenter, P.R., & Langeloh, A. (2003). The teratogenic potential of the herbicide glyphosate-Roundup in Wistar rats. *Toxicology Letters*, *142*(1–2), 45–52. Retrieved from http://www.ncbi.nlm.nih.gov/pubmed/12765238

De Roos, A.J., Blair, A., Rusiecki, J.A., Hoppin, J.A., Svec, M., Dosemeci, M., . . . Alavanja, M.C. (2005). Cancer incidence among glyphosate-exposed pesticide applicators in the Agricultural Health Study. *Environmental Health Perspectives*, *113*(1), 49–54. Retrieved from http://www.pubmedcentral.nih.gov/articlerender.fcgi?artid=1253709&tool=pmcentrez&rendertype=abstract

Delborne, J.A. (2008). Transgenes and transgressions: Scientific dissent as heterogeneous practice. *Social Studies of Science*, *38*(4), 509–541. doi:10.1177/0306312708089716

ECLAM, E.C.L.A. de M.C. (2010). *XXXXI Reunion Anual del Estudio Colaborativo Latinoamericano de Malformaciones Congenitas* (pp. 1–97). Rio de Janeiro.

EUROCAT, E.S. of C.A. (2012). *Congenital Anomalies Prevalence Data Tables*. (pp. 1–97). Retrieved from http://www.eurocat-network.eu/accessprevalencedata/prevalencetables

Folgado, C. (2013, September 17). A luta constante contra os agrotóxicos. *Brasil de Fato*. Retrieved from http://www.brasildefato.com.br/node/11533

Frickel, S., Gibbon, S., Howard, J., Kempner, J., Ottinger, G., & David, H.J. (2010). Undone science: Charting social movement and civil society challenges to research agenda setting. *Science, Technology and Human Values*, *35*(4), 444–473.

Group, P. (2014). Estudio de Mercado de Fitosanitarios 2013. CASAFE.

Hardell, L., Eriksson, M., & Nordstrom, M. (2002). Exposure to pesticides as risk factor for non-Hodgkin's lymphoma and hairy cell leukemia: pooled analysis of two Swedish case-control studies. *Leukemia & Lymphoma*, *43*(5), 1043–1049. Retrieved from http://www.ncbi.nlm.nih.gov/pubmed/12148884

Hess, D. (2007). *Alternative pathways in science and industry* (p. 344). Cambridge: MIT Press.

Hess, D.J. (2009). The potentials and limitations of civil society research: Getting undone science done. *Sociological Inquiry*, 306–327.

Hess, D.J. (2010). Social movements, publics, and scientists. *Invited Lecture, Japanese Society for Science and Technology Studies, Tokyo*. Retrieved from http://www.davidjhess.org/

Huergo, H. in E.C.T.V.S. (2009, May 4). Interview with Minister of Science and Technology Lino Barañao. Argentina: Private TV Channel. Retrieved from http://www.youtube.com/watch?v=h5m8fqJ7hUQ

Izaguirre, M.F., Lajmanovich, R.C., Peltzer, P.M., Soler, A.P., & Casco, V.H. (2000). Cypermethrin-induced apoptosis in the telencephalon of Physalaemus biligonigerus tadpoles (Anura: Leptodactylidae). *Bulletin of Environmental Contamination and Toxicology*, *65*(4), 501–507. Retrieved from http://www.ncbi.nlm.nih.gov/pubmed/10960142

James, C. (2014). *Global status of commercialized biotech/GM Crops: 2013* (No. 46). Ithaca, NY: ISAAA.

Jasanoff, S. (1990). *The fifth branch: Science advisers as policymakers* (p. 302). Cambridge, MA: Harvard University Press.

Lajmanovich, R.C., Attademo, A.M., Peltzer, P.M., Junges, C.M., & Cabagna, M.C. (2011). Toxicity of four herbicide formulations with glyphosate on Rhinella arenarum (anura: bufonidae) tadpoles: B-esterases and glutathione S-transferase inhibitors. *Archives of Environmental Contamination and Toxicology*, *60*(4), 681–689. doi:10.1007/s00244–010–9578–2

Lajmanovich, R.C., Sánchez-Hernández, J.C., Stringhini, G., & Peltzer, P.M. (2004). Levels of serum cholinesterase activity in the rococo toad (Bufo paracnemis) in agrosystems of Argentina. *Bulletin of Environmental Contamination and Toxicology*, 72(3), 586–591. doi:10.1007/s00128–001–0284–5

Lorenzatti, E., Maitre, M.I., Lenardon, A., Lajmanovich, R., Peltzer, P., & Anglada, M. (2004). Pesticide residues in immature soybean in Argentina croplands. *Fresen. Environ. Bull.*, *13*, 675–678.

Mañas, F., Peralta, L., Gorla, N., Bosh, B., & Aiassa, D. (2009). Aberraciones cromosómicas en trabajadores rurales de la Provincia de Córdoba expuestos a plaguicidas. *BAG. Journal of Basic and Applied Genetics*, *20*(1). Retrieved from http://www.scielo.org.ar/scielo.php?script=sci_arttext&pid=S1852-62332009000100002&lng=es&nrm=iso&tlng=es

Marc, J., Bellé, R., Morales, J., Cormier, P., & Mulner-Lorillon, O. (2004). Formulated glyphosate activates the DNA-response checkpoint of the cell cycle leading to the prevention of G2/M transition. *Toxicological Sciences*, *82*(2), 436. doi:10.1093/toxsci/kfh281

Marc, J., Le Breton, M., Cormier, P., Morales, J., Bellé, R., & Mulner-Lorillon, O. (2005). A glyphosate-based pesticide impinges on transcription. *Toxicology and Applied Pharmacology*, *203*(1), 1–8. doi:10.1016/j.taap.2004.07.014

Marc, J., Mulner-Lorillon, O., & Bellé, R. (2004). Glyphosate-based pesticides affect cell cycle regulation. *Biology of the Cell / under the Auspices of the European Cell Biology Organization*, *96*(3), 245–249. doi:10.1016/j.biolcel.2003.11.010

Martin, B. (1999). Suppression of Dissent in Science. *Research in Social Problems and Public Policy*, *7*, 105–135.

McDuffie, H.H., Pahwa, P., McLaughlin, J.R., Spinelli, J.J., Fincham, S., Dosman, J.A., . . . Choi, N.W. (2001). Non-Hodgkin's lymphoma and specific pesticide exposures in men: cross-Canada study of pesticides and health. *Cancer Epidemiology, Biomarkers & Prevention : A Publication of the American Association for Cancer Research, Cosponsored by the American Society of Preventive Oncology*, *10*(11), 1155–1163. Retrieved from http://www.ncbi.nlm.nih.gov/pubmed/11700263

Montenegro, R. (2002). *Ituzaingo, plaguicidas en suelo. Informe de prensa.* Cordoba.

Montenegro, R. (2003). *Informe sobre los posibles contaminantes que habrían provocado la alta morbi-mortalidad registrada en barrio ituzaingo anexo. Establecimiento de los contaminantes principales y de sus rutas.* (p. 56). Córdoba.

Moore, K., Kleinman, D.L., Hess, D., & Frickel, S. (2011). Science and neoliberal globalization: a political sociological approach. *Theory and Society*, *40*(5), 505–532. doi:10.1007/s11186-011-9147-3

Moreira, J.C., Peres, F., Pignati, W.A., & Dores, E.F.G.C. (2010). *Avaliação do risco à saúde humana decorrente do uso de agrotóxicos na agricultura e pecuária na região Centro Oeste* (Relatório de Pesquisa No. CNPq 555193/2006-3.). Brasília.

Motta, R. (2014). Transnational Discursive Opportunities and Social Movement Risk Frames Opposing GMOs. *Social Movement Studies*, (August), 1–20. doi:10.1080/14742837.2014.947253

Motta, R., & Alasino, N. (2013). Medios y política en la Argentina: las disputas interpretativas sobre la soja transgénica y el glifosato. *Question*, *1*(38), 323–335. Retrieved from http://perio.unlp.edu.ar/ojs/index.php/question/article/view/1787

Municipalidad de Córdoba—Secretaría de Salud—Equipo de trabajo UPAS 28. (2013). El caso de Barrio Ituzaingó Anexo. Córdoba, Argentina. *Revista Cuestiones de Población Y Sociead*, *3*(3), 125–152.

Neto, M. de L.F. (2010). *Análise dos parâmetros agrotóxicos da Norma Brasileira de Potabilidade de Água: uma abordagem de avaliação de risco*. Escola Nacional de Saúde Pública, Rio de Janeiro.

Paganelli, A., Gnazzo, V., Acosta, H., López, S.L., & Carrasco, A.E. (2010). Glyphosate-based herbicides produce teratogenic effects on vertebrates by impairing retinoic acid signalling. *Chemical Research in Toxicology*, *23*(10), 1586–1595. doi:10.1021/tx1001749

Paula, F. (2015, January 25). A opção do país pelo agronegócio faz o brasileiro consumir 5,2 litros de agrotóxicos por ano. *Carta Maior*. Retrieved from http://cartamaior.com.br/?/Editoria/Meio-Ambiente/A-opcao-do-pais-pelo-agronegocio-faz-o-brasileiro-consumir-5-2-litros-de-agrotoxicos-por-ano/3/32594

Pelaez, V., Silva, L.R. da, & Araújo, E.B. (2013). Regulation of pesticides: A comparative analysis*. *Science and Public Policy*. doi:10.1093/scipol/sct020

Pelaez, V., Terra, F.H.B., & Silva, L.R. da. (2010). A regulamentação dos agrotóxicos no Brasil: entre o poder de mercado e a defesa da saúde e do meio ambiente. *Revista de Economia*, *2'36*(1), 27–48.

Peltzer, P.M., Lajmanovich, R.C., & Beltzer, M.A. (2003). The effects of habitat fragmentation on amphibian species richness in the floodplain of the middle Paraná River. *Herpetol*, *13*, 95–98.

Peltzer, P.M., Lajmanovich, R.C., Sánchez-Hernandez, J.C., Cabagna, M.C., Attademo, A.M., & Bassó, A. (2008). Effects of agricultural pond eutrophication on survival and health status of Scinax nasicus tadpoles. *Ecotoxicology and Environmental Safety*, *70*(1), 185–197. doi:10.1016/j.ecoenv.2007.06.005

Pignati, W.A., Machado, J.M.H., & Cabral, J.F. (2007). Major rural accident: The pesticide 'rain' case in Lucas do Rio Verde city—MT. *Ciência & Saúde Coletiva*, *12*(1), 105–114. doi:10.1590/S1413-81232007000100014

Porto, M.F., & Milanez, B. (2009). Eixos de desenvolvimento econômico e geração de conflitos socioambientais no Brasil: desafios para a sustentabilidade e a justiça ambiental. *Ciência & Saúde Coletiva*, *14*(6), 1983–1994.

Ramírez, M.L., Belingheri, B., Nicoli, M.B., Seveso, M. del C., Ramírez, L., & Garcete, M. (2012). *Relación enre el uso de agroquímicos y el estado sanitario de la población en localidades de los Departamentos Bermejo, Independencia y Tapenaga de la Provincia de Chaco* (p. 68). Resistencia, Chaco.

REDUAS—Médicos de Pueblos Fumigados. (2010). *1° Encuentro Nacional de Médicos de Pueblos Fumigados* (pp. 1–40).

REDUAS, M. de P.F. (n.d.). Objetivos. Retrieved January 2, 2015, from http://www.reduas.fcm.unc.edu.ar/

Richard, S., Moslemi, S., Sipahutar, H., Benachour, N., & Séralini, G.-E. (2005). Differential effects of glyphosate and roundup on human placental cells and aromatase. *Environmental Health Perspectives*, *113*(6), 716–720. Retrieved from http://www.questia.com/googleScholar.qst?docId=5009957048

Rigotto, R.M. (2010). *Estudo epidemiológico da população da região do Baixo Jaguaribe exposta à contaminação ambiental em área de uso de agrotóxicos*. Fortaleza. Retrieved from http://www.memorialapodi.com.br/linha-do-tempo/docs/2010/08/Pesquisa, Estudo Epidemiologico da Populacao do Baixo Jaguaribe, Doc Sintese dos Resultados Parciais da Pesquisa, 08.2010.pdf

Rigotto, R.M., Porto, M.F., Folgado, C., Faria, N.M., Augusto, L.G., Bedor, C., . . . Tygel, A. (2012). *Agrotóxicos, conhecimento científico e popular: construindo a ecologia de saberes*. Porto Alegre: ABRASCO. Retrieved from http://www.abrasco.org.br/UserFiles/File/ABRASCODIVULGA/2012/DossieAGT.pdf

Seralini, G., Clair, E., Mesnage, R., Gress, S., Defarge, N., Malatesta, M., . . . de Vendomois, J. (2012). Long term toxicity of a Roundup herbicide and a Roundup-tolerant genetically modified maize. *Food Science & Technology Toxicology*, *50*(11), 4221–4231.

Simoniello, M.F., Kleinsorge, E.C., Scagnetti, J.A., Grigolato, R.A., Poletta, G.L., & Carballo, M.A. (2008). DNA damage in workers occupationally exposed to pesticide mixtures. *Journal of Applied Toxicology (JAT)*, *28*(8), 957–965. doi:10.1002/jat.1361

Simoniello, M.F., Kleinsorge, E.C., Scagnetti, J.A., Mastandrea, C., Grigolato, R.A., Paonessa, A.M., & Carballo, M.A. (2010). Biomarkers of cellular reaction to pesticide exposure in a rural population. *Biomarkers: Biochemical Indicators of Exposure, Response, and Susceptibility to Chemicals*, *15*(1), 52–60. doi:10.3109/13547500903276378

Trombotto, G. (2009). *Tendencia de las Malformaciones Congénitas Mayores en el Hospital Universitario de Maternidad y Neonatología de la Ciudad de Córdoba en los años 1972–2003*. National University of Cordoba.

Tubino, N. (2013, January 24). Agrotóxicos: o perigo eterno. *Carta Maior*. Retrieved from http://cartamaior.com.br/?/Editoria/Meio-Ambiente/Agrotoxicos-o-perigo-eterno-/3/29058

UNCTAD. (2012). *The state of commodity dependence 2012*. New York and Geneva: UNCTAD. Retrieved from http://unctadxiii.org/en/SessionDocument/suc2011d8_en.pdf

Vara, A.M. (2005). *Argentina, GM natio. Chances and choices in uncertain times. Project on International GMO Regulatory Conflicts*. (p. 205). New York.

Vara, A.M., Piaz, A., & Arancibia, F. (2012). Biotecnología agrícola y 'sojización' en la Argentina: controversia pública, construcción de consenso y ampliación del marco regulatorio. *Política & Sociedade*, *11*(20), 135–170. doi:10.5007/2175-7984.2012v11n20p135

Woodhouse, E., Hess, D., Breyman, S., & Martin, B. (2002). Science studies and activism: possibilities and problems for reconstructivist agendas. *Social Studies of Science*, *32*(2), 297.

# 10 Changing Discourses of Risk and Health Risk

## A Corpus Analysis of the Usage of *Risk* Language in the *New York Times*

*Jens O. Zinn and Daniel McDonald*

## INTRODUCTION

In recent decades, with the development of social media, mobile devices and advancements in the digitisation and storage of text, *Big Data* are offering new opportunities for social science research. It is not only the production of new data in the present but the digitisation of old data such as (historical) newspaper archives which open unprecedented opportunities for sociologists to examine long-term social change. This is of particular interest for the sociology of risk and uncertainty, where different approaches compete to explain social change towards risk. Though the cultural approach (Douglas & Wildavsky 1982; Douglas 1990, 1992), the risk society perspective (Giddens 1990, 2000; Beck 1992, 2009), governmentality (Ewald 1986; Dean 1999; Rose 1999; O'Malley 2004), and modern systems theory (Luhmann 1989, 1993) have all made significant contributions describing social risk phenomena, there have been few attempts to examine the relative explanatory power of different approaches for an overall shift towards risk in public debates or how different social domains and events have contributed to the dynamics of societal risk discourse.

This is surprising, given that the media have been identified as crucial for social risk awareness. Many risks are only experienced through the reporting in the media. They might happen at different places or require research to be identified. Therefore, the media shape societal risk awareness. At the same time, the media report on issues considered relevant and thereby reflect typical social issues at the time and how they are understood. Language is a key element in this process. How a risk is reported, which words and grammatical constructions are used reflect a deeper social reality, expresses a particular *Zeitgeist*, institutional set up and sociocultural context.

Our study capitalises on the increased availability of digitised newspaper archives in order to examine discursive changes in the meaning and use of risk, focusing on data from the *New York Times* (NYT) between 1987–2014. In contrast to most risk studies, we do not examine a particular risk but how the risk semantic—or more concretely—how risk as a lexical item occurs, in which forms and in which contexts. We make use of a combination of corpus linguistic methods and systemic functional linguistic theory (Halliday & Matthiessen 2004) to analyse the lexical and grammatical patterns in clauses containing a risk word, identifying key areas of change.

This chapter has two purposes. First, we aim to demonstrate the viability of corpus linguistic methods as a means of empirically observing longitudinal change in risk discourse. Second, we test some key hypotheses in risk research.

We begin our contribution with the proposition that examining the use of the term risk in media coverage can be a useful approach to understand long-term social change and the explanatory power of different social science approaches to risk. Next we outline a number of key hypotheses from risk theories more generally, and for the health domain in particular, considering how these hypotheses might manifest in language. We then outline the methodological foundations of our study, which utilises systemic functional linguistics and frame semantics' conceptualisation of the 'risk frame' as a theoretical framework and practices from corpus and computational linguistics as an approach to data analysis. In the results, we show that the growing institutionalisation of risk practices can be clearly found in changing linguistic forms. Among other findings, we demonstrate that there is a clear trend towards the negative side of risk and, increasingly, a representation of risk as uncertain rather than controlled. Everyday people are increasingly presented as bearers of risk, while powerful institutions and actors remain the most common risk takers. Furthermore, we highlight the strong relationship of risk and health-related news in particular. This is evidenced by very high peaks in the co-occurrence of risk and single health-related events and/or ongoing health issues such as chronic illnesses or cancer. Also within the area of health risks, we find an increase in reference to scientific research and experts. We finish with concluding remarks highlighting some key issues and perspectives for further research.

## STATE OF RESEARCH AND SOME KEY QUESTIONS

Mainstream social science theories conceptualise 'risk' relatively independent of empirical linguistic evidence. For example, Douglas does not emphasise the difference of a risk discourse compared to danger or threat. Instead she outlines the functional equivalence of earlier notions of *sin* and *taboo* compared to the modern notion of *risk*. From this perspective, risk becomes synonymous with danger; more risk would equate to more danger (Douglas 1990, Lupton 1999). She argues that risk and danger respectively were transformed through sociocultural worldviews into challenges for a particular institutional set up of a social unit.

In the governmentality perspective, risk has often been associated with calculative technologies. In many studies, reference is made to the application of technical or formal techniques, such as probability analysis and statistics, which usually use risk as a technical or jargon term, rather than threat or possible harm or danger. Ewald suggested when discussing insurance that a risk becomes only a risk through being part of a statistic probabilistic calculation (Ewald 1991). Bernstein (1997) has shown that risk as a concept is linked to the development and application of statistics in different areas of society, as Hacking (1990, 1991) has argued, risk has been central in new ways of governing populations. At the same time, scholars emphasise the importance of the normative contexts, which determines how calculative technologies are set up and used in social practice. Scholars in the governmentality perspective often emphasise the influence of neoliberalism for the pervasiveness of risk discourse (Dean 1999; Rose 1999; Kelly 2006). More generally Kemshall (2002) observed an increased *responsibilisation* of the individual in institutional practices in the UK, while Hacker (2006) stated *The Great Risk Shift* from social institutions to the individual in the US.

In contrast to the partly rather 'technical' understanding of risk in the governmentality perspective, Luhmann, in his analysis of social structure and semantics, has claimed, that the risk semantic stands for a historical new social experience that required a new expression (1993: 10/1):

> Certain advantages are to be gained only if something is at stake . . . It is a matter of a decision that, as can be foreseen, will be subsequently regretted if a loss that one had hoped to avert occurs.

However, Luhmann's argument mainly refers to the shift from stratified differentiation in the Middle Ages to functional differentiation in modern industrialised societies. Beck, instead, claims that the more recent increase of risk communication would be a result of a shift within modernisation in particular after WW2.

According to Beck, the significant increase of risk in public debates would be the result of the unexpected side effects of modernisation that had produced new risks, uncertainties and new unknown spheres in contrast to the modern myth of increasing control and predictability (e.g. Weber 1948). As a result of difficulties in controlling and predicting events in the natural and social world (even the distinction between both becomes questionable), the modern myth of increased rationality has been challenged. However, the erosion of scientific authority caused by the lacking ability to solve social conflicts through the provision of true knowledge has not lead to a loss of importance of scientific expertise. Instead, Beck claims that science has become even more significant to strengthen one's argument (1992). Scientific expertise is still a crucial resource in social claims making processes and is still one of the most trustworthy sources in particular that the media rely on.

In Beck's view, the increasing worries about risk and uncertainty would be caused by the quality of new risks and mega risks (Beck 1992, 2009) but also processes of institutional individualism linked to detraditionalisation (Beck 1992, Beck & Beck-Gernsheim 2002). The assumption is that traditions and old institutions would lose their power to guide decision making and to protect against risks. Individuals would increasingly have to make decisions and to reinvent themselves in a context of decreasing control and predictability. The freedoms we gain from detraditionalisation would be replaced by risks and uncertainties to be dealt with individually. Late or reflexive modernity would be characterised by the *risky freedoms*, which expose individuals to new decision-making situations. Some scholars claim that in particular people in powerful positions and the privileged middle class are among the individualisation winners, while many are among the individualisation losers being mainly made responsible for what happens to them without much opportunity to plan their lives (Beck & Beck-Gernsheim 2002: 47).

While there is a plethora of empirical risk studies addressing a large number of risk issues, there is comparatively little work which reconstructs particular risk issues in a long-term perspective, such as the introduction of social insurance in France (Ewald 1986), the introduction of life insurance in the US (Zelizer 1983), the development of environmental risk debates (Strydom 2002) or the shift from danger to risk in psychiatry (Castel 1991).

There is also little research that systematically examines how different areas relate to each other or to what extent particular social domains contribute to the general risk awareness and/or public discourses. Many media studies refer to particular risk issues or relatively short periods of attention cycles in media coverage when examining the dynamics of risk discourses in the media (Grundmann et al. 2013; Holland et al. 2012). They often refer to a particular risk such as climate change, infectious disease or a new technology and distinguish positive from negative or supportive and critical discourses or reconstruct dynamics of risk reporting (Grundmann & Krishnamurthy 2010; Holland et al. 2012; Grundmann & Scott 2014).

There is very little work in the vein of Mairal (2011), who examines more generally how past experiences with risk influence and structure the ways in which we think about unknown and uncertain risks of the future. A good example is how the so-called swine flu (H1N1) in 2009 was perceived against the background of the deadly Spanish flu pandemic from 1918 to 1920, which killed more than an estimated 50 million people worldwide.

Mairal's research also developed an interesting argument about the development of a particular genre in journalism that places risk in its centre. He used Defoe's work on the Plague in London in 1665 as a case study to show how an emerging practice of evidence-based reporting developed into a new 'narrative matrix' that remains dominant in the reporting of risk in mass media today. If risk is part of such a new genre of journalism, Skolbekken's observation of a risk epidemic in scholarly articles in medical journals in the US, Britain and Scandinavia from 1967 to 1991 might be crucial for understanding increased usage of the risk semantic in the health area. He suggests that the shift towards risk cannot be explained by a change in terminology only, and he hypothesises that the shift results from a particular social culture that developed historically and is linked to the development of probability statistics, focus on risk management and health promotion and computer technology. However, he does not provide evidence of how the risk epidemic connects to public discourse.

Coming from a discourse studies perspective, in recent decades, applied linguists have become interested in incorporating sociological dimensions into the study of language (e.g. Van Dijk 1997, Wodak & Meyer 2001). To date, however, this stream of research has contributed little to the reconstruction of the historical development of discourses (Brinton 2001; Carabine 2001; Harding 2006) although many linguists are interesting in examining long-term semantic changes (e.g. Nerlich & Clarke 1988, 1992, 2000; Traugott & Dasher 2002).

Regarding risk, corpus linguists have shown that sociologists' assumptions about the usage of risk are often informed by everyday life knowledge rather than systematic empirical analysis of how the term *risk* is actually used (Hamilton et al. 2007). Frame Semantics (Fillmore & Atkins 1992) has provided a detailed analysis of the available risk frames;[1] but neither approach examines historical changes of the usage and notion of risk.

## TOWARDS A USAGE-DRIVEN ACCOUNT OF RISK

It is not clear what the relationship between linguistic changes in the media and broader institutional and socio-structural changes are. In media studies, there is vast research on agenda-setting studies (grounded in the traditional media effects tradition) that explores the relationships between the media and the public agendas (e.g. McCombs 2004; McCombs & Shaw 1972). Yet there are very few studies which systematically examine what forces set the media agenda (one exception: Collistra 2012) and how the media agenda is influenced by broader societal developments or how more general historical ideas (Koselleck 1989) influence and change media coverage.

Conceptualisations of language change within linguistics and history have tended to focus more on broader social transformations than on the role played by single events and particular institutional changes. The recent emergence of large, well-structured digital datasets, as well as tools and methods capable of analysing them, however, makes such studies possible, both on the scale of evolution of jargon terms within a single online community (Danescu-Niculescu-Mizil et al., 2013) to research utilising Google's database of millions of digitised books, chronologically arranged (Michel et al. 2011).

In a discourse analytic perspective, a contrasting argument would emphasise that we can only change a future in a particular way when we can imagine that the future is different from the past. Or, we could say that a society always produces discourses about more possible futures than can be realised (Luhmann 1980). This implies that thinking and talking about possible futures might change discursive practices even before institutional changes manifest or before unique disasters such as in Chernobyl or the September 11 terrorist attack took place. Changing discourses might be responsible, for disasters are experienced as unique and path-breaking.

## SIGNIFICANT INCREASE OF THE USAGE OF RISK IN THE *NEW YORK TIMES* AFTER WW2

Previous research (Zinn 2010) has proven that the increasing usage of the term *risk* in media coverage of NYT is one of the most outstanding developments compared to similar phrases after WW2. Figure 10.1 shows the number of articles where *risk* and other related words such as threat or danger were mentioned at least once. *Danger* has significantly decreased after WW2 while *threat* became common during the Great Depression and since then remained on a relatively stable level. Only recently, after September 11 and the Iraq War, have the number of articles using *threat* again increased in usage. *Risk* had a turbulent trajectory after WW2 with no clear direction but with the late 1968s and early 1970s the trajectory is a steep increase where major disasters such as Chernobyl and the terror attack of September 11 were preceded by an increase in risk communication in the NYT.

The preceding increase of articles using risk language shows that already before these iconic events happened, social risk communication had increased, which might imply a heightened social sensitivity for risk issues

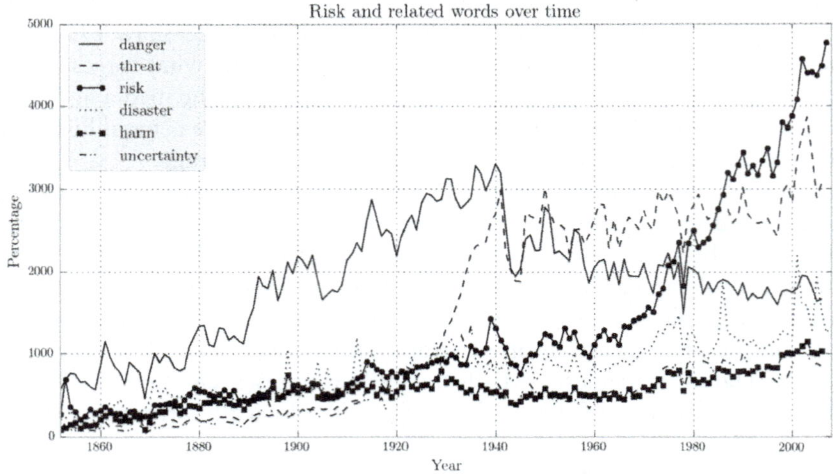


*Figure 10.1* Number of articles in the *New York Times* with at least one risk token 1852–2008 (source: Zinn 2010)

before these disasters took place. We take this as a first indication of how the analysis of large collections of digitised text might be able to discover unexpected insights into risk. That said, we can draw only limited conclusions from this kind of data, as it provides little possibility of discovering the co-text and context in which *risk* and related words appear.

## HYPOTHESES: GENERAL TREND TOWARDS RISK

Many scholars claim that there is a strong tendency towards negative connotations of risk and an increasing synonymy with words denoting negative outcomes, such as danger or harm (Douglas 1992; Lupton 1999). Risk less and less refers to the risk-taking process, which involves opportunities as well as possible negative outcomes. Public debates about risk would increasingly focus on the negative side only, the possible dangers and threats. Linguistically, evidence for increasing synonymy of risk and negative outcomes could be observed by looking at the functional role of risk words: when risk is a participant in discourse ('The risk was real'), synonymy with negative outcomes is greater than when risk is a process ('They risked their safety'). This can be demonstrated by contrasting *risk* in both roles with explicit positive outcomes:

a) The risks outweighed the rewards; the risk/benefit ratio
b) He risked alienating voters, but it paid off
c) The risks had rewards

Note that in process-range configurations, though risk is nominal, it conforms semantically to the role of process, rather than participant:

c) They ran/took the risk and were rewarded

For example, Beck (1992) has claimed that risk would increasingly escape individual control. They cannot be calculated. Instead, we now have to deal with the experience of possible risks—the general worry that things go wrong or what might happen to us—rather than with the notion of calculated risks indicating that risks are under control. Reporting that has an increasingly possibilistic approach to risk would support his claim of increased concerns about risk. Linguistically, calculatedness of risk could be examined by locating the kinds of modifiers of nominal risks ('A calculated/potential risk.').

At the same time, different approaches in risk studies (e.g. Beck 1992; Dean 1999) have in different ways emphasised a shift towards greater responsibility of the individual reflecting other US scholars who have criticised growing individualism in the USA (Putnam 2000; Slater 1970), which has also manifested in a recent institutional risk shift of responsibility in public and social policy towards the individual (Hacker 2006). We expect that such a shift would be detectable in the NYT through, for example, a stronger mentioning of everyday life people rather than social institutions and organisation in relation to risk.

## THE CENTRALITY OF THE HEALTH SECTOR IN DRIVING PUBLIC RISK DEBATES

When risk research developed within sociology in the 1980s, the focus was mainly on new technologies and in particular nuclear power (Douglas & Wildavsky 1982, Perrow 1984, Luhmann 1989, Beck 1992). However, there had also been indications that risk thinking is entering society on different levels and in different areas. In particular, Skolbekken had indicated a shift towards risk in health in his article about a risk epidemic in medical science journals though not examining to what extent the scientific debates have entered public debates and news media.

In order to get a better feeling for the relative relevance of risk in different social domains, Zinn (2011) conducted an explorative study in which he compared the news coverage in the volume 1900 with 2000 of the *New York Times* to see to what extent reporting using the risk semantic has changed historically. The study took samples from the 1900 volume (n=209; N=622) and the 2000 volume (n=409; N=5188). The areas were thematically coded regarding the domains they are referring to. For example, technological risks referred to risks which were caused by, at the time, relatively new technologies. Health refers to health issues more generally, while medicine refers to organised/institutionalised medicine. Similarly reporting on war is distinguished from reports on the military as an organisation (Zinn 2011). Assuming that what is newsworthy reflects to a large extent the reality of a society at a particular time and not only a specific mode of news production seems supported by the areas connected to risk in the earlier volume compared with the later (e.g. the stronger prominence of war, the military, transport/infrastructure, social order, and disaster; compare Figure 10.2). It supports the recent occurrence of risk in the context of new technologies and the environment, but it also shows the outstanding importance of health and medicine as sectors of risk discourses in the media. It indicates that the risk semantic entered increasingly a broader range of different social domains in the more recent volume and draws attention to often-neglected areas in societal risk debates, such as sport and arts. If confirmed by more rigorous research, the picture drawn by this exploration suggests placing health-related issues more centrally in theorising on a recent shift towards a risk society.

## HYPOTHESES—HEALTH DOMAIN

There are a number of assumptions about developments in the area of health and illness that have not yet been examined empirically. There is a well-known

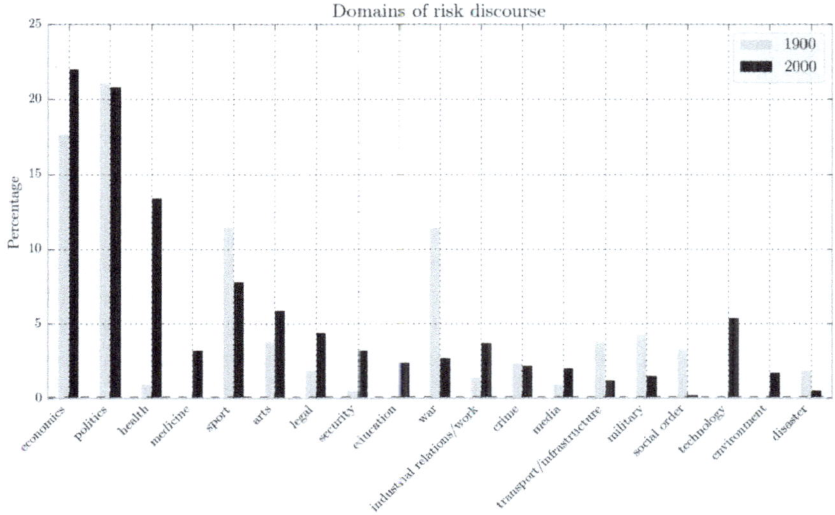


*Figure 10.2* Number of articles in the *New York Times* containing at least one risk token by topics/domains, 1900 versus 2000 (source: Zinn 2011)

general trend of civilisation illnesses and chronic illnesses becoming more dominant in health and illness, while infectious diseases lose relative importance but do not disappear (e.g. Kuryłowicz & Kopczyński 1986). Our interest is in how such trends are reflected in the usage of the risk semantic in the health domain.

A number of scholars have claimed scientific research entering news reporting (Mairal 2011), the importance of research for claims making (Beck 1992), while Skolbekken (1995) has found a risk epidemic in health journals in the US medical journals, among others. Therefore, we sought to determine whether the increasing usage of the risk semantic in news coverage is indeed increasingly referring to scientific studies and experts.

We also wanted to test whether the trend towards individualism (Beck 1992; Putnam 2000) manifests in issues reported in the health domain. It was of interest, for example, what role common terms for people in everyday life (woman, man, person, child, etc.) played in the landscape of risk and how this differed from the role played by institutions or influential people.

## METHODOLOGY AND METHODS

There is no doubt that the media and newspaper coverage is an important part of social reality, constituting an arena for social discourses and influencing individual comprehension (e.g. Gamson 1989; Stuart et al. 2000; Flynn et al. 2001; Pidgeon et al. 2003). This happens simultaneously on the content plane of discourse-semantics and on the expression plane of lexis and grammar. For example, functional linguistic theories such as frame semantics and systemic functional linguistics support the view that social changes and language changes are connected and assume that meaning can be made only with reference to a structured background of experience, beliefs or practices (Fillmore & Atkins 1992, Halliday & Matthiessen 2004).

Since media coverage relies on the social knowledge and language of a society, it contributes to and reflects changes in social symbols, norms, values and institutions. Thus media coverage can be used to examine social change, although there are some restrictions. The media follows a specific logic of news-production and risk-management strategies. Changes in the readership, the ideological stance and the specific socially stratified audience may influence results (Kitzinger 1999; Boyne 2003, p. 23–41) and have to be carefully controlled by analysis of changes in the organisational context of the NYT (e.g. changes in leadership, publisher and editors, corporate identity) and its position in the history of US journalism.

The Glasgow approach in media studies has emphasised the need to research the media production process in much more detail. However, the study approaches the risk semantic from a different perspective. It is informed by the sociology of risk, sociological analysis of historical social change, discourse analysis and corpus linguistics.

From a media studies perspective, the argument supported by Fürsich (2009) for text-focused analysis of media discourses comes closest to our approach. This perspective interprets the text as a structure produced in complex processes, which involve a range of players, including journalists, readerships and media moguls and open a number of different, but not arbitrary, interpretations. It is unlikely that the power struggle in a newspaper's management or a shift in journalism can fully determine the usage of a specific semantic, even in democratic countries with a relatively independent press (Tulloch & Zinn 2011). Far more reasonable is the assumption that the instantiation of particular discourses in news plays a role in both the construction and reflection of more general social changes. Considering these concerns, an explorative examination of possible differences in news coverage of the NYT and the *Washington Post* supports this assumption (Zinn 2010, p. 115). Only relatively minor differences in the number of articles using 'risk' but very similar long-term developments were found. Thus we assumed that the long-term historical changes are sufficiently general (Koselleck 2002; Luhmann 1980) that they can be traced even through a single newspaper.

In the following we outline the risk frames identified by Fillmore and Atkins (1992, p. 76f.) we use as a starting point for understanding the kinds of participant roles in the process of risking. We then outline our use of systemic functional linguistics for our analyses.

## RISK IN FRAME SEMANTICS

Frame semantics can serve as a general blueprint to understand the common risk frame in use. Developed through the analysis of a large text corpus, it is claimed to represent the complete structure of the risk frame. This includes an actor, a valued object, a goal, a deed, possible harm and a victim, which may not necessarily be the actor.

Hamilton et al. (2007) use a frame semantics approach to understand the behaviour of *risk* in two corpora: the 56-million-word Collins WordBanksOnline Corpus and the 5 million word CANCODE. They find that risk is commonly nominal in contemporary language use and that risk co-occurs with negative semantic prosody. Further, they find that health risks are a more salient semantic domain than has been commonly understood in risk research.

We depart from their methods in a number of respects, however. First, they use general corpora, while we used a specialised corpus of NYT articles. Second, our study is diachronic, while theirs is largely monochronic. Third, we differ dramatically in the number of risk words analysed (approx. 300 vs. 240,082). Fourth, they relied on collocation, while we parsed the data for linguistic structure and performed specific queries of the lexicogrammar of clauses containing risk words. Finally, we augment the frame-semantic approach to risk with core tenets of systemic-functional grammar. Though the components of the risk frame are semantically clear, they are often difficult to automatically extract from corpora, even when the corpus has been annotated for grammatical structure: even in prototypical risk processes, whether or not the valued object or the possible harm is often grammatically unmarked (*I risked my life/I risked death*). When risk is a modifier, or a participant, things become less clear still, with fewer of the components of the frame being mentioned overtly at all. Furthermore, when risk is not the process or participant, the extent to which the risk frame is being instantiated is difficult to assess:

a) In 1999, we sold the company, and the next year, we moved to the United States with our two children—a third was born in 2003—so I could pursue my idea of helping low-income, at-risk youth.
b) Mr. Escobedo said that Vioxx was especially dangerous to Mr. Garza because of his other risk factors and that he should never have been prescribed the drug.

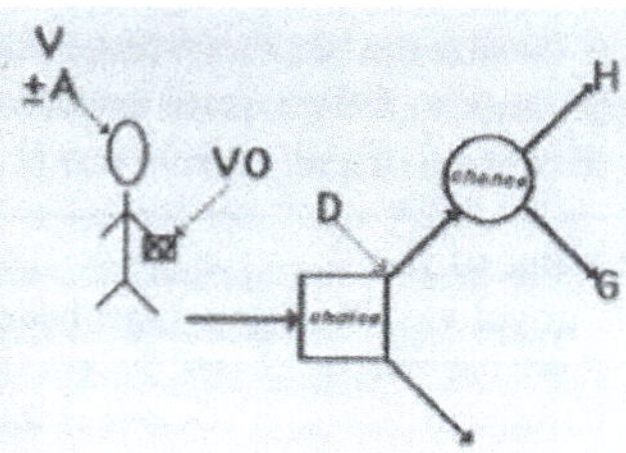


FIG. 2.3. H = Harm, G = Goal, D = Deed, VO = Valued Object, V = Victim, A = Actor.

*Figure 10.3* Risk Frame (from Fillmore & Atkins, 1992)

## SYSTEMIC FUNCTIONAL LINGUISTICS AND THE SYSTEMIC-FUNCTIONAL GRAMMAR

We utilise systemic functional linguistics as both an English grammar and a means of connecting lexical and grammatical phenomena to their meaning and function in news discourse. Unlike frame semantics, it is not a cognitive-semantic theory, instead prioritising lexis and grammar as delicate meaning-making resources and arguing that context is often embedded within the linguistic choices made in a text (Eggins 2004). These ideas are particularly helpful affordances in analyses of texts within a one-way medium such as print news, especially in diachronic contexts, where access to writers and readers for follow-up interviews is extremely limited.

In systemic functional linguistics, the transitivity system is considered the means through which experiential meanings are made—that is, meanings designed to represent events and happenings in the social world (as opposed to the mood system, which is responsible for the negotiation of interpersonal meanings). It is here that we situate our analysis of risk (though forthcoming work provides a treatment of risk according to mood choices too).

Within the transitivity system, the three main functional roles are *participant*, *process* and *circumstance*. These roles pattern to some extent with formal word classes. Verbs and verb phrases congruently represent processes. Nouns and noun phrases typically represent participants, and prepositional phrases and adverbs typically represent circumstances. The example below shows a basic transitivity analysis of a clause from our data with the *heads* of the participants and process in bold.

Using these categories, we divide risk semantically into *risk-as-participant* (where risk is the head of an argument of the verb), *risk-as-process* (where risk is the semantic 'head' of the main verbal group) and *risk-as-modifier* (where risk is an adjective modifying a participant, within a circumstance, etc.).

Adding complexity to the systemic functional grammar (and, therefore, any potential analysis of language use) is the fact that meanings are often made in incongruent ways: nominalisation (*decline* → *declination*), as well as the ability for similar meanings to be made at different levels (*'the risk was big' vs. 'the big risk')*. A key distinction between our work and that of both Fillmore & Atkins (1992) and Hamilton et al. (2007) is a heightened

*Table 10.1* Example of a transitivity analysis of a clause containing risk (NYT, 2005)

| But | the bang of the gavel | can hold | risk | for novices |
|---|---|---|---|---|
| | Participant: Carrier | Process: relational attributive | Participant: attribute | Circumstance: extent |

sensitivity to incongruent forms of risk words: while the earlier studies investigate differences in the function of risk words according to the grammatical form, we instead focus on a functional definition. A key example of this difference is in our treatment of *run risk* and *take risk* as kinds of risk processes, despite the risk word itself being nominal, due to closer synonymy with verbal risk and relatively empty semantic content of the verb.

## RESEARCH STRATEGY

The *New York Times* (NYT) was selected as case study because of the central role of the US in the world and the prestige and clout of the NYT. The NYT is a historically central institution of media coverage (Chapman 2005) with a continuously high status and standard of coverage. It is a worldwide influential, highly circulated and publicly acknowledged news media. It contains extensive coverage of both national and international developments, and its digital archive covers all years since WW2 and it is relatively easy to access. A detailed analysis of available newspapers' archives found that, in the US, only the *Washington Post* provides a comparable archive, while access and data management has proven easier and more reliable with the NYT.

Our approach is three-pronged. Following on from earlier work, we simply begin by counting the number of articles containing risk words. Second, we use Stanford CoreNLP's parsers (see Manning et al. 2014) to annotate paragraphs containing a risk word between 1987 to mid-2014 with grammatical information and use this information to perform nuanced querying of clauses containing risk words in order to look for lexical and grammatical sites of change.

For these analyses, we built a text corpus (general) and a subcorpus (health domain) of digitised texts from NYT editions between 1987 and 2014. These texts (defined here as individual, complete chunks of content) are predominantly news articles but, depending on archiving practices, also included in our corpus is text-based advertising, box scores, lists, classifieds, letters to the editor, and so on. More specifically, we were interested in any containing at least one 'risk word'—any lexical item whose root is risk (risking, risky, riskers, etc.) or any adjective or adverb containing this root (e.g. at-risk, risk-laden, no-risk). We relied on two sources for our data. The *New York Times Annotated Corpus* (Sandhaus 2008) was used as the source for all articles published between 1987 and 2006. ProQuest was used to search for and download articles containing a risk word from 2007–2014, alongside some metadata, in HTML format (Zinn & McDonald 2015).

A particular focus is on determining common actors/agents of risk in health articles and using linear regression to sort these results by their longitudinal trajectory. By comparing these results with frequency counts for

*Table 10.2* Text corpus (general) and subcorpus (health domain) of digitised texts from NYT editions between 1987 and 2014

| | Words | Articles | Risk words |
|---|---|---|---|
| Full corpus | 153,828,656 | 149,504 | 240,082 |
| Health subcorpus | 8,524,023 | 6,944 | 36,547 |

noun phrases in our corpus, we can observe trends toward general involvement in risk discourse and involvement in risk discourse as the agent behind the process of risk. Using thematic categorisation, we abstract the significance of these results, uncovering the general kinds of social actors (humans, institutions, illnesses, research, etc.) increasingly or decreasingly are agents and/or experiencers of risk.

## RESULTS

For a better understanding of the recent shifts in the utilisation of risk words in the NYT we analysed the lexical and grammatical features surrounding all risk words used in NYT articles between 1987 and mid-2014. This allowed us a more fine-grained window into the behaviour of risk words.

Due to limitations of space, we cannot always provide lengthy contextualised examples of the lexical or grammatical phenomena under investigation or being plotted. Researchers can, however, navigate to https://www.github.com/interrogator/risk, which functions as the main repository for the code and findings generated by our investigation. At this address, we have both static documents that present key findings in more detail, as well as a Python-based toolkit that can be used to manipulate and visualise the NYT corpus itself.

## GENERAL CHANGES IN THE BEHAVIOUR OF RISK WORDS

Most generally, we found evidence for an increasingly rich and nuanced behaviour of risk, as well as divergence from the prototypical risk scenario and the associated 'risk frame'.

As a starting point, we used part-of-speech annotation to determine the distribution of adjectival, nominal and verbal risk words over time.

We noted increased usage of risk as a noun. In order to determine whether or not nominalisation is a general trend in the NYT over our sampling period, we calculated the percentage of each of the four word classes

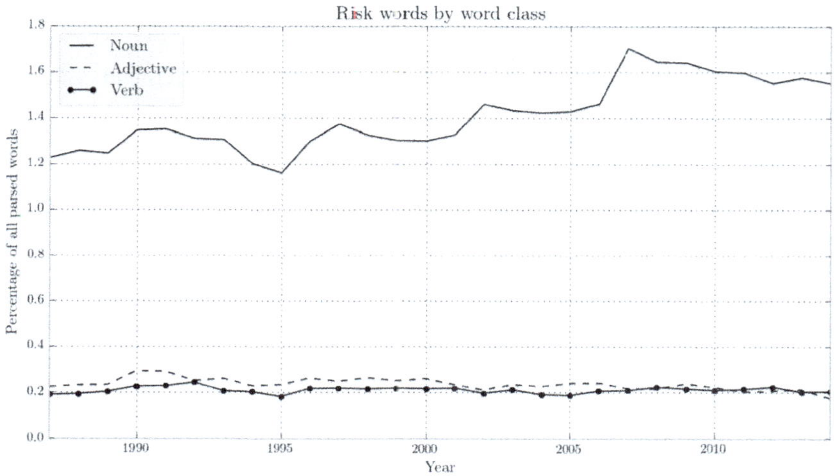


*Figure 10.4* Risk words by word class (general corpus)

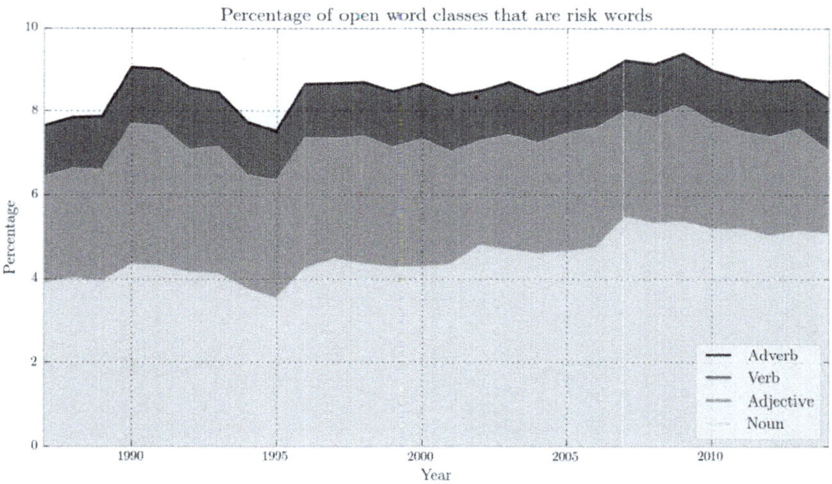


*Figure 10.5* Percentage of open word classes that are risk words (general corpus)

in each year that are risk words. This confirmed that the nominalisation of risk is not simply a part of a more general trend.

As discussed earlier, nominal risks are often synonymous with negative outcomes, while verbal risks typically denote the entire process (an agent making the process occur, the change for negative or positive outcomes, etc.). Accordingly, trends toward nominalisation can be seen as evidence for the argument that risk more and more resembles only the negative components of the risk frame.

Formal word class categories are not necessarily reliable means of determining which kind of risk semantic is being instantiated, however. Risk is nominal in 'risk management', but is serving a modifier function. Risk is also nominal in 'to take a risk', but is really a part of the process, as in 'to take a break' or 'to have a shower'. Accordingly, we used Stanford CoreNLP's dependency parser to categorise risk words by experiential function rather than grammatical form.

We find here a more accurate picture of the increasing synonymy of risk and negative outcomes, the shift away from the standard risk frame and, finally, a greater implicitness of risk. In SFL, the process is the central part of experiential meaning. The process and participants coupled together form the nucleus of the clause—they are what is effectively being discussed. Modifiers and circumstances, on the other hand, provide ancillary information, describing these participants or the manner in which the process occurred. Shifts toward modifier forms thus suggest an increased implicitness of risk within the texts, where risk permeates discussion of an ever-growing set of domains but less and less forms the propositional nub of what is being focally represented in the discourse.

## FROM CALCULATED TO POSSIBILISTIC RISK

We can, for example, look at the kinds of adjectives modifying risk-as-participants in order to better understand the ways in which risks are judged or

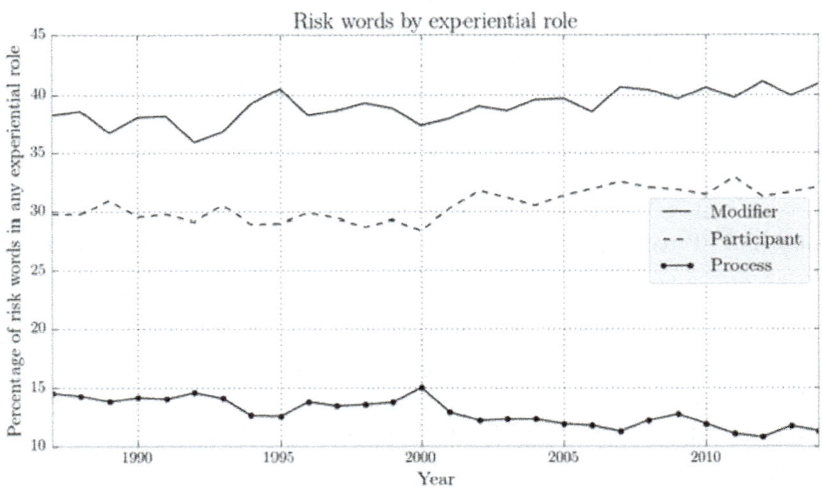


*Figure 10.6* Risk-as-Participant, Process and Modifier (general corpus)

appraised in the NYT. As Max Weber has stated, rationalisation as a core characteristic of the modernisation process goes along with the belief that things should be rationally managed. Exactly this modern dream has been set under pressure in late modernity. As Beck has emphasised, the modern techniques such as insurance would fail when dealing with new mega risks. Unexpected side effects, high complexity and contradictory knowledge might create an unexpected feeling of being exposed to all kinds of risks without the ability to calculate and control them. It might be difficult to pin such a complex shift down easily. With this conceptualisation in mind, we examined the modifiers of risk used in the volumes of the NYT. Very dominant was the expression 'high risk' with a clear peak during the H5N1 Asian Flu outbreak. It is interesting that we could found a clear trend in the last 25 years away from using risk in the context of the *calculability* of risk towards a general *potentiality* of risk.

## DECREASING AGENCY IN RISK PROCESSES

Subdividing risk processes (Figure 10.8), we can see that the 'base' risk process is declining steadily in frequency, with newer risk processes such as *put at risk* and *pose risk* overtaking *running risk* in frequency. Like the trend toward risk-as-participant, the changing climate of risk-as-process points to movement away from the standard risk frame.

While *risking*, *taking risks* and *running risks* all conform more or less to the semantic frames mapped out by Fillmore & Atkins (1992), with a risker and positive and negative outcomes, this is not the case with *posing* and *putting at risk*. In neither of these constructions does the actor take the

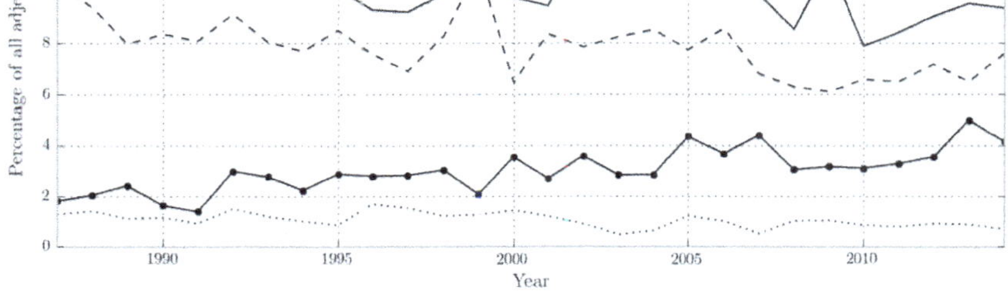


*Figure 10.7* Adjectives modifying nominal risk (general corpus)

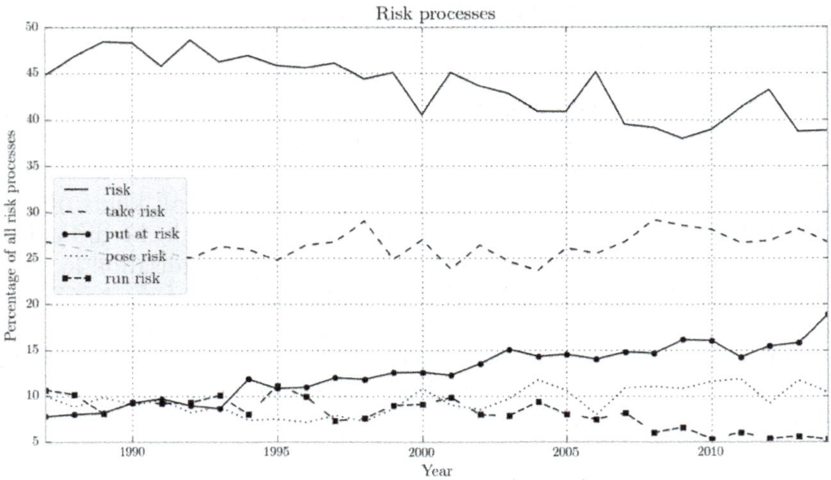


*Figure 10.8* Risk processes (general corpus)

role of the risker. In the *pose risk* construction, the risker here is optionally encoded in a circumstance beginning with the preposition 'to'. From 2006:

> The industry has also denied that electromagnetic emissions from overhead power lines **pose any health risks.**
>
> But if the newer antidepressants **posed a significant suicide risk**, suicide attempts would probably rise, not fall, after treatment began, Dr. Simon said.
>
> Those deemed by a judge to **pose a greater risk** to themselves or others are housed at the Bergen County Jail in Hackensack.
>
> The ministry said the workers **posed no risk** to others and had the A (H5N2) virus, a milder strain than A (H5N1) which has killed more than 70 people.
>
> Finance ministers from the world's richest countries and Russia said Saturday that "high and volatile" energy prices **posed a risk** to global economic growth that otherwise appeared solid.

This same distinction is even clearer in *put at risk*, whose actor tends to be an inanimate of abstract noun, and whose experiential object is generally a broad group of everyday people, such as women, children or citizens. The following examples are from NYT articles on health topics from 2012:

> Pharmacists also overlooked or approved cases in which medications were prescribed at questionable levels or in unsafe combinations that could **put patients at risk** of seizures, accidents or even death, according to the public health department.

> It also cited studies showing that women with unintended pregnancies are more likely to be depressed and to smoke, drink and delay or skip prenatal care, potentially harming fetuses and **putting babies at increased risk** of being born prematurely and having low birth weight.
>
> Last September, Qualitest Pharmaceuticals, a unit of Endo Pharmaceuticals, voluntarily recalled "multiple lots" of contraceptive pills—also because of a "packaging error" that could **put women at risk** for pregnancy.
>
> Representative Chris Smith, a New Jersey Republican and leader of the House anti-abortion forces, said the latest announcement demonstrated that the president "will use force, coercion and ruinous fines that **put faith-based charities, hospitals and schools at risk** of closure, harming millions of kids, as well as the poor, sick and disabled that they serve, in order to force obedience to Obama's will."
>
> The Japanese government's failure to warn citizens about radioactive danger **put the entire city of Tokyo at health risk**—and the rest of us as well.

These results support the hypothesis of degreasing agency in risk reporting.

## THE INSTITUTIONALISATION OF RISK PRACTICES

Risk-as-modifier is very common because they encompass a number of diverse subcategories: risk may be (among other things) an adjectival modifier (*a risky decision*), an adverbial modifier (*he riskily chose*), a nominal modifier (*risk management*) or the head of a nominal group inside a prepositional phrase, serving the role of modifying the main verb of the clause (*They were appalled by the risk*).

By charting these different forms, an interesting picture emerges: adjectival modifiers decline gradually in frequency, while nominal modifiers (examples from 2012 below) rise.

> "That's why more companies are turning to certified **financial risk managers**," the ad continues.
>
> Many clients asked Teresa Leigh, owner of **Household Risk Management**, a North Carolina-based advisory service for wealthy households, to explain just what all the headlines are about.
>
> Rather than downsizing their lifestyles, "they're spending more money on protecting their homes," said Paul M. Viollis Sr., the chief executive of **Risk Control Strategies**, a security advisory firm based in New York City, whose clients have an average net worth of more than $100 million.
>
> A recent survey by the Spectrem Group found that "while somewhat more moderate in **risk tolerance** than in 2009, investors remain more interested in protecting principal than growing their assets."

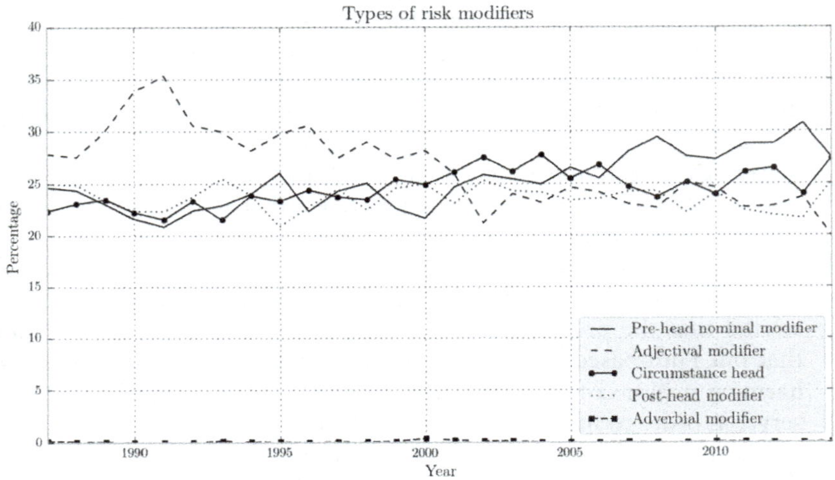


*Figure 10.9* Types of risk modifiers (general corpus)

> Mr. Munson suggested a more enlightened view that looks at "**risk budgeting,**" or gauging how much risk you can take, and design a portfolio that tracks your tolerance—or intolerance—for stock market exposure.

Foremost, this supports the idea that institutions increasingly devote special attention to risk. Importantly, adjectives attach to nouns very freely, but nominal modification of nouns requires some kind of codification within the culture: a novel situation may be described as a risky one, but *risk arbitrage* is an activity created explicitly to handle the phenomenon of risk. As such, nominal modifiers are an important signifier that risk has taken on a more and more central and tangible role within institutions.

## RISK TAKERS AND RISK BEARERS

We have seen that expressions of active risk taking are in decrease, while more 'technocratic' expressions (to pose/put at risk) express that less agency expressions are on the rise. This is surprising, considering hypothesis of governmentality or individualisation theorists that institutions would increasingly expect that individuals manage risks themselves. If this is expected, we would at least expect that terms such as person, man and woman are addressed in risk reporting even when they are not in power but exposed to risk. Individualisation processes would then be reflected in the news coverage of the NYT in reporting the opposite of what is desirable, the exposure to risk of the vulnerable.

Grammatical annotation can be used to look for the subjects of risk processes whose subject is the agent behind the risk (*to risk, to run risk, to take risk, to put at risk*). By focusing on the most common grammatical riskers, we can see that person/people, companies, banks, states, investors, governments, man/men and leaders are leading the riskers overall in the NYT. The list thus contains both powerful institutions and terms often used for everyday people.

To examine the role of risker more closely, we created a list of all heads of nominal groups in the corpus and determined the percentage of the time that noun occurs as the actor in a risk process. This involves determining a sensible threshold for the minimum number of total occurrences, lest the top results be simply words that only appeared once, as a risker, in the dataset. Thus words appearing fewer than 750 times in the corpus were excluded.

The division between powerful people in government and law, compared to everyday terms for average people, is startling:

> Today, George W. **Bush**, with his dauphin's presumption that the Presidency is his for the taking and his cocky refusal to depart from his canned stump speech, **may risk** repeating Dewey's error and give his opponents the sentimental underdog's advantage.
>
> After months of giving President Fox the cold shoulder, Mr. **Bush**'s action on immigration may foretell an end to the tensions, particularly since Mr. Bush is **taking a political risk** by angering anti-immigration Republicans.

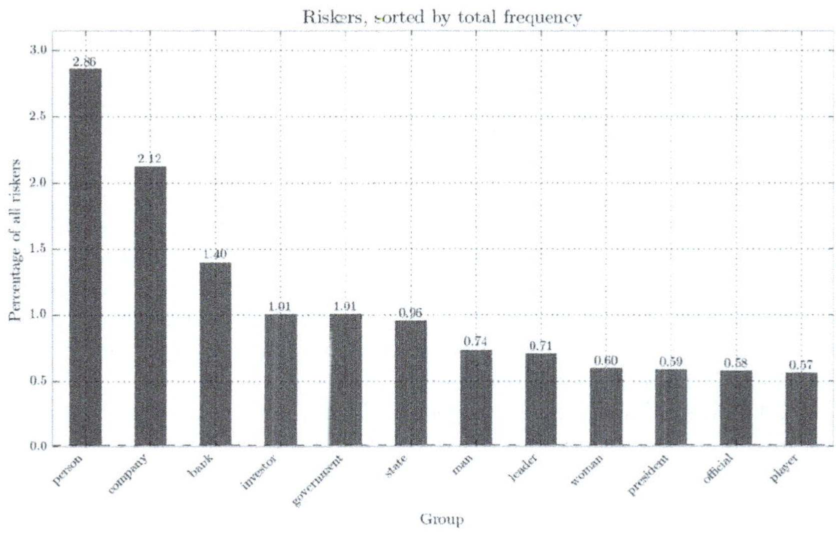


*Figure 10.10* Most common riskers (general corpus)

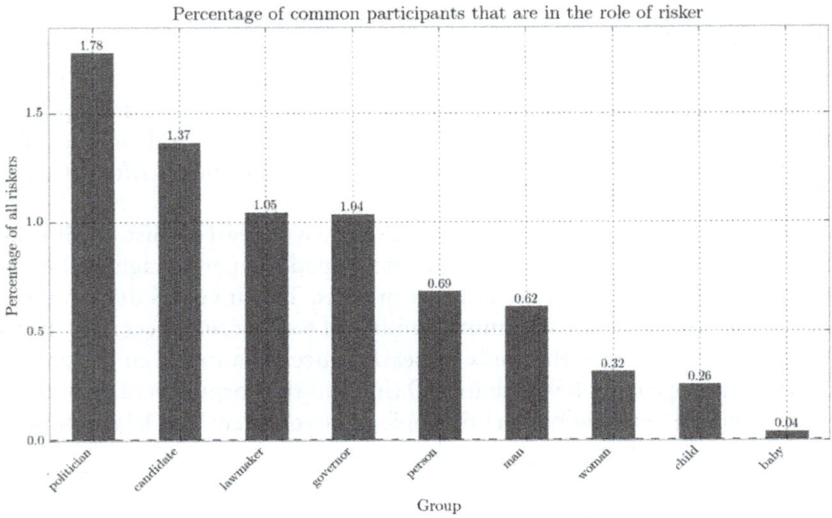


*Figure 10.11* Percentage of common participants that are in the role of risker (general corpus)

> By raising the question of his role in the Iran arms-for-hostages deal, even to decry those questions as part of a "Democrat-run" witchhunt, Mr. **Bush risked** appearing defensive and risked prolonging news coverage of a six-year-old scandal that has already eaten up one of his last four days of campaigning.
>
> Longtime Washington observers question if Mr. Obama would risk a battle over his secretary of state
>
> Ignoring the fact that it's her beloved Tea Party dragging the country to ruin, Palin suggested on Facebook that if the country defaults on its debt, Obama is risking impeachment.
>
> Perfectly normal **men** and **women** were risking prison by making a pass at someone
>
> "Some **people** will clearly **risk death** to reach Europe," said Israel Díaz Aragón, who captains one of the boats of Spain's maritime rescue services.
>
> Even those **women** who become cam models of their own free will take on serious risks associated with sex work
>
> People who were lactose intolerant could have risked losing water from diarrhea, Dr. Tishkoff said.
>
> The humiliating result, six workers said in separate interviews, was that men were sometimes forced to urinate in their pants or risk heat exhaustion.

Thus, in comparison to influential people, everyday people are rarely agents of risk processes. In the few cases where everyday people do function as grammatical agents, negative outcomes are grave, often concerning sickness or death, while influential figures risk negative outcomes to do with facets of their careers.

We will see later on when examining health articles that the terms 'women', 'person', 'man', 'child', 'consumer' and 'baby' all occur regularly as participants but, as we have seen here, they are presented with less agency than powerful institutional actors. 'Banks', 'companies', 'firms' and 'agencies' are increasingly reported as riskers, while 'person', 'man' and 'woman' are on an upwards slope (compare Zinn & McDonald 2015).

## THE RISK SEMANTIC IN HEALTH DISCOURSES

Findings from an earlier investigation have shown that health plays a larger role in risk discourse in 2000 than it did in 1900. We were interested in both whether we can confirm the significance of health through linguistic analysis and whether a richer picture of the relationship between risk and health could be provided. Given the attention paid by Beck to the status of science and research in reflexive modernity, a particular focus was on the ways in which risk, health and research co-occur.

The salience of health topics is clear: in their most prominent years, *AIDS*, *Vioxx* and *Merck* comprise over 1.6 per cent of all proper nouns that co-occur with a risk word. This is higher than *Clinton*, *Bush* or *Obama* at their peaks, as well as *Soviet Union* in 1987 or *Europe* during the Eurozone crisis in 2011.

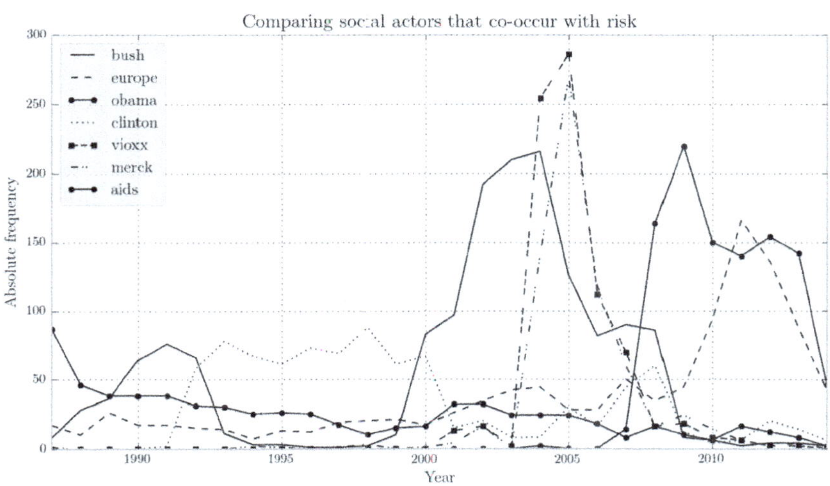


*Figure 10.12* Comparing social actors that co-occur with risk

| | | |
|---|---|---|
| . . . of a crucial clinical trial of the painkiller | **Vioxx** | to play down its heart risks . . . |
| . . . he questioned her about the details of data about | **Vioxx** | risks of causing heart attacks . . . |
| . . . popular painkillers like Pfizer's Celebrex or Merck's | **Vioxx** | increased the risk of heart attacks . . . |
| Yet the United States and | **Europe** | face the risk that their problems will feed on . . . |
| There is a risk over time that democracy will lead | **Europe** | to splinter . . . |
| In addition | **Europe** | is ailing, there is a risk that oil prices will . . . |

Further evidence for the salience of health topics when compared to others was found by searching for nominal modification of risk-as-participant (e.g. *the cancer risk/the risk of cancer*) to uncover more explicit marking of the negative outcomes in the corpus of all risk tokens.

Concordancing these examples revealed the sharp rise in 'risk of attack' has very little to do with war or terrorism but, instead, is almost always referring to the increased risk of heart attack discovered in those who take Vioxx. From 2004, for example:

> It reported that both drugs appeared to increase the **risk of heart attack** and stroke, but that the danger from Vioxx appeared higher.

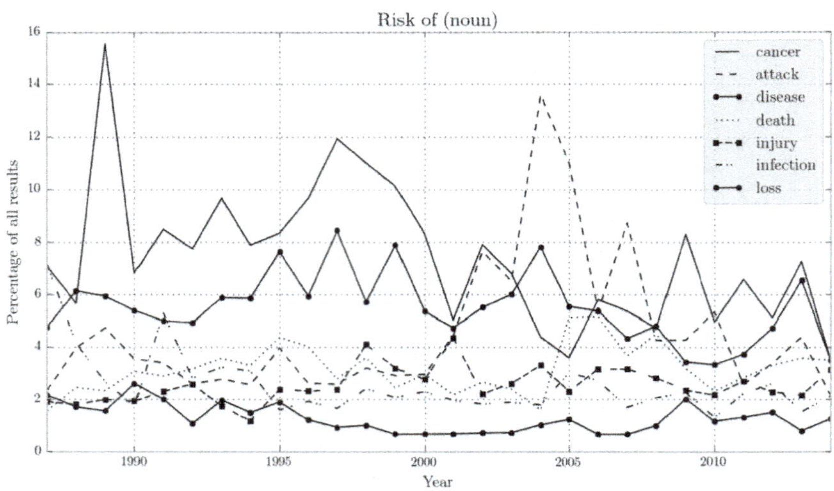


*Figure 10.13* Risk of (noun) (general corpus)

In an April 2004 study in the journal Circulation, researchers from Harvard Medical School found that Vioxx raised the **risk of heart attacks** relative to Celebrex; two months later, several of the same researchers reported in another journal that Vioxx increased the risk of hypertension.

## THE SHIFT TOWARDS INDIVIDUALISM IN HEALTH DISCOURSE

By locating all participants in the health subcorpus, and sorting by those on increasing and decreasing paths, we can see broad shifts in the climate of health risks that are responsive to both events and broader social change: heightened discussion of health insurance in the USA in the early 1990s is related to the Clinton Healthcare Plan (1993), for example. That said, despite the more recent US healthcare reform (beginning with the Affordable Care Act of 2009), insurance-related participants do not re-emerge in the later samples of the corpus, potentially indicating broader shifts in health/risk discourse that require further attention.

The bill, which became law on April 1, forces commercial insurance companies to accept any small-business applicant and to charge uniform rates, regardless of risk of illness, as **Empire** does.

**Empire** used the false data in its successful lobbying campaign last year for changes in state insurance law intended to force competitors to accept some high-risk customers.

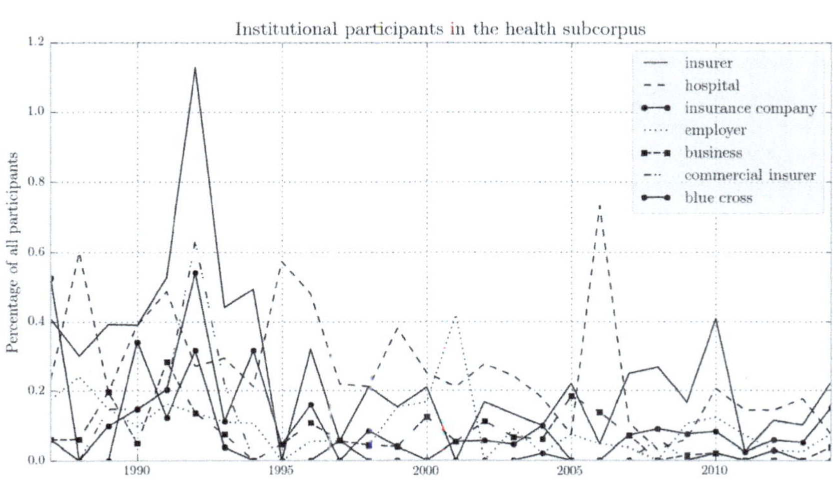


*Figure 10.14* Institutional participants (health subcorpus)

In contrast, most of the everyday participants in the health subcorpus are on the rise. That means that the trends in the health subcorpus might in some respects differ from the overall trend. Risk is increasingly communicated with vulnerable social groups such as women, children and babies but also with persons more generally, men and consumers.

Our analysis of n-grams (recurring occurrence of two-word combinations from open word classes) showed that a number of civilisation illnesses

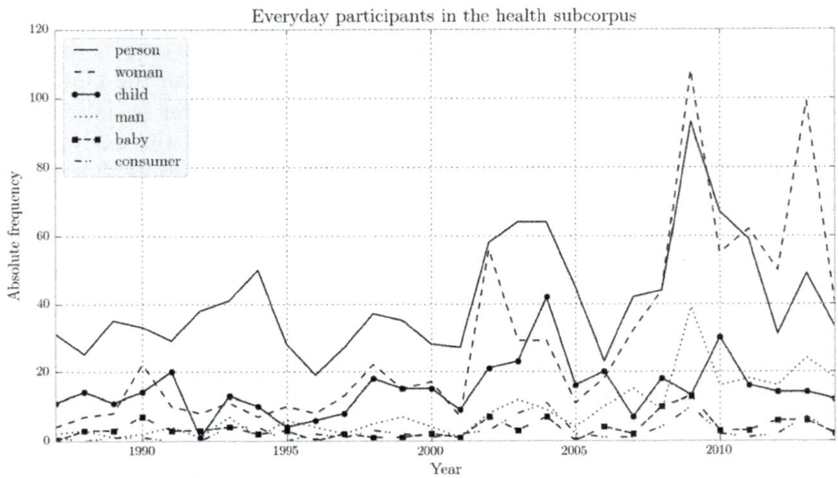


*Figure 10.15* Everyday participants (health subcorpus)

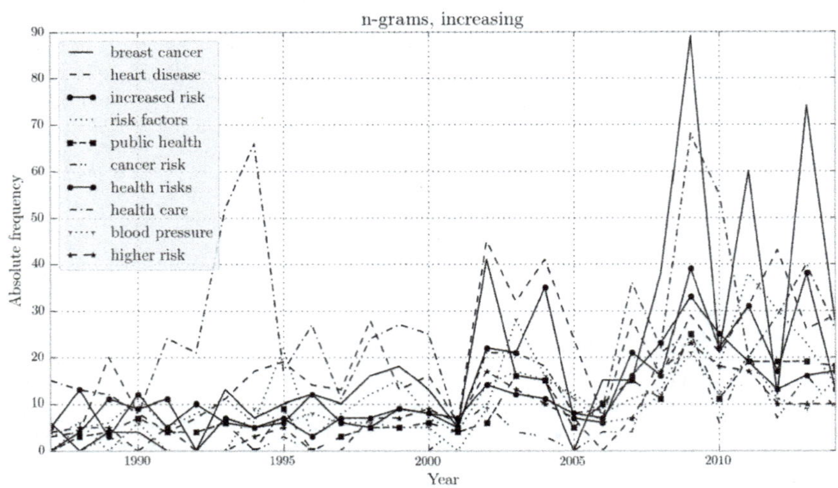


*Figure 10.16* N-grams, increasing (health subcorpus)

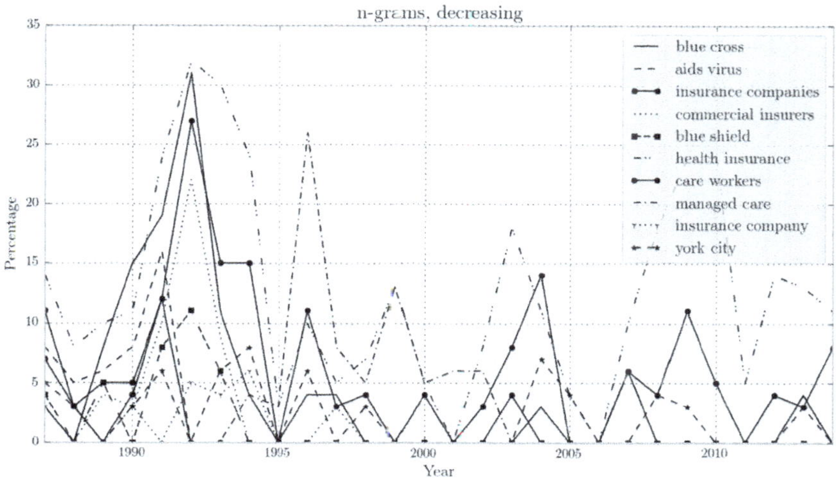


*Figure 10.17* N-grams decreasing (health subcorpus)

and related health issues, such as heart disease, heart attack, prostate cancer, ovarian cancer, lung cancer, blood clots and mental health, giving evidence of the prominence of cancer, heart disease and mental health issues in media coverage of recent debates. At the same time, debates about health insurance, health plan, commercial insurer and insurance company decrease, indicating (as with the analysis of participants in the health corpus) that these debates exist no longer reference to risk as a significant concept. The use of the risk semantic in the health sector is increasingly used in relation to everyday life people presented as vulnerable groups and decreasingly in the context of organisations.

## HEALTH DISCOURSE IS DRIVEN BY INCREASING REFERENCE TO SCIENTIFIC EXPERTISE

There is large support from different scholars that risk reporting is driven by journalism that refers to scientific experts and empirical evidence. While Mairal (2011) claimed that this is characteristic for a particular genre of journalism that developed in journalism during modernisation. Also, Beck's claim that the loss of scientific expertise does not lead to a decrease but increase of importance of scientific evidence supported the view that we should expect more reference to scientific expertise whether to research, scientific evidence or experts. Skolbekken's study on the risk epidemic in medical journals has shown that at least for scientific journals the increase in risk communication has manifested but the question remained to what extent this shift towards risk has also affected reporting in news media.

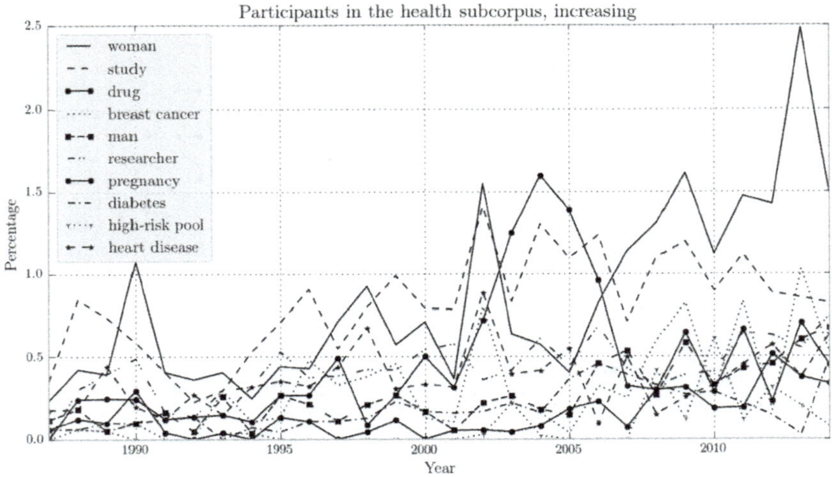


*Figure 10.18* Participants increasing (health subcorpus)

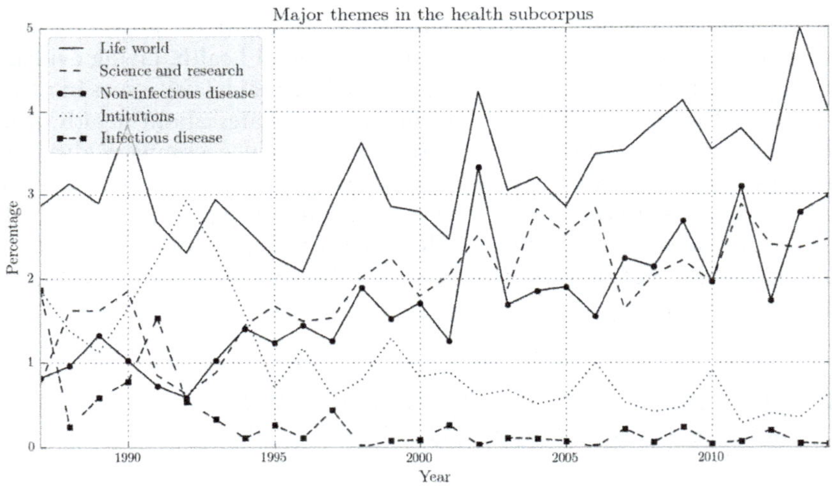


*Figure 10.19* Major themes (health subcorpus)

Our analysis of participants in the health subcorpus supports the assumption that research-related participants in the discourses have increased over the last decades. Of the top 11 increasing participants, two are explicitly associated with science and research (*study*, *researcher*), while other terms can be concordanced to reveal strong associations with this topic (*factor, test*, *level*).

In summary, of the overall trends in the health subcorpus we have grouped the different infectious diseases (*aids, aids virus, aids patient, transmission, flu, influenza*), everyday people (*person, man, woman, child, baby, consumer*), institutions (*empire, hospital, commercial, business, insurance company, HMO/health maintenance organisation, blue cross, disease control, employer, insurer, health insurance association, insurance industry, office*) and non-infectious diseases (*breast cancer, cancer, heart disease, diabetes, heart attack, prostate cancer, stroke, ovarian cancer, obesity*) as well as science and research (*study, researcher, finding, new study, author, university, expert*).

The overview shows the clear trend of decreasing reporting on infectious diseases and institutions related to the risk semantic in the *New York Times* coverage. It also shows the risk of everyday life people referred to when using the risk semantic, the importance of science and research for driving the usage of the risk semantic as well as the non-infectious diseases such as cancer and lifestyle diseases.

## CONCLUDING REMARKS

The analyses have shown a number of clear linguistic trends in media discourses utilising the risk semantic which indicate the growing institutionalisation of risk practices but can also be used to examine and test hypotheses from risk studies.

Our data show an interesting ambivalence in the reporting of the NYT, similar to what was suggested in Beck's individualisation thesis (1992): A culture of institutional individualism takes place at a time when individuals can increasingly less control decision-making outcomes. As a result, we find a shift towards greater emphasis on everyday life social groups (e.g. women, men, children) in stories but, at the same time, less agency in the linguistic expressions related to everyday people. Concurrently, the notion of risk calculation decreases in favour of a general sense of exposure to risk. These results altogether support the assumption that in advanced modern societies, all the advancement in science and technology—including medical technologies—has not supported discursive forms of control but discourses of uncertainty and potential risk. However, presentations differ regarding social groups. The emphasis on everyday life people in news coverage is increasing, while it is mainly powerful people and organisations which are presented as decision makers. Everyday life people are usually presented as risk bearers in news reporting of the NYT.

There is also good evidence that risk words increasingly occur in the context of scientific studies as a technical term. This shows that the general trend Skolbekken (1995) observed in the 1980s and 1990s towards risk studies in medical sciences has found its way into media coverage. It also supports the view of Mairal (2011) that risk enters the media as part of a new, evidence-based genre of news reporting.

We also found evidence that risk as a semantic process is in consistent decline, becoming steadily displaced by risk as a participant in discourse or risk as a modifier of other kinds of processes and participants. In part, this is an expression of the institutionalisation of risk practices in social institutions, the kind of modifier on the sharpest upward trajectory is pre-head nominal modification—a form closely associated with occupations (e.g. financial risk managers), organisations (e.g. risk budgeting) or practices (e.g. risk arbitrage).

We were also able to show a number of clear trends in the health sector. Reporting of infectious diseases decreased after the AIDS crisis in the USA, while non-infectious diseases gain prominence alongside greater focus on terms for everyday people. This mainly reflects ongoing issues such as different forms of cancer and how to deal with it and the so called civilisation illnesses, which tend to occupy more space in news coverage over decades.

Our research is only the beginning, at this point intended to determine whether we can find compelling linguistic evidence for institutional change in print news archives. Though our present analysis appears to have demonstrated that this is methodologically feasible, we have yet to triangulate our results with sustained, contextualised interpretation of individual texts within the corpus.

Accordingly, further research should focus on detailed qualitative institutional analysis, examining how discursive shifts in prototypical articles across the corpus are linked to specific institutional and sociocultural changes. The increasing use of the 'at-risk' modifier, or the strong increase of the notion of the 'risk factor' (Zinn & McDonald 2015), seems in different ways linked to broader social changes of the organisational regulation of the social. To reconstruct this connection would allow a more fundamental understanding of how social and linguistic changes are connected.

We faced a number of difficulties. To begin with, the challenge of translating and connecting sociological thinking with corpus linguistic research strategies and elaborate functional grammars is by no means a simple task. Corpus linguistics, in seeking to distil the content of very large collections of text, may be at odds with a sociological tradition of sustained analysis of smaller, well-contextualised samples. Though the goal within the emerging field of *corpus-assisted discourse studies* is to use quantitative and qualitative methods as a methodological synergy (Baker et al. 2008), such a goal is difficult to operationalise when working with a very large corpus consisting of many subcorpora. Furthermore, shortcomings in the availability of digital tools for doing quantitative functional linguistic research mean that the accuracy and/or usefulness of software used to automatically annotate data remains a serious issue. CoreNLP's existing dependency parser, for example, does not distinguish grammatically between process-range configurations (*She took a risk)* and transitive processes (*She took an apple*), despite important differences in meaning. This limits what can be automatically located or adds considerable complexity to the process of querying the corpus and manipulating the results.

Finally, systemic functional linguistics encompasses a theory of the relationship between text and context that in many respects clashes with mainstream sociological theory: the notion that context is *in* text is hard to reconcile with sociological analyses of texts that centre on highlighting relationships between texts and the broader social changes that may inform the production of texts, while leaving little trace in the lexical and grammatical choices made therein.

Though the analyses show results that are certainly an expression of broader social changes, there are a number of potential future avenues we hope to explore: comparison of newspapers by location, political orientation or language is indeed possible using the methods developed for this project and may prove insightful. Having more data available will also allow us to conduct more fine-grained analysis of developments in different social domains such as politics, economics, health, sports and life world. On this basis, we will start with comparative international analysis.

We are also particularly keen to engage with the question of how related terms such as danger, threat, chance and security relate to the identified shifts in health risk discourse. Sustained focus on particular kinds of health risks, such as cancer or obesity, could do much to elucidate longitudinal transitions toward or from risk.

## NOTE

1. These are cognitive-semantic schemata used by interactants to communicate and understand the process of risk.

## REFERENCES


Baker, P., Gabrielatos, C., Khosravinik, M., Krzyżanowski, M., McEnery, T., & Wodak, R. (2008). A useful methodological synergy? Combining critical discourse analysis and corpus linguistics to examine discourses of refugees and asylum seekers in the UK press. *Discourse & Society*, *19*(3), 273–306.

Beck, U. & Beck-Gernsheim, E. (2002). *Individualization: Instititutionalized individualism and its social and political consequences*. Los Angeles, London, New Delhi, Singapore: Sage.

Beck, U. (1992). *Risk society: Towards a new modernity*. London: Sage.

Beck, U. (2009). *World at risk*. Cambridge, Malden (MA): Polity Press.

Bernstein, P.L. (1997). *Against The Gods*. New York: John Wiley.

Boyne, R. (2003). *Risk*. Buckingham, Philadelphia: Open University Press.

Brinton, L.J. (2001). Historical discourse analysis. In D. Schiffrin, D. Tannen & H.E. Hamilton (Eds.), *Handbook of discourse analysis* (pp. 138–160). Malden (MA): Oxford: Blackwell Publishers.

Carabine, J. (2001). Unmarried motherhood 1830–1990: A genealogical analysis. In M. Wetherell, S. Taylor & S.J. Yates (Eds.), *Discourse as data. A guide for analysis* (pp. 267–310). London: Sage.

Castel, R. (1991). From dangerousness to risk. In G. Burchell, C. Gordon & P. Miller (Ed.), *The Foucault effect. Studies in governmentality* (pp. 281–298). London: Harvester/Wheatsheaf.

Chapman, J. (2005). *Comparative media history: An introduction: 1789 to the present*. Cambridge, Malden (MA): Polity Press.

Collistra, R. (2012). Shaping and cutting the media agenda: Television's reporters' perceptions of agenda frame building and agenda cutting influences. *Journalism and Mass Communication Monographs, 14*(2): 85–146.

Danescu-Niculescu-Mizil, C., West, R., Jurafsky, D., Leskovec, J., & Potts, C. (2013, May 13–17). No country for old members: User lifecycle and linguistic change in online communities. In *Proceedings of the 22nd International Conference on World Wide Web* (pp. 307–318). Republic and Canton of Geneva, Switzerland: International World Wide Web Conferences Steering Committee.

Dean, M. (1999). *Governmentality: Power and rule in modern society.* London: Sage.

Douglas, M. & Wildavsky, A.B. (1982). *Risk and culture: An essay on the selection of technical and environmental dangers.* Berkeley: University of California Press.

Douglas, M. (1990). Risk as a Forensic Resource. *DAEDALUS, 119*(4), pp. 1–16.

Douglas, M. (1992). *Risk and blame: Essays in cultural theory.* London, New York: Routledge.

Eggins, S. (2004). *Introduction to systemic functional linguistics.* New York: Continuum International Publishing Group.

Ewald, F. (1986). *L'Etat providence.* Paris: B. Grasset.

Ewald, F. (1991). Insurance and risks. In: Burchell, G., Gordon, C. & Miller, P. (Eds.), *The Foucault effect: Studies in governmentality* (pp. 197–210). London: Harvester Wheatsheaf.

Fillmore, C.J. & Attkins, B.T. (1992). Towards a frame-based lexicon: The semantics of RISK and its neighbors. In Lehrer, A. & Kittay, E. (Eds.), *Frames, fields & contrasts: New essays in semantic & lexicon organization* (pp. 75–102). Hillsdale (NJ): Lawrence Erlbaum.

Flynn, J., Slovic, P. & Kunreuther, H. (2001). *Risk, media, and stigma: Understanding public challenges to modern science and technology.* London, Sterling (VA): Earthscan.

Fürsich, E. (2009). In defense of textual analysis: Restoring a challenged method for journalism and media studies. *Journalism Studies, 10*, 238–252.

Gamson, W.A. (1989). Media discourse and public opinion on nuclear power: A constructions approach', *American Journal of Sociology, 95*(1), 1–37.

Giddens, A. (1990). *The consequences of modernity.* Cambridge: Polity in association with Blackwell.

Giddens, A. (2000). *Runaway world.* New York: Routledge.

Grundmann, R. & Krishnamurthy, R. (2010). The discourse of climate change: A corpus-based approach', *CADAAD Journal*, 4(2), 125–146.

Grundmann, R. & Scott, M., (2014). Disputed climate science in the media: Do countries matter? *Public Understanding of Science*, 23(2), pp. 220–235.

Grundmann, R., Scott, M. & Wang, J., (2013). Energy security in the news: North/South perspectives. *Environmental Politics*, 22(4), 571–592.

Hacker, J. (2006). *The great risk shift: The assault on American jobs, families, health care, and retirement.* New York: Oxford University Press.

Hacking, I. (1990). *The taming of chance.* Cambridge [England]: Cambridge University Press.

Hacking, I. (1991). How should we do the history of statistics? In G. Burchell, C. Gordon & P. Miller (Eds.), *The Foucault Effect. Studies in Governmentality* (pp. 181–195). London, Toronto, Sydney, Tokyo, Singapore: Harvester Wheatsheaf.

Halliday, M. & Matthiessen, C. (2004). *An introduction to functional grammar.* London: Routledge.

Hamilton, C., Adolphs, S. & Nerlich, B. (2007). The meanings of 'risk': a view from corpus linguistics. *Discourse & Society, 18*, 163–181.

Harding, R. (2006). Historical representations of aboriginal people in the Canadian news media', *Discourse & Society, 17*(2), 205–235.

Holland, K., Blood, R. W., Imision, M., Chapman, S. & Fogarty, A. (2012). Risk, expert uncertainty, and Australian news media: Public and private faces of expert opinion during the 2009 swine flu pandemic. *Journal of Risk Research, 15*(6), 657–671.
Kelly, P. (2006). The entrepreneurial self and 'youth at-risk': Exploring the horizons of identity in the twenty-first century. *Journal of Youth Studies, 9*(1), 17-32.
Kemshall, H. (2002). *Risk, social policy and welfare.* Buckingham: Open University.
Kitzinger, J. (1999). Researching risk and the media. *Health, Risk & Society, 1,* 55–69.
Koselleck, R. (1989). Linguistic change and the history of events. *The Journal of Modern History, 61*(4), 649-666.
Koselleck, R. (2002). *The practice of conceptual history: Timing history, spacing concepts (cultural memory in the present).* Stanford (CA): Stanford University Press.
Kuryłowicz, W. & Kopczyński, J. (1986). Diseases of civilization, today and tomorrow. *MIRCEN Journal of Applied Microbiology and Biotechnology 2*(2), 253–265.
Luhmann, N. (1980). Gesellschaftstruktur und Semantik. *Studien zur Wissenssoziologie der modernen Gesellschaft.* Frankfurt a. M.: Suhrkamp.
Luhmann, N. (1989). *Ecological communication.* Cambridge, UK: Polity Press.
Luhmann, N. (1993). *Risk: A sociological theory.* New York: A. de Gruyter.
Lupton, D., (1999). *Risk.* London: Routledge.
Mairal, G. (2011). The history and the narrative of risk in the media. *Health, Risk & Society 13*(1), 65-79.
Manning, C.D., Surdeanu, M., Bauer, J., Finkel, J., Bethard, S.J., & McClosky, D. (2014, June). The Stanford CoreNLP natural language processing toolkit. In *Proceedings of 52nd Annual Meeting of the Association for Computational Linguistics: System Demonstrations* (pp. 55–60). Baltimore, MA: Association for Computational Linguistics.
McCombs, M.E. & Shaw, D.L. (1972). The agenda-setting function of mass media. *Public Opinion Quarterly, 36,* 176–187.
McCombs, M.E. (2004). *Setting the agenda: The mass media and public opinion.* Cambridge: Polity.
Michel, J.B., Shen, Y.K., Aiden, A.P., Veres, A., Gray, M.K., Pickett, J.P., . . . & Aiden, E.L. (2011). Quantitative analysis of culture using millions of digitized books. *Science, 331*(6014), 176–182.
Nerlich, B. & Clarke, D. D. (1988). A dynamic model of semantic change. *Journal of Literary Semantics, 17,* 73–90.
Nerlich, B. & Clarke, D. D. (1992). Semantic change: Case studies based on traditional and cognitive semantics. *Journal of Literary Semantics, 21,* 204–225.
Nerlich, B. & Clarke, D. D. (2000). Semantic fields and frames: Historical explorations of the interface between language, action, and cognition. *Journal of Pragmatics, 32,* 125–150.
O'Malley, P. (2004). *Risk, uncertainty and government.* London: Glashouse Press.
Perrow, C. (1984). *Normal Accidents. Living with High-Risk Technologies.* Princeton, NJ: Princeton University Press.
Pidgeon, N.F., Kasperson, R.E. & Slovic, P. (2003). *The social amplification of risk.* Cambridge, New York: Cambridge University Press.
Putnam, R.D. (2000). *Bowling alone: The collapse and revival of American community.* New York, NY: Simon & Schuster.
Rose, N. (1999). *The powers of freedom.* Cambridge: Cambridge University Press.
Sandhaus, E. (2008). *The New York Times Annotated Corpus LDC2008T19.* Linguistic Data Consortium.
Skolbekken, J. (1995). The risk epidemic in medical journals. *Social Science & Medicine, 40*(3), 291–305.

Slater, P.E. (1970). *The pursuit of loneliness. American culture at the breaking point.* Boston: Beacon Press.
Strydom, P. (2002). *Risk, environment and society: Ongoing debates, current issues and future prospects.* Buckingham: Open University Press.
Stuart, A., Adam, B. & Cynthia, C. (Eds.) (2000). *Environmental risks and the media.* London, New York: Routledge.
Traugott, E.C. & Dasher, R.B. (2002). *Regularity in semantic change.* Cambridge: Cambridge University Press.
Tulloch, J. & Zinn, J.O. (2011). Risk, health and the media. *Health, Risk and Society, 40*(1), 1–16.
van Dijk, T.A. (1997). *Discourse as structure and process. A multidisciplinary introduction.* London: Sage.
Weber, M. (1948). Science as a Vocation. In H.M.C.W. Gerth (Ed.), *Weber, Max: Essays in Sociology* (pp. 129–156). London: Routledge & Kegan Paul LTD.
Wodak, R. & Meyer, M. (2001). *Methods of critical discourse analysis.* London: Sage.
Zelizer, V.A.R. (1983). *Morals and markets: The development of life insurance in the United States.* New Brunswick: Transaction Books.
Zinn, J.O. & McDonald, D. (2015). *Discourse-semantics of risk in the New York Times, 1963, 1987–2014: A corpus linguistic approach.* Melbourne. www.github.com/interrogator/risk.
Zinn, J. O. (2010). Risk as discourse: Interdisciplinary perspectives. *Critical Approaches to Discourse Analysis across Disciplines,* 4(2) 106–124.
Zinn, J.O. (2011). *Changing risk semantics—A comparison of the volumes 1900 and 2000 of the New York Times*, RN22 Sociology of Risk and Uncertainty at the 10th European Sociological Association (ESA) Conference "Social Relations in Turbulent Times", Geneva, Switzerland, 7–10 September, 2011.

# Contributors

**Andy Alaszewski** is emeritus professor of health studies at the University of Kent. He is an applied social scientist who has examined the ways in which social policy making has shaped the ways health- and social-care professionals deliver health and social care and the role and nature of risk in health and social care. He edits *Health, Risk & Society*, an international peer-reviewed journal published by Taylor and Francis. He is author of *Using Diaries for Social Research* (2006, Sage Publications) and coauthor with B. Heyman of *Risk, Safety and Clinical Practice: Healthcare through the Lens of Risk* (2010 Oxford University Press), as well as with P. Brown of *Making Health Policy: A Critical Introduction* (2012, Polity Press).

**Florencia Arancibia** is a post-doctoral researcher at CENIT—STEPS Latin America Centre, for the National and Scientific Research Council (CONICET), Argentina. Her research areas include social movements, environmental controversies, risk governance and social studies of science and technology. Her dissertation focuses on new forms of collective action in the arena of "regulatory science", as well as novel relationships between social movements and expertise. She holds a *Licenciatura* in Sociology from the National University of Buenos Aires, Argentina; a MA in Education from the University of San Andrés, Argentina; and a PhD in Sociology from the State University of New York at Stony Brook, United States. She was a Fulbright scholar and an IAF-IIE Grassroots Development fellow.

**Patrick Brown** is assistant professor at the Department of Sociology and member of the Centre for Social Science and Global Health at the University of Amsterdam. His research explores various social processes of decision making and action amidst uncertain health-care contexts, not least of those involving medicines. His recently published books are, with Mike Calnan, *Trusting on the Edge* (2012, Policy Press,) and with Andy Alaszewski, *Making Health Policy* (2012, Polity Press).

**John Martyn Chamberlain** is a senior lecturer in criminology and social policy in the Department of Social Science at Loughborough University. His research interests include the profiling and risk management of violent and sex offenders as well as health- and social-care professional regulation in relation to medical malpractice and acts of criminality. He is author of *Doctoring Medical Governance: Medical Self-Regulation in Transition* (2009, New York: Nova Science Publishers Inc.), *The Sociology of Medical Regulation: An Introduction (*2012, Springer: New York and Amsterdam), and *Medical Regulation, Fitness to Practice and Medical Revalidation: A Critical Introduction* (2015, Bristol: Policy Press and Chicago: Chicago University Press).

**Nadav Even Chorev** is a PhD candidate at the Department of Politics and Government, Ben-Gurion University of the Negev, Israel. His research interests include political sociology, political and social theory, science and technology studies, politics and sociology of medicine and information systems research. In his research, he aims at understanding how risk and uncertainty are configured, managed and understood in the field of personalized medicine, with a particular focus on the role information technology artifacts play in this. He holds an MA degree in Sociology from the Hebrew University of Jerusalem, as well as an MSc degree in Information Systems Management from the London School of Economics and Political Science.

**Jeremy Dixon** is a lecturer in social work in the Department of Social and Policy Sciences of the University of Bath, UK. His research interests include the sociology of mental health and illness, the sociology of risk and uncertainty and socio-legal decision making. His recent research focuses on mentally disordered offenders' views of their own offending, risk assessments and supervision in the community.

**Fiorella Mancini** is a researcher at the Social Research Institute, National University of Mexico (IIS-UNAM), whose research interests include uncertainty and social risks, work and labor markets in Latin America, as well as social inequalities and life course.

**Daniel McDonald** is a PhD student in linguistics at the University of Melbourne. His thesis research involves combining corpus and computational linguistic methods with systemic functional linguistics as a theory of language in order to investigate large datasets.

**Gemma Mitchell** is a sociology PhD student at the University of Leicester. She is also a qualified social worker. Her research interests include risk and uncertainty, child and family social work, knowledge translation and the sociology of scientific knowledge (SSK). The children and families she has worked with professionally have inspired her to challenge her preconceptions and ask: how do child and family social workers, as experts in the 'risk society', translate and navigate risk knowledges within their expert practice? She seeks to address this question in her research.

**Renata Motta** is a teaching and research assistant and post-doctoral researcher in sociology at the Institute for Latin American Studies at the Free University of Berlin. The topic of her dissertation is social disputes over GMOs in Argentina and Brazil. Her teaching areas include social movements and environmental conflicts. Her research is located at the intersection of political sociology, political economy, risk sociology and media studies; and she has published in *Social Movement Studies, Sociology Compass Revista Brasileira de Ciências Sociais* and written for the United Nations Economic Commission for Latin America and the Caribbean (ECLAC). Her chapter in the book *Balancing between Trade and Risk*, edited by van Asselt, Versluis and Vos (Routledge 2013), analyzes the trade dispute between the European Union and the USA, Canada, and Argentina on GMOs. She holds a BA in International Relations from PUC-MG, Brazil; a MA in Social Sciences from the University of Brasília, Brazil, and a PhD in Sociology from the Free University of Berlin, Germany.

**Jens O. Zinn** is T.R. Ashworth associate professor in sociology at the University of Melbourne. He is the founder of the international research networks on the Sociology of Risk and Uncertainty (SoRU) within the European Sociological Association (ESA) and the International Sociological Association (ISA). He is a board member of the international journal *Health, Risk & Society*. He was recently awarded the Friedhelm-Wilhelm Bessel Award by the Alexander von Humboldt Foundation for his achievements in the sociology of risk and uncertainty. His research in the risk domain focuses on conceptual work, historical social change related to risk and biographical risk management, among other topics such as risk governance, social policy, risk communication and corpus assisted approaches to risk.